ENDOCRINE DISRUPTION AND HUMAN HEALTH

ENDOCRINE DISRUPTION AND HUMAN HEALTH

Edited by

PHILIPPA D. DARBRE, BScHons, PhD

School of Biological Sciences, University of Reading, Reading, UK

AMSTERDAM • BOSTON • HEIDELBERG • LONDON
NEW YORK • OXFORD • PARIS • SAN DIEGO
SAN FRANCISCO • SINGAPORE • SYDNEY • TOKYO

Academic Press is an imprint of Elsevier

Academic Press is an imprint of Elsevier
125 London Wall, London EC2Y 5AS, UK
525 B Street, Suite 1800, San Diego, CA 92101-4495, USA
225 Wyman Street, Waltham, MA 02451, USA
The Boulevard, Langford Lane, Kidlington, Oxford OX5 1GB, UK

Notices
Knowledge and best practice in this field are constantly changing. As new research and experience broaden our understanding, changes in research methods, professional practices, or medical treatment may become necessary.

Practitioners and researchers must always rely on their own experience and knowledge in evaluating and using any information, methods, compounds, or experiments described herein. In using such information or methods they should be mindful of their own safety and the safety of others, including parties for whom they have a professional responsibility.

To the fullest extent of the law, neither the Publisher nor the authors, contributors, or editors, assume any liability for any injury and/or damage to persons or property as a matter of products liability, negligence or otherwise, or from any use or operation of any methods, products, instructions, or ideas contained in the material herein.

ISBN: 978-0-12-801139-3

British Library Cataloguing-in-Publication Data
A catalogue record for this book is available from the British Library.

Library of Congress Cataloging-in-Publication Data
A catalog record for this book is available from the Library of Congress.

For Information on all Academic Press publications
visit our website at http://store.elsevier.com/

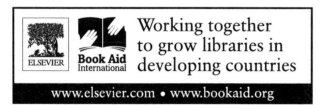

Working together
to grow libraries in
developing countries

www.elsevier.com • www.bookaid.org

Publisher: Mica Haley
Acquisition Editor: Kristine Jones
Editorial Project Manager: Molly McLaughlin
Production Project Manager: Caroline Johnson
Designer: Maria Inês Cruz

Typeset by MPS Limited, Chennai, India
www.adi-mps.com

Contents

3

CONCERNS FOR HUMAN HEALTH

8. Endocrine Disruption and Female Reproductive Health
PHILIPPA D. DARBRE

9. Endocrine Disruption and Male Reproductive Health
PHILIPPA D. DARBRE

4
PUBLIC POLICY AND REGULATORY CONSIDERATIONS

List of Contributors

Gerard M. Cooke PhD   Regulatory Toxicology Research Division, Bureau of Chemical Safety, Food Directorate, Health Canada, Ottawa, ON, Canada

Philippa D. Darbre BScHons, PhD   School of Biological Sciences, University of Reading, Reading, UK

Rodney R. Dietert PhD   Department of Microbiology and Immunology, College of Veterinary Medicine, Cornell University, Ithaca, NY, USA

Rowena H. Gee BScHons, PhD   National Centre for Environmental Toxicology, WRc plc, Swindon, Wiltshire, UK

Philip W. Harvey BSc, PhD, ERT, CBiol, FSB, Fellow ATS   Department of Toxicology, Covance Laboratories, Harrogate, UK

John D. Meeker MS, ScD   Department of Environmental Health Sciences, University of Michigan School of Public Health, Ann Arbor, MI, USA

Rekha Mehta BSc, PhD   Regulatory Toxicology Research Division, Bureau of Chemical Safety, Food Directorate, Health Canada, Ottawa, ON, Canada

Jenny Odum BSc, MSc, PhD   Regulatory Science Associates, Coventry, UK

Leon S. Rockett BScHons   National Centre for Environmental Toxicology, WRc plc, Swindon, Wiltshire, UK

Paul C. Rumsby BTech, PhD, ERT   National Centre for Environmental Toxicology, WRc plc, Swindon, Wiltshire, UK

J. Thomas Sanderson PhD   INRS-Institut Armand-Frappier, Université du Québec, Laval, QC, Canada

Monica K. Silver MPH   Department of Environmental Health Sciences, University of Michigan School of Public Health, Ann Arbor, MI, USA

Catherine Sutcliffe BSc(Agr)Hons, MA, VetMB, MS, MRCVS   Department of Pathology, Covance Laboratories, Harrogate, UK

Laura N. Vandenberg PhD   University of Massachusetts – Amherst, School of Public Health, Division of Environmental Health Science, Amherst, MA, USA

Graeme Williams BSc, BAppSc, MBBS   School of Biological Sciences, University of Reading, Reading, UK

Preface

I alone cannot change the world, but I can cast a stone across the waters to create many ripples. Mother Teresa

Endocrine disruption was introduced as a term only at the turn of the millennium, but in less than two decades, it has become not only an acknowledged scientific phenomenon, but also a concept known to the general public. Experimental, clinical, and epidemiological studies have documented effects of environmental endocrine-disrupting chemicals (EDCs) on animal and human well-being, and endocrine disruption is set to become a worldwide environmental issue and human health concern of the twenty-first century. This book aims to provide the first comprehensive textbook on endocrine disruption as it relates to human health. Over 19 chapters, information is provided on basic mechanisms of action and the latest research: if it opens readers' eyes to the magnitude of the issues, then this book will have served its purpose. It explains how EDCs that enter the human body through oral, inhalation, and dermal routes threaten the normal functioning of hormones and how exposures at early life stages may influence endocrine-dependent processes later in life: if the science described here moves readers into action, then the effort given to writing the book will have been worthwhile.

The book is divided into four sections. The first section provides an introduction to the sources of EDCs and the broad issues surrounding their presence in human tissues. The second section provides overviews of mechanisms by which EDCs can interfere in normal endocrine function, outlining the implications of their targeted effects through biological receptors and describing current assays used in defining their pathways of action. The third section reviews current areas of concern for human health, including evidence about the consequences of exposure to EDCs at differing life stages for human reproductive tissues, thyroid and adrenal actions, the immune system, and metabolism. Evidence for causal links to impaired reproductive function, cancer, and metabolic diseases is discussed as well. The final section outlines principles of risk assessment and current regulatory approaches to EDCs in food, water, and personal care products. The evidence base is set to continue to grow, and it seems inevitable that in the future, other different pathways of EDC action will be added to those described herein. A major need for the immediate future will be to develop ways of assessing the effects of long-term, low-dose exposure to chemical mixtures rather than short-term actions of relatively high doses (i.e., high compared to environmental exposures) of single chemicals. The environmental reality is that the human body is not exposed to only one, but to hundreds or even thousands of chemicals on a daily basis. These chemicals are present over the long term and may be present at only low doses individually, but they act together in an additive or complementary manner to interfere with normal endocrine function. The ability to identify the specific mixtures of greatest consequence for human health and to translate the published science into preventative measures will remain major challenges for national and international regulatory bodies.

I would like to thank all those who have contributed to this book. First, I would like to acknowledge the willing contributions by the other authors, without which the scope of this book would have been much more limited. I would also like to acknowledge the many scientists who have contributed to this field but who are too numerous to give due credit in the references cited. From a more personal angle, I would like to thank my scientific colleagues who have guided me along the way, the members of nongovernmental organizations (NGOs) who have challenged me out of my academic comfort zone, and the members of the general public who have taken the time to write me letters of encouragement. Finally, I am immensely grateful to my family: to my parents, who ensured my sound scientific education and brought me up with a healthy respect for the sparing use of chemicals outside a laboratory; to my children, who have endured and followed; and to my very dear husband, who has changed from skeptic to convinced scientist, and without whose supportive daily walk by my side, my scientific career would never have been possible.

Philippa D. Darbre
**School of Biological Sciences,
University of Reading, Reading, UK**

OVERVIEW AND SCOPE

CHAPTER

1

What Are Endocrine Disrupters and Where Are They Found?

Philippa D. Darbre

OUTLINE

Endocrine Disruption and Human Health.
DOI: http://dx.doi.org/10.1016/B978-0-12-801139-3.00001-6

Abstract

This chapter provides an introduction to the importance of hormones to the healthy functioning of the human body and an overview of the varied types and sources of environmental chemicals that can interfere in their action. Such compounds, termed *endocrine-disrupting chemicals (EDCs)*, may occur naturally, but the majority are artificial compounds that have been released into the environment without prior knowledge of their impact on human health. The chapter begins with some historical background, especially related to the endocrine-disrupting effects of EDCs in wildlife, and then outlines general mechanisms by which EDCs may disrupt hormone activity. Descriptions are then given of the range of compounds that are EDCs, their chemical structures, and the sources of exposure for the human population.

1.1 INTRODUCTION

An endocrine disrupter is an exogenous substance that causes adverse health effects in an intact organism, and/or its progeny, consequent to changes in endocrine function [1].

Human health depends on a functional endocrine system in which hormones act as chemical messengers to regulate and coordinate bodily functions. The hormones are secreted by glands distributed around the body and are then carried by the blood to act on cells of distant target organs. Their ability to act at the target organs is determined by binding to specific cellular receptors, which then relay signals to the target cells. The healthy functioning of the human body depends on the coordinated actions of a balanced network of hormones, each at the correct concentration and all acting in synchrony with one another at exactly the appropriate times. It is now recognized that many chemicals present in the environment have the ability to interfere in the action of human hormones and therefore are termed *endocrine-disrupting chemicals (EDCs).* They can act to disrupt the balance and coordination of the normal homeostatic processes of hormone activity. Some of these compounds are present in nature, but the majority are artificial and released into the environment by the activities of humans without any prior knowledge of their impact on ecosystems, animal welfare, or human health. Therefore, there is now the potential for long-term harm to human health. This book will seek to provide the current state of evidence linking exposure to EDCs with specific human health issues.

1.2 HISTORICAL BACKGROUND

Although endocrine disruption has been receiving high-profile attention only since the 1990s, the phenomenon has been known for considerably longer than that (Figure 1.1). In the 1920s, pig farmers in the United States became concerned about the lack of fertility in swine herds fed with moldy grain [2]; this was exacerbated in the 1940s, when sheep farmers in Western Australia reported infertility in their sheep after grazing on specific fields of clover [3]. More recent research has showed that the underlying reasons were consumption of estrogenic compounds contained within the mold (mycoestrogens) or plant material (phytoestrogens), which were disrupting fertility through their potent estrogenic activity.

In the 1950s, chemists in London led by Sir Charles Dodds were synthesizing a range of chemicals with estrogenic properties [4] for the purpose of studying the mechanisms of

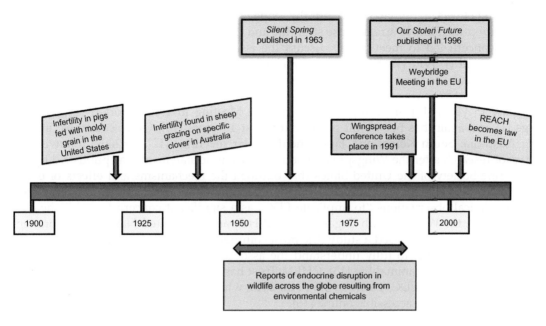

FIGURE 1.1   Historical landmarks in the recognition of endocrine disruption.

estrogen action. Therefore, a potential medical value of such compounds was realized [5] and a new industry of synthetic hormones was born, ultimately leading to the development of oral contraceptives and hormone replacement therapy. The 1950s and 1960s heralded a new culture of sexual freedom, and oral contraceptives were widely adopted as a result. As this same generation grew older, these women wanted to control menopausal symptoms as well, and hormone replacement therapy became a normal expectation of the population as a whole. The long-term consequences of the desire to control reproductive hormone exposures have still to be fully understood, in terms not only of effects on the individual person, but also of the consequences of releasing so many synthetic hormones and their metabolites into the environment.

In 1962, the book *Silent Spring* by Rachel Carson was published [6], warning of the long-term consequences of environmental contamination with artificial chemicals, most notably from the liberal agricultural use of pesticides and herbicides. She described the already evident loss of wildlife from chemical contamination of the land and predicted worse to come if chemical use continued to increase unchecked. In the following decades, endocrine-disrupting properties of the pesticide dichlorodiphenyltrichloroethane (DDT) and its metabolites were reported in birds [7] and mammals [8,9], which coincided with controversial warnings of more widespread consequences of pollution for wildlife populations from organochlorine compounds. Carson died in 1964, so she never lived to see that the impact of her book sparked an international environmental movement to champion the issues raised. The book *Our Stolen Future* was published by Theo Colborn and colleagues in 1996, and it is considered a follow-up publication describing even more serious environmental warnings [10]. Many questioned whether the effects reported in wildlife might be predictive of the impending effects on human health, but the scope of the proof needed for invoking any precautionary principle was an immense scientific and clinical task.

This concern led to meetings to discuss the issues, the first of which was the World Wildlife Fund (WWF) Wingspread Conference in Wisconsin in the United States in 1991. Here, the term *endocrine disrupter* was first proposed, and the consensus statement published the next year was insightful and still relevant today [11] and has been built on over the past 15 years [12]. In Europe, the Weybridge Meeting in 1996 reported similar findings [1] and again has been built on over the past 15 years [13]. Other countries, including Australia, South Korea, and Japan, held similar meetings [12]. In 2009, following 18 years of research after the Wingspread meeting, a scientific statement was published by the Endocrine Society of the United States that outlined the mechanisms and effects of endocrine disrupters and showed how experimental and epidemiological studies converge with human clinical observations "to implicate EDCs as a significant concern to public health" [14]. In 2013, the World Health Organization (WHO) and the United Nations Environment Programme (UNEP) released a study (the most comprehensive report on EDCs to date) calling for more research to fully understand the association between EDCs and the risks to health of human and animal life [15]. CHEM Trust has collated an annotated list of key scientific statements on EDCs between 1991 and 2013, which provides more useful chronological information and is accessible online [16].

In 1998, the US Environment Protection Agency (EPA) announced the Endocrine Disrupter Screening Program, which was given a mandate under the Food Quality Protection Act and Safe Drinking Water Act to establish a framework for priority setting, screening, and testing of more than 85,000 chemicals in commerce. The basic concept behind the program was that prioritization would be based on existing information about chemical uses, production volume, structure activity, and toxicity. Through the Registration, Evaluation, Authorisation and restriction of CHemicals (REACH) legislation, which became law in the European Union (EU) in 2007 and will be implemented gradually over the next decade, some EDCs now require a portfolio of safety information prior to being released into the environment, rather than waiting for problems to emerge afterward.

1.3 EVIDENCE FOR ENDOCRINE DISRUPTION IN WILDLIFE POPULATIONS AND HOW THIS MAY PREDICT EFFECTS ON HUMAN HEALTH

Over the past 50 years, cases of endocrine disruption in wildlife have been increasingly documented and linked to specific environmental exposures to EDCs [1,6–13,15]. In particular, exposure of aquatic wildlife to chemicals in the water in which they live has been linked to many reproductive problems and population declines. Early work in this field showed extensive loss of bivalves and gastropods in harbor waters caused by tributyltin (TBT) from the antifouling paints used on the underside of ships (see Section 1.3.1). A spill of dicofol into Lake Apopka near Orlando, FL, caused extensive damage to the lake's wildlife, particularly the alligator population (discussed further in Section 1.3.2). In the United Kingdom, feminization of male fish was reported downstream of sewage effluent works (see Section 1.3.3). Loss of bird populations due to eggshell thinning has been extensively reported as resulting from pesticide exposure (see Section 1.3.4). The strongest evidence of the causality of the link has been the demonstration of the reversal of problems following reduction in chemical exposure [15]. The long-debated question remains as to whether such effects might also occur in the human population in response to the same chemicals, and therefore whether the wildlife effects might be a forewarning of consequences for human health.

1.3.1 TBT and Imposex in Mollusks

One of the highly documented effects of chemicals on wildlife has been the formation of imposex in mollusks following exposure to TBT. *Imposex* is the acquisition of male sex organs, including the penis and vas deferens, by female snails, which has been shown to lead to reproductive failure in over 150 species worldwide [17]. TBT is a biocide that was introduced into antifouling paints in the 1970s for treating the underside of ships, but the release of this compound into harbor waters led to the wide-scale masculinization of bivalves and gastropods and consequent population declines [18]. Due to these effects, use of TBT was restricted in some countries during the 1990s, leading to subsequent recovery of multiple marine snail populations [19].

1.3.2 Dicofol and Reproduction of Alligators

In 1980, there was an accidental spill of the pesticide dicofol into a tributary of Lake Apopka. This had serious consequences for the alligator population, and genital abnormalities were reported in both male and female alligators [20]. Female alligators in the lake were reported to have abnormal ovarian morphology, large numbers of polyovular follicles, and raised plasma estradiol levels [20].

1.3.3 Feminization of Male Fish in the UK Rivers

Studies of feminization of male fish in UK rivers has highlighted issues of estrogenic components in sewage effluent. Exposure of male fish to sewage effluent has been reported to cause the induction of vitellogenin (which is an exclusively female protein) and the appearance of ovarian tissue in the testes [21]. A gradient of effect exists, with fish at the closest proximity to the sewage outflow responding the most severely [22]. Although initial studies came from the United Kingdom, the phenomenon has now been reported globally [15]. Studies using caged fish have confirmed the sewage effluent to be responsible for these responses; and chemical fractionation has shown the presence of natural and synthetic estrogens in biologically relevant concentrations, but no single compound has been implicated [15].

1.3.4 Eggshell Thinning in Birds

Reports of eggshell thinning in predatory birds has been reported as associated with organochlorine pesticide exposure since the 1960s [23–25]. The banning of DDT in North

America and Europe led to reduced body burdens in birds, improved eggshell thickness, and recovery of many populations, but other compounds such as dioxins and polybrominated diphenylethers (PBDEs) continue to be found in wildlife near urban areas causing toxic effects [26], including eggshell thinning; embryonic deformities of the foot, bill, and spine; and chick deaths and retarded growth [27].

1.4 WHICH HORMONES ARE DISRUPTED BY EDCs?

Three broad classes of hormone can be identified in humans according to their chemical structure (amines, peptide/proteins, and steroids), and Figure 1.2 lists the main hormones of the human body and where they are synthesized. Much of the disruptive activity by EDCs has been reported in relation to the action of steroid hormones, most notably, but not exclusively, estrogens, androgens, and thyroid hormones. This is not surprising because many environmental pollutants are organic, with some key structural similarities to these steroid and thyroid hormone molecules, which then enables them to compete for binding to the hormone receptors in the target cells (see Chapters 3–6). The steroid receptors are part of a family of related nuclear hormone receptors that bind organic, steroid, or fatty acid compounds: disruption has been reported through the receptor types listed in Figure 1.3, and time may yet reveal actions through other receptors of this large superfamily. In addition, many organic pollutants can act through the aryl hydrocarbon receptor (AhR), which is a member of another nuclear receptor family (see Chapter 6).

1.5 HOW DO EDCs DISRUPT HORMONE ACTION?

Hormones act in the body by an endocrine mechanism, which means that they are secreted by cells of an endocrine gland and carried by the blood to the target cells in the distant organ (Figure 1.4). This is distinct from paracrine mechanisms, where factors can be secreted locally in a tissue to act on neighboring cells, and autocrine mechanisms, in which factors act on the same cells that secreted them. The hormones are then often both modified for transport in the blood by conjugation (sulfation of glucuronidation) and bound to carrier proteins. At target sites, the free (bioavailable) hormone binds to cellular receptors, which then relay the signal to the cell to enable the response. Endocrine disruptors can disturb any of these processes (Figure 1.4). The first studies of EDCs identified their ability to compete with the hormone for binding to hormone receptors in the target cells, and in so doing, either mimic or antagonize the action of the hormone. Further studies have shown that EDCs can also act by altering synthesis of the hormones in the endocrine gland and by altering bioavailability through either interfering with activity of conjugation enzymes or competing for binding to carrier proteins. Some EDCs can also alter hormone metabolism, excretion, or both. More recent work has shown that they can act to modify receptor levels in the target cells, and since the number of receptors per cell is critical to determining signal response by the target cell, any alteration to receptor numbers (either more or less) will alter the usual hormone action.

Gland	Hormone
Hypothalamus	
	❖ Corticotrophin-releasing hormone
	❖ Dopamine
	❖ Gonadotrophin-releasing hormone
	❖ Growth hormone releasing hormone
	❖ Somatostatin
	❖ Thyrotrophin-releasing hormone
Anterior pituitary	
	❖ Adrenocorticotropic hormone
	❖ Follicle-stimulating hormone
	❖ Growth hormone
	❖ Luteinizing hormone
	❖ Prolactin
	❖ Thyroid-stimulating hormone
Posterior pituitary	
	❖ Oxytocin and vasopressin
Pineal	
	❖ Melatonin
Thyroid	
	❖ Calcitonin
	❖ **Triiodothyronine and thyroxine**
Parathyroid	
	❖ Parathyroid hormone
Adrenal cortex	
	❖ Aldosterone
	❖ Cortisol
Adrenal medulla	
	❖ Epinephrine (adrenalin) and norepinephrine (noradrenalin)
Stomach	
	❖ Gastrin
Pancreas	
	❖ Glucagon, insulin, and somatostatin
Duodenum	
	❖ Cholecystokinin and secretin
Kidney	
	❖ **Calcitriol** and erythropoietin
Ovary	
	❖ Oestrogens and progesterone
	❖ Activin and inhibin
Testis	
	❖ Androstenedione and testosterone
	❖ Activin, inhibin, and Anti-Mullerian hormone

FIGURE 1.2   Principal human endocrine glands and the hormones they produce. Hormones may be steroid (red), nonsteroidal organic (black), amine (blue), or peptide/protein (green).

Hormone	Cellular Receptor	Principal Function
Androgen (testosterone)	AR	Male sexual development
Estrogen (estradiol)	ERα, ERβ	Female sexual development
Progesterone	PR	Female sexual development
Glucocorticoid (cortisol)	GR	Regulation of glucose metabolism, stress response, inflammation, body fluid homeostasis
Mineralocorticoid (aldosterone)	MR	Salt and water balance
Thyroid hormones (triiodothyronine, thyroxine)	TRα, TRβ	Regulation of metabolism
Retinoic acid (vitamin A)	RARα, RARβ, RARγ RXRα, RXRβ, RXRγ	Growth and development
Lipids/fatty acids	PPARα, PPARβ, PPARγ	Lipid homeostasis, glucose metabolism
Foreign compounds	PXR	Elimination of foreign compounds
Foreign compounds (no known endogenous ligand)	AhR	Elimination of foreign compounds

FIGURE 1.3 Human nuclear receptors to which EDCs are known to be able to bind and, by binding, may mimic or antagonize hormone action.

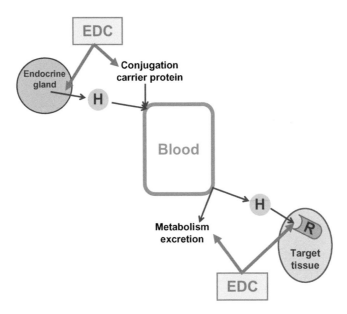

FIGURE 1.4 Mechanisms by which endocrine disrupters can act. A hormone (H) is secreted by an endocrine gland and then enters the bloodstream, where it may be conjugated and bound to a carrier protein. A free hormone may enter the target tissue, where it recognizes target cells by the presence of a receptor (R). Alternatively, hormones may be metabolized and excreted. EDCs may interfere with hormone secretion, conjugation, binding to carrier protein, and metabolism. They may also interfere at the target cells by competing for the binding to receptors or by modifying receptor levels.

Levels of hormones are tightly regulated in synchrony with physiological needs or changes to the external environment, but environmental chemicals enter human tissues in an unregulated manner, so they can cause inappropriate responses at inappropriate times (see Chapter 2). Such responses may involve either increase or decrease in endogenous hormone activity. A particularly vulnerable time for exposure is prior to birth, where disruption of endocrine regulation in the developing embryo or fetus can have implications for the health in adult life not only of reproductive organs, but also of brain function and immunity (see Chapters 8–15). Furthermore, some of the alterations caused by environmental chemicals can have long-lasting effects, even transgenerational ones that pass on to progeny without need for further chemical exposure (see Chapter 2).

1.6 WHICH CHEMICALS ARE SOURCES OF HUMAN EXPOSURE TO ENDOCRINE DISRUPTERS?

Humans are exposed to environmental chemicals with endocrine-disrupting properties not only through specific occupational circumstances, but nowadays more generally also from the ordinary day-to-day domestic and workplace lifestyles of the twentieth and twenty-first centuries. Occupational exposures, such as of agrochemicals on farms or of plastics in manufacturing plants, can cause specific high exposures, but the general population also uses pesticides and herbicides around the home, and plastics are abundant in domestic environments. A main ubiquitous route of exposure is through intake of food, water, and air. In water, it may consist of trace contaminants inadequately removed by water treatment processes themselves (see Chapter 18). In food, it may occur through the consumption of endogenous estrogenic components of plant material (phytoestrogens), through trace residues of herbicides and pesticides on fruits and vegetables, through trace lipophilic pollutants passing up the food chain in animal fat, or through food additives and supplements (see Chapter 17). Air contains increasing numbers of contaminants, not only outdoors but also indoors, because opening of windows is less frequent these days due to dependence on central heating and air conditioning systems. In addition, many consumer products that are used in workplace, living, and domestic environments contain EDCs, not least through extensive use of flame-retardant and stain-resistant coatings.

Use of personal care products, including cosmetics, is another source of exposure to EDCs. This occurs mainly through dermal application, but some substances may enter the system orally or via the inhalation of sprays. The growing dependence of the population on pharmaceuticals is another exposure route, most notably the increased consumption of painkillers such as paracetamol. Another source of EDC exposure is through nutraceuticals, food or food products that are promoted as providing health or medical benefits through the prevention or treatment of disease.

1.6.1 Persistent Organic Pollutants—"The Dirty Dozen"

Persistent organic pollutants (POPs) are organic compounds that are stable and do not degrade easily. For this reason, they tend to persist in the environment and to bioaccumulate in animal and human tissues. Many are lipophilic and therefore tend to lodge in fatty

TABLE 1.1   POPs Classified as "The Dirty Dozen" by the Stockholm Convention on Persistent Organic Pollutants in 2001 [28]

POP	Use	Source of human exposure	Evidence for endocrine disrupting activity
Aldrin	Insecticide	Dietary animal fat	Yes
Chlordane	Insecticide	Air pollution	Yes
DDT	Insecticide (malaria)	Food	Yes and metabolites
Dieldrin	Pesticide	Food	Yes
Endrin	Insecticide	Food	Yes
Heptachlor	Pesticide	Food	Yes
Hexachlorobenzene	Fungicide	Food	Yes
Mirex	Insecticide or flame retardant	Animal meat, fish, wild game	Yes
Polychlorinated biphenyls (PCBs) (209 congeners)	Electrical products	Food	Yes for some congeners
Polychlorinated dibenzodioxins (PCDDs) (75 congeners)	Incomplete combustion of waste	Dietary animal fat, air pollution	Yes for some congeners
Polychlorinated dibenzofurans (PCDFs) (135 congeners)	Incomplete combustion of waste	Dietary animal products	Yes for some congeners
Toxaphene	Insecticide	Food	Yes

The Stockholm Convention on POPs was signed in 2001 and entered into force in 2004. Cosignatories agreed to limit the use of DDT to malaria control, to reduce the inadvertant production of dioxins and furans, and to ban the remaining nine chemicals.

tissues and pass up the food chain in animal fat. Many have been used as pesticides or herbicides, and others in industrial processes. Some POPs can be generated by volcanic activity and vegetation fires, but most are artificial, either intentionally or as by-products. Many POPs have been shown to be EDCs. The effect of POPs on environmental and human health was discussed by the international community at the Stockholm Convention on POPs in 2001 with the intention to eliminate or restrict their production. The results of the Stockholm Convention were adopted by the UNEP, and a list of the top 12 chemicals for regulating, nicknamed the "dirty dozen," was devised; it is shown in Table 1.1 [28]. The Stockholm Convention on POPs was signed in 2001 and entered into force in 2004. The co-signatories agreed to ban 9 of the 12 chemicals, to limit the use of DDT to malaria control, and to reduce inadvertent production of dioxins and furans. The EU adopted this position in Regulation (EC) number 850/2004.

Many of these compounds in Table 1.1 have been used as pesticides or herbicides across agricultural and urban lands. DDT [29] (Figure 1.5), synthesized in the late 1800s, was first used as a pesticide against the Colorado beetle on potato crops in 1936. After World War II, it was approved for more general agricultural and domestic use and used especially against

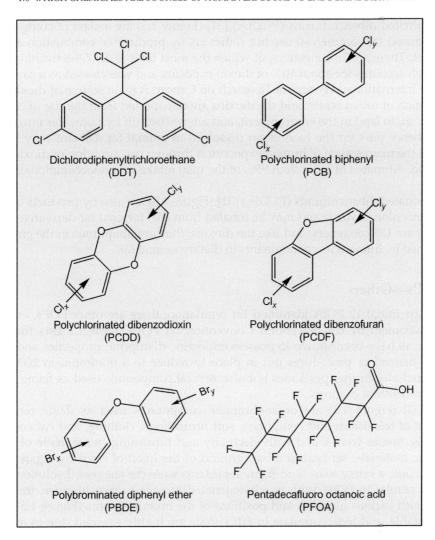

FIGURE 1.5 Chemical structures of POPs. Cl_x, Cl_y, Br_x, and Br_y indicate that there may be varied numbers and positions of chloride (Cl) or bromide (Br) atoms on the organic ring.

mosquitoes in the fight against malaria. Carson's book *Silent Spring* [6] catalogued the environmental impacts of indiscriminate DDT spraying, and a public outcry led to a ban in the United States in 1972, but it took until the Stockholm Convention of 2001 for a worldwide ban to be formalized.

Polychlorinated biphenyls (PCBs) [30] (Figure 1.5) are a class of chlorinated hydrocarbons with 209 congeners according to the number and configuration of the chlorines. They were used as industrial lubricants and coolants, particularly in transformers and capacitors and other electrical products. They were first manufactured commercially in 1927 and sold under trade names such as Arochlor, but their production was largely stopped in the 1970s.

Polychlorinated dibenzodioxins (PCDDs) [31] (Figure 1.5) are a class of compounds that are not produced for commercial use but rather are by-products of combustion and chemical processes. There are 75 congeners, of which the most toxic is 2,3,7,8-tetrachlorodibenzo-dioxin, which accounts for about 10% of dioxin exposure and was classed as a carcinogen in 1997 by the International Agency for Research on Cancer. A main source of dioxins is from the incineration of urban waste, and the dioxins are transported from the site of combustion through the air, to land in the environment, and are washed off by rainwater into rivers and lakes and thence pass up the food chain dissolved in animal fat. Dioxins may be inhaled directly, but the main source of human exposure is through consumption of dioxin contaminants in food, estimated at more than 95% of the total intake for nonoccupationally exposed people [32].

Polychlorinated dibenzofurans (PCDFs) [31] (Figure 1.5) are also by-products of incineration of organochlorine waste and may be inhaled from coal tar, coal-tar derivatives, and creosote. There are 135 congeners, and like the dioxins, they are ubiquitous in the environment and consumed by humans as contaminants in dietary animal fat.

1.6.2 POPs—Others

Beyond the initial 12 POPs identified for regulation, there are other POPs, and there is ongoing assessment by the Stockholm Convention on POPs. Table 1.2 lists further compounds that all have been shown to possess endocrine-disrupting properties and that have been either banned or procedures put in place to reduce to a minimum in 2009, 2011, or 2013. This includes further pesticides but also several compounds used as flame retardants and for stain-resistant coatings.

PBDEs [33] (Figure 1.5) are organobromine compounds used as flame retardants in plastic cases of televisions and computers, soft furnishings, clothing, and car components. By the 1960s, homes were wired with electricity and furnishings were made of combustible synthetic materials: set against a background of the habit of smoking cigarettes, home fires had become a safety issue, and flame retardants were the suggested solution. They are structurally similar to PCBs, with two halogenated aromatic rings; likewise, there are 209 congeners with various numbers and positions of the bromine atoms (Figure 1.5). They are lipophilic, stable, and bioaccumulate in fat. People are highly exposed due to their prevalence in common household items. Some of the PBDEs have been now classed as POPs with limited production (Table 1.2).

Perfluorooctanoic acid (PFOA) (Figure 1.5) has been used in the manufacture of consumer goods since the 1940s most notably as polytetrafluoroethylene (Teflon) and Gore-Tex. It is used as a water and oil repellent in fabrics and leather, floor waxes, insulators, and fire-fighting foam. As a salt, the dominant use is as an emulsifier for the emulsion polymerization of fluoropolymers such as Teflon.

Perfluorooctanesulfonic acid (PFOS) is a fluorosurfactant used most notably as the key ingredient in the fabric protector Scotchgard. Production of PFOS began in 1949, but by 2000, the primary US manufacturer announced that it was to be phased out, and it was added to the Annex B of the Stockholm Convention on POPs in 2009 (Table 1.2). Although attention has been focused on the commercially produced straight-chain heptadecafluoro-1-octane sulfonic acid, there are another 89 linear and branched-chain isomers with varied

TABLE 1.2 Further POPs with Endocrine-Disrupting Properties for Which Production Has Been Either Stopped or Reduced Under the Stockholm Convention from 2009 to 2013

Date added	POP	Use	Source of human exposure
2009	Chlordecone	Insecticide	Insecticide use, contamination of food
2009	α-Hexachlorocyclohexane	By-product of manufacture of lindane	
2009	β-Hexachlorocyclohexane	By-product of manufacture of lindane	
2009	Lindane (γ-hexachlorocyclohexane)	Pesticide	Pesticide use, contamination of food
2009	Pentachlorobenzene	None	Municipal waste incineration
2009	Tetrabromodiphenylether	Flame retardant	From use on consumer products
2009	Pentabromodiphenyl ether	Flame retardant	
2009	Hexabromodiphenyl ether	Flame retardant	
2009	PFOS	Stain resistance	Consumer products
2009	PFOSF	Used in the manufacture of PFOS	
2011	Endosulphan	Insecticide and acaricide	Insecticide and acaricide use, contamination of food
2013	Hexabromocyclododecane	Flame retardant	Consumer products

physical, chemical, and toxicological properties. Both PFOS and PFOA are highly stable compounds that persist in the environment and can bioaccumulate.

1.6.3 The Herbicides Atrazine and Glyphosate

Atrazine and glyphosate both possess endocrine-disrupting properties and are widely used herbicides, both listed in the 2004 Organisation for Economic Co-operation and Development (OECD) list of high-production-volume (HPV) chemicals [34]. The OECD lists chemicals produced at levels greater than 1000 tons per year in at least one member country or state. In 2004, there were 4843 chemicals in this list [34].

Atrazine (Figure 1.6) is a herbicide used widely for broadleaf crops such as maize and sugarcane, as well as on golf courses and residential lawns. It was banned in the EU in 2004, but it remains in use in many other parts of the world. In the United States as of 2014, atrazine remains the second-most-applied herbicide, after glyphosate. Its endocrine-disrupting properties were first described in amphibians [35].

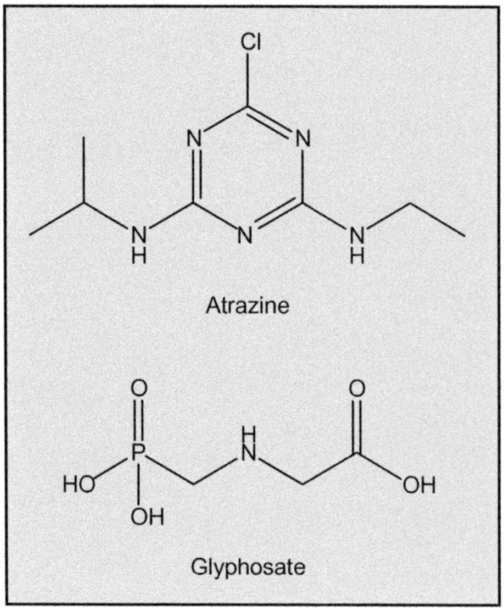

FIGURE 1.6   Chemical structures of atrazine and glyphosate.

Glyphosate [N-(phosphonomethyl)glycine] [36] (Figure 1.6) is a broad-spectrum systemic herbicide used to kill broadleaf weeds and grasses. It was first marketed in the 1970s under the trade name of Roundup, and was widely adopted in conjunction with glyphosate-resistant crops to enable farmers to kill weeds more effectively without killing the crops. However, it is now also in wide use in the urban environment, including domestic gardens. Its action is to inhibit the enzyme 5-enolpyruvylshikimate-3-phosphate synthase required for the synthesis of aromatic amino acids tyrosine, phenylalanine, and tryptophan. Recent work has shown that it has endocrine-disrupting properties [37].

1.6.4 Bisphenol A

Bisphenol A (BPA) [38,39] (Figure 1.7) was first synthesized by a Russian chemist, A. P. Dianin, in 1891 and is now used for its cross-linking properties in the manufacture of polycarbonate plastics and epoxy resins, which are now ubiquitous in our daily lives. BPA-based plastic is clear and tough; it is used in a range of consumer products such as water bottles, sports equipment, and CDs and DVDs. BPA-containing epoxy resins are used to line water pipes, as coatings on food and beverage cans and in thermal paper. It is also used in dental sealants. It has been in commercial use since 1957 and is listed in the 2004 OECD list of HPV chemicals with a production volume in excess of 1000 tons each year in at least one member country [34]. It is estimated that more than 8 billion pounds of BPA are produced annually and approximately 100 tons released into the atmosphere each year [38]. Because of its incomplete polymerization and degradation of the polymers by exposure to

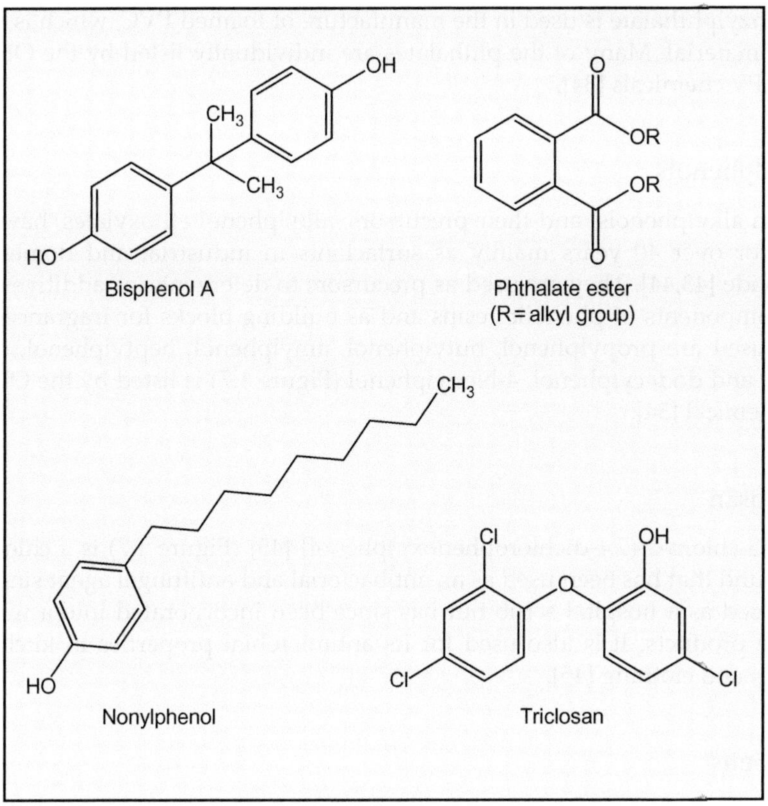

FIGURE 1.7   Chemical structures of BPA, phthalate esters, nonylphenol, and triclosan.

high temperatures, BPA can leach out of plastic containers, [40] and such containers are now used ubiquitously for food and drink storage [38,39].

1.6.5 Phthalates

Phthalates [41,42] (Figure 1.7) are esters of phthalic acid and are used mainly as plasticizers to increase flexibility, transparency, and durability of plastic materials. They are found in many plastic consumer products, including adhesives and glues, paints, packaging, children's toys, electronics, flooring, medical equipment, personal care products, air fresheners, food products, pharmaceuticals, and textiles. Phthalate exposure may be either direct, or from leaching from the product or plastic containers in which the product is stored. The phthalates are physically bound to the plastics, but not by covalent bonding; therefore, some leaching out can occur, especially by heat or solvents. The most widely used phthalates are di(2-ethylhexyl) phthalate (DEHP), diisodecyl phthalate, and diisononyl phthalate. DEHP is the dominant plasticizer used in polyvinyl chloride (PVC) due to its low cost. Butylbenzylphthalate is used in the manufacture of foamed PVC, which is used mostly as a flooring material. Many of the phthalates are individually listed by the OECD in their 2004 list of HPV chemicals [34].

1.6.6 Alkylphenols

Long-chain alkylphenols, and their precursors, alkylphenol ethoxylates, have been used in industry for over 40 years mainly as surfactants in industrial and domestic applications worldwide [43,44]. They are used as precursors to detergents, as additives in fuel and lubricants, components of phenolic resins and as building blocks for fragrances. The main compounds used are propylphenol, butylphenol, amylphenol, heptylphenol, octylphenol, nonylphenol, and dodecylphenol. 4-Nonylphenol (Figure 1.7) is listed by the OECD in 2004 as an HPV chemical [34].

1.6.7 Triclosan

Triclosan [5-chloro-2-(2,4-dichlorophenoxy)phenol] [45] (Figure 1.7) is a chlorinated aromatic compound that has been used as an antibacterial and antifungal agent since the 1970s. It was first used as a hospital scrub but has since been incorporated into a wide range of personal care products. It is also used for its antimicrobial properties in kitchen utensils, toys, bedding, and clothing [45].

1.6.8 Parabens

The alkyl esters of *p*-hydroxybenzoic acid (parabens) (Figure 1.8) are used as antimicrobial agents for the preservation of foods, pharmaceuticals, and cosmetics. More recently, they have been used in the preservation of paper products [46]. The main parabens used in personal care products are methylparaben, ethylparaben, *n*-propylparaben, *n*-butylparaben, isobutylparaben, and benzylparaben.

1.6.9 UV Filters

Many compounds are now used to absorb ultraviolet (UV) light in consumer products [47]. They were used initially primarily in suncare products to protect the skin of the user from sunburn, but they are now used in a range of personal care products to protect the product itself from damage by UV light during storage. They are also finding uses in the clothing industry. Compounds with endocrine-disrupting properties that are used include the benzophenones, 2-ethylhexyl 4-methoxy cinnamate, 3-(4-methyl-benzilidene) camphor, and homosalate [47]. Benzophenone (Figure 1.8) is listed in the 2004 OECD list of HPV chemicals [34].

1.6.10 Organometals and Metals

⁻BT is an organotin compound [48] composed of three butyl groupings covalently ⁴ to a tetrahedral tin center. For 40 years, TBT was added as a biocide to antifouling

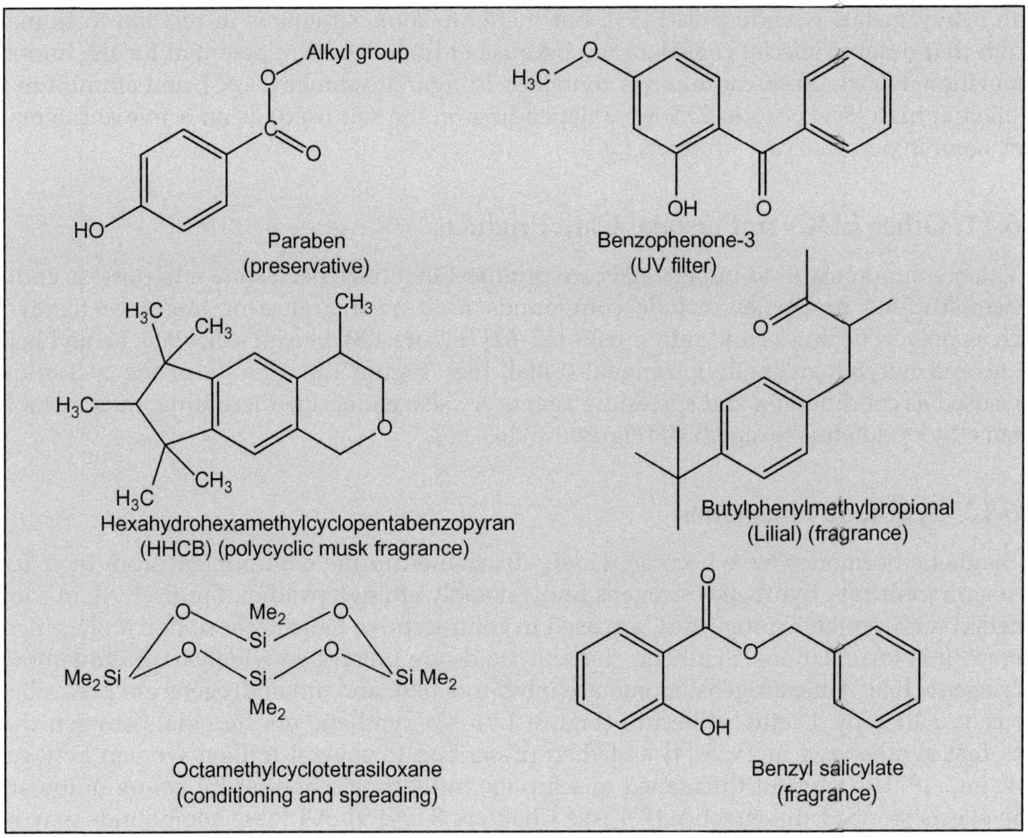

FIGURE 1.8   Chemical structures of compounds used in personal care products. The function in the product is indicated in brackets.

paints used to protect the hulls of ships from growth of organisms. The antifouling properties of TBT were first identified in the 1950s in the Netherlands, and due to its efficacy and low cost, it had become the most popular antifouling paint worldwide by the mid-1960s. The paints gave fuel efficiency to the ships and delayed costly ship repairs. Unfortunately, over widespread use with time, the TBT leached into the water, causing widescale toxicity to aquatic organisms. It has now been banned by several international organizations, including the Rotterdam Convention of the UNEP in 2009, [49] but its long life in sediment makes it a continued environmental pollutant.

Although most EDCs have an organic component, some metal ions have also been shown capable of interfering in estrogen action and these inorganic xenoestrogens have been termed metalloestrogens [50]. These include both cations and anions. Some of the metals have known physiological functions, but others, like aluminum [51], have no role in biology and have simply been unleashed from the earth by the activities of humans. The metalloestrogens include aluminum, antimony, arsenite, barium, cadmium, chromium [Cr(II)], cobalt, copper, lead, mercury, nickel, selenite, tin, and vanadate [52]. Pollution of the ecosystem with heavy metals is widespread [53], but there are some situations in relation to human health that deserve special consideration because of high exposure potential for the human population. For example, cadmium is contained in cigarette smoke [54,55], and aluminum is applied at high levels (up to 25% w/v depending on the salt used) as an active antiperspirant agent in personal care products [56].

1.6.11 Other EDCs in Personal Care Products

Other compounds used in personal care products that have been shown to possess endocrine-disrupting properties include compounds used as fragrance or fragrance fixatives such as polycyclic musks and nitromusks [57–61] (Figure 1.8), benzyl salicylate, benzyl benzoate, and butylphenylmethylpropional (Lilial) [62] (Figure 1.8). Certain of the cyclosiloxanes used as conditioning and spreading agents are also endocrine-disrupting, most notably octamethylcyclotetrasiloxane (D4) (Figure 1.8) [63–65].

1.6.12 Synthetic Hormones

Synthetic hormones have become widely distributed in the environment from their use as pharmaceuticals. Synthetic estrogens [most notably ethinylestradiol (Figure 1.9)], in combination with synthetic progestins, are used in contraceptive [66] and hormone replacement therapy [67] formulations. Synthetic glucocorticoids are prescribed widely as antiinflammatory agents [68]. Antiestrogens, aromatase inhibitors [69], and antiandrogens are prescribed for cancer therapy. Diethylstilbestrol (Figure 1.9) is a synthetic nonsteroidal estrogen that was first synthesized in 1938 [4] and then prescribed to several million women between 1940 and 1971 to prevent threatened miscarriage in the first trimester [5] before untoward side effects stopped this practice [70] (see Chapters 8 and 9). All these compounds may be released into the environment not only as the parent compound, but also as the metabolites in the urine and feces of people who use them as medications.

1.6.13 Paracetamol

N-Acetyl-p-aminophenol (paracetamol) (Figure 1.9) is widely used as an analgesic (pain reliever) and antipyretic (fever reducer). It has been freely available to purchase without a prescription since the 1950s, so it has become a common household drug. Its mode of action is at least partly through the inhibition of cyclooxygenase enzymes, notably COX-2 [71]. In 1997, it was estimated to have a production volume of 30,000–35,000 tons in the United States which is about half the world's consumption [72,73]. It has recently been shown to possess endocrine-disrupting properties [74].

1.6.14 Mycoestrogens

Mycoestrogens are compounds produced by fungi that possess estrogenic activity. A main example is zearalenone, a fungal metabolite (Figure 1.10), and this caused infertility in swine in the 1920s (as discussed earlier). Mycoestrogens are found commonly in stored grain, so they can be consumed in food [75].

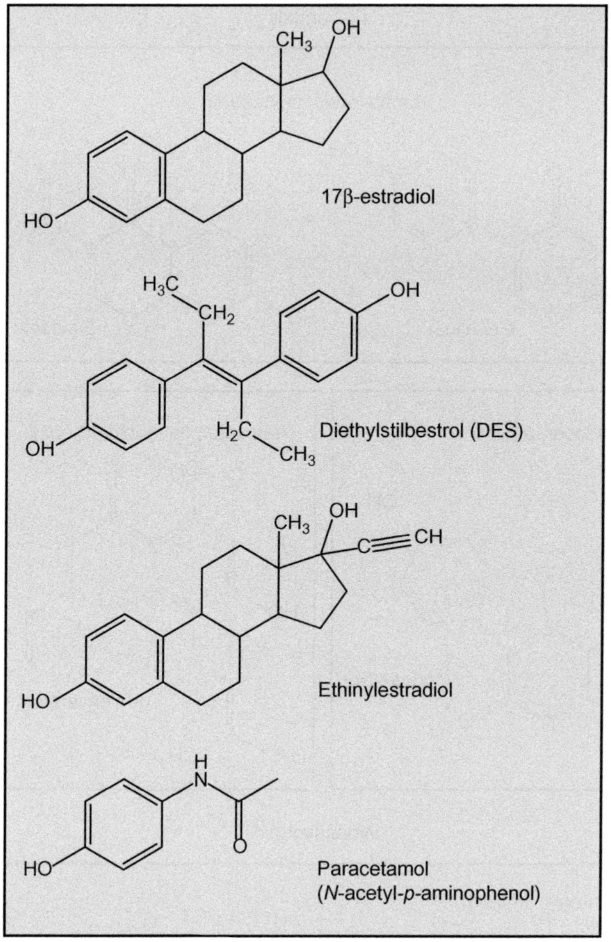

FIGURE 1.9   Chemical structures of pharmaceutical products.

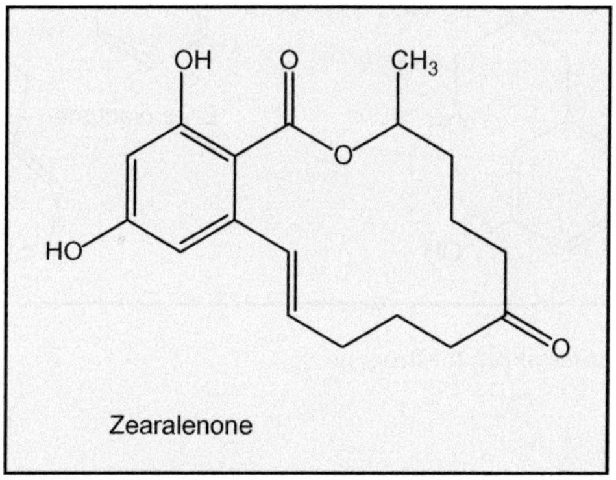

FIGURE 1.10   Chemical structure of zearalenone, a mycoestrogen.

1. OVERVIEW AND SCOPE

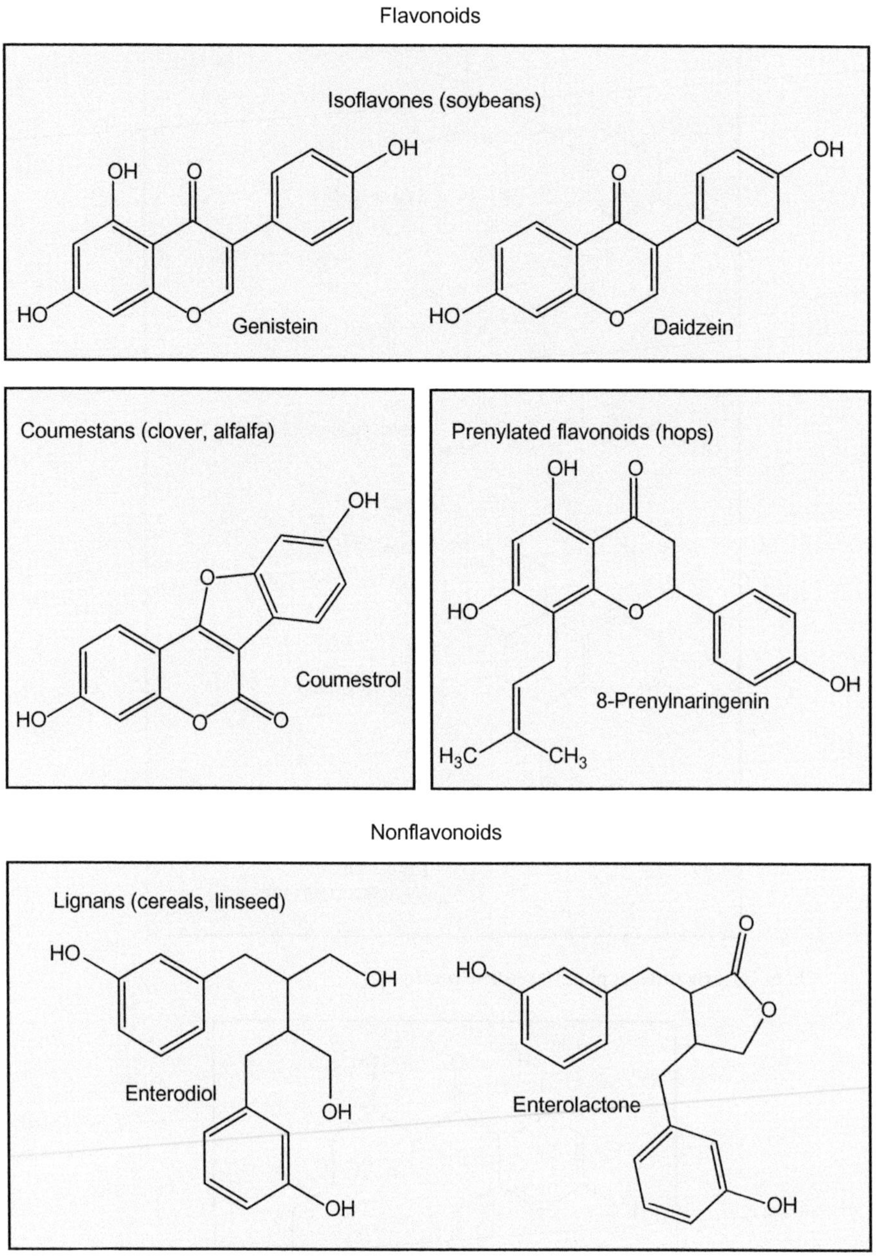

Flavonoids

FIGURE 1.11   Chemical structures of phytoestrogens.

1.6.15 Phytoestrogens

Phytoestrogens (*phyto*; from the Greek word for *plant*) are organic compounds produced naturally by plants that have the ability to mimic or interfere in the action of estrogens. They are found in over 300 different plant species and can be ingested by humans in the diet through the consumption of plant materials [76]. There are two main chemical types: flavonoids and nonflavonoids (Figure 1.11). Flavonoids include isoflavones, such as genistein and daidzein, found in soybeans, legumes, lentils, and chickpeas; coumestans, such as coumestrol found in young sprouting legumes, clover, and alfalfa sprouts; and prenylflavonoids, such as 8-prenylnaringenin, found in hops. Lignans are the most prevalent nonflavonoids, of which enterodiol and enterolactone are the principal estrogenic metabolites, and these are found in most cereals, linseed, fruits, and vegetables. On the basis that compounds of natural origin are assumed to be beneficial whereas artificial compounds are automatically assumed to be adverse, society has responded in opposing ways to the plant-based phytoestrogens from the artificial pollutant xenoestrogenic contaminants. Although both phytoestrogens and xenoestrogens display estrogenic activity in in vitro and animal models, society has generally chosen to positively embrace use of the phytoestrogens while mistrusting the xenoestrogens. With this background, it is likely that the potential benefits of phytoestrogens often have been overstated and adverse effects underappreciated.

1.6.16 Nutraceuticals

Nutraceuticals are a relatively new form of consumer product whose name is coined from the words *nutrition* and *pharmaceutical.* They include a range of nutrients, herbal products, and dietary supplements taken on the basis that they provide health benefits. Some of these products contain EDCs, most notably phytoestrogens (as discussed previously).

References

[1] Report of the European workshop on the impact of endocrine disrupters on human health and wildlife. Weybridge, UK. Report EUR17549 of the Environment and Climate Change Research Programme of DGXII of the European Commission; 1996.
[2] McNutt SH, Purwin P, Murray C. Vulvo-vaginitis in swine: preliminary report. J Am Vet Med Assoc 1928;73:484.
[3] Bennets H, Underwood EJ, Shier FL. A specific breeding problem of sheep on subterranean clover pasture in Western Australia. Aust Vet J 1946;22:2–12.
[4] Dodds EC, Goldberg L, Lawson W, Robinson R. Estrogenic activity of certain synthetic compounds. Nature 1938;141:247–8.
[5] Smith OW. Diethylstilboestrol in the prevention and treatment of complications of pregnancy. Am J Obstet Gynecol 1948;56:821–34.
[6] Carson R. Silent spring. Boston, MA: Houghton Mifflin; 1962.
[7] Burlington H, Linderman VF. Effect of DDT on testes and secondary sex characteristics of white leghorn cockerels. Proc Soc Exp Biol Med 1950;74:48–51.
[8] Bitman J, Cecil HC, Harris SJ, Fries GF. Estrogenic activity of o,p′-DDT in the mammalian uterus and avian oviduct. Science 1968;162:371–2.
[9] Welch RM, Levin W, Conney AH. Estrogenic action of DDT and its analogs. Toxicol Appl Pharmacol 1969;4:358–67.
[10] Colborn T, Dumanoski D, Myers JP. Our stolen future. New York, NY: Dutton; 1996.
[11] Colborn T, Clement C. Chemically-induced alterations in sexual and functional development: the wildlife/human connection. Princeton, NJ: Princeton Scientific Publishing Co Inc; 1992.

[12] Hotchkiss AK, Rider CV, Blystone CR, Wilson VS, Hartig PC, Ankley GT, et al. Fifteen years after "Wingspread"—environmental endocrine disrupters and human and wildlife health: where we are today and where we need to go. Toxicol Sci 2008;105:235–59.

[13] European Environment Agency (EEA) The impacts of endocrine disrupters on wildlife, people and their environments. The Weybridge + 15 (1996–2011) report. Luxemburg: Publications Office of the European Union; 2012. ISBN 978-92-9213-307-B.

[14] Diamanti-Kandarakis E, Bourguignon JP, Giudice LC, Hauser R, Prins GS, Soto AM, et al. Endocrine-disrupting chemicals: an endocrine society scientific statement. Endocrine Rev 2009;30:293–342.

[15] Bergman A, Heindel JJ, Jobling S, Kidd KA, Zoeller RT, editors. The state of the science of endocrine disrupting chemicals—2012. United Nations Environment Programme (UNEP) and World Health Organisation (WHO); 2013. <http://unep.org/pdf/9789241505031_eng.pdf>.

[16] CHEMTrust. CHEMTrust overview of key scientific statements on endocrine disrupting chemicals (EDCs) 1991–2013. January 2014. <http://www.chemtrust.org.uk/wp-content/uploads/Scientific-Statements-on-EDCs-V2-Dec20132.pdf>.

[17] Horiguchi T. Masculinization of female gastropod mollusks induced by organotin compounds, focusing on mechanism of actions of tributyltin and triphenyltin for development of imposex. Environ Sci 2006;13: 77–87.

[18] Matthiessen P. Historical perspective on endocrine disruption in wildlife. Pure Appl Chem 2003;75:2197–206.

[19] Jorundsdottir K, Svavarsson J, Leung KM. Imposex levels in the dogwhelk Nucella lapillus (L.)—continuing improvement at high latitudes. Mar Pollut Bull 2005;51:744–9.

[20] Guillette Jr LJ, Gunderson MP. Alterations in development of reproductive and endocrine systems of wildlife populations exposed to endocrine-disrupting contaminants. Reproduction 2001;122:857–64.

[21] Jobling S, Nolan M, Tyler CR, Brighty G, Sumpter JP. Widespread sexual disruption in wild fish. Environ Sci Technol 1998;32:2498–506.

[22] Harries JE, Janbakhsh A, Jobling S, Mattiessen P, Sumpter JP, Tyler CR. Estrogenic potency of effluent from two sewage treatment works in the United Kingdom. Environ Toxicol Chem 1999;18:932–7.

[23] Ratcliff DA. Decrease in eggshell weight in certain birds of prey. Nature 1967;215:208–10.

[24] Ratcliff DA. Changes attributable to pesticides in egg breakage frequency and eggshell thickness in some British birds. J Appl Ecol 1970;7:67–115.

[25] Lundholm CE. DDE-induced eggshell thinning in birds: effects of p,p'-DDE on the calcium and prostaglandin metabolism of the eggshell gland. Comp Biochem Physiol Part C Pharmacol Toxicol Endocrinol 1997;118:113–28.

[26] Bosveld ATC, van den Berg M. Reproductive failure and endocrine disruption by organohalogens in fish-eating birds. Toxicology 2002;181:155–9.

[27] Bowerman WW, Best DA, Grubb TG, Sikarskie JG, Giesy JP. Assessment of environmental endocrine disruptors in bald eagles of the Great Lakes. Chemosphere 2000;41:1569–74.

[28] Publications of the secretariat of the Stockholm convention on persistent organic pollutants. <www.pops.int>.

[29] World Health Organisation. DDT and its derivatives. Environmental Health Criteria 1979; Number 9.

[30] World Health Organisation. Polychlorinated biphenyls and terphenyls. Environmental Health Criteria 1992; Number 140.

[31] World Health Organisation. Polychlorinated dibenzo-p-dioxins and dibenzofurans. Environmental Health Criteria 1989; Number 88.

[32] Parzefall W. Risk assessment of dioxin contamination in human food. Food Chem Toxicol 2002;40:1185–9.

[33] World Health Organisation. Brominated diphenyl ethers. Environmental Health Criteria 1994; Number 162.

[34] Organisation for Economic Cooperation and Development (OECD) The 2004 OECD list of high production volume chemicals. Paris, France: Environment Directorate; 2004.

[35] Hayes TB, Anderson LL, Beasley VR, de Solla SR, Iguchi T, Ingraham H, et al. Demasculinization and feminization of male gonads by atrazine: consistent effects across vertebrate classes. J Steroid Biochem Mol Biol 2011;127:64–73.

[36] World Health Organisation. Glyphosate. Environmental Health Criteria 1994; Number 159.

[37] Walsh LP, McCormick C, Martin C, Stocco DM. Roundup inhibits steroidogenesis by disrupting steroidogenic acute regulatory (StAR) protein expression. Environ Health Perspect 2000;108:769–76.

[38] Rubin BS, Bisphenol A. An endocrine disruptor with widespread exposure and multiple effects. J Steroid Biochem Mol Biol 2011;127:27–34.

[39] Rochester JR. Bisphenol A and human health: a review of the literature. Reprod Toxicol 2013;42:132–55.

[40] Krishnan AV, Stathis P, Permuth SF, Tokes L, Feldman D. Bisphenol-A: an estrogenic substance is released from polycarbonate flasks during autoclaving. Endocrinology 1993;132:2279–86.

[41] Kamrin MA. Phthalate risks, phthalate regulation and public health: a review. J Toxicol Environ Health Part B 2009;12:157–74.

[42] Huang PC, Liou SH, Ho IK, Chiang HC, Huang HI, Wang SL. Phthalates exposure and endocrinal effects: an epidemiological review. J Food Drug Anal 2012;20:719–33.

[43] Nimrod AC, Benson WH. Environmental estrogenic effects of alkylphenol ethoxylates. Crit Rev Toxicol 1996:335–64.

[44] Kovarova J, Blahova J, Divsova L, Svobodova Z. Alkylphenol ethoxylates and alkylphenols—update information on occurrence, fate and toxicity in aquatic environment. Pol J Vet Sci 2013;16:763–72.

[45] Dann AB, Hontela A. Triclosan: environmental exposure, toxicity and mechanisms of action. J Appl Toxicol 2011;31:285–311.

[46] Darbre PD, Harvey PW. Parabens can enable hallmarks and characteristics of cancer in human breast epithelial cells: a review of the literature with reference to new exposure data and regulatory status. J Appl Toxicol 2014;34:925–38.

[47] Krause M, Klit A, Blomberg-Jensen M, Søeborg T, Frederiksen H, Schlumpf M, et al. Sunscreens: are they beneficial for health? An overview of endocrine disrupting properties of UV-filters. Int J Androl 2012;35: 424–36.

[48] World Health Organisation. Tin and organotin compounds. Environmental Health Criteria 1980; Number 15.

[49] The Rotterdam Convention of the United Nations Environment Programme, 2009. <www.pic.int>.

[50] Safe S. Cadmium's disguise dupes the estrogen receptor. Nat Med 2003;9:1000–1.

[51] World Health Organisation. Aluminium. Environmental Health Criteria 1997; Number 194.

[52] Darbre PD. Metalloestrogens: an emerging class of inorganic xenoestrogens with potential to add to the oestrogenic burden of the human breast. J Appl Toxicol 2006;26:191–7.

[53] Jarup L. Hazards of heavy metal contamination. Br Med Bull 2003;68:167–82.

[54] World Health Organisation. Cadmium. Environmental Health Criteria 1992; Number 134.

[55] Rani A, Kumar A, Lal A, Pant M. Cellular mechanisms of cadmium-induced toxicity: a review. Int J Environ Health Perspect 2014;24:378–99.

[56] Darbre PD, Mannello F, Exley C. Aluminium and breast cancer: sources of exposure, tissue measurements and mechanisms of toxicological actions on breast biology. J Inorg Biochem 2013;128:257–61.

[57] Bitsch N, Dudas C, Korner W, Failing K, Biselli S, Rimkus G, et al. Estrogenic activity of musk fragrances detected by the E-screen assay using human MCF-7 cells. Arch Environ Contam Toxicol 2002;43:257–64.

[58] Gomez E, Pillon A, Fenet H, Rosain D, Duchesne MJ, Nicolas JC, et al. Estrogenic activity of cosmetic components in reporter cell lines: parabens, UV screens and musks. J Toxicol Environ Health A 2005;68:239–51.

[59] Schreurs RH, Sonneveld E, Jansen JH, Seinen W, van der Burg B. Interaction of polycyclic musks with the estrogen receptor (ER), androgen receptor (AR) and progesterone receptor (PR) in reporter gene assays. Toxicol Sci 2005;83:264–72.

[60] Mori T, Iida M, Ishibashi H, Kohra S, Takao Y, Takemasa T, et al. Hormonal activity of polycyclic musks evaluated by reporter gene assay. Environ Sci 2007;14:195–202.

[61] Van der Burg B, Schreurs R, Linden S, Seinen W, Brouwer A, Sonneveld E. Endocrine effects of polycyclic musks: do we smell a rat? Int J Androl 2008;31:188–93.

[62] Charles AK, Darbre PD. Oestrogenic activity of benzyl salicylate, benzyl benzoate and butylphenylmethylpropional (Lilial) in MCF7 human breast cancer cells in vitro. J Appl Toxicol 2009;29:422–34.

[63] Hayden JF, Barlow SA. Structure–activity relationships of organosiloxanes and the female reproductive system. Toxicol Appl Pharmacol 1972;21:68–79.

[64] McKim JM, Wilga PC, Breslin WJ, Plotzke KP, Gallavan RH, Meeks RG. Potential estrogenic and antiestrogenic activity of the cyclic siloxane ocatamethylcyclotetrasiloxane (D4) and the linear siloxane hexamethyldisiloxane (HMDS) in immature rats using the uterotrophic assay. Toxicol Sci 2001;63:37–46.

[65] He B, Rhodes-Brower S, Miller MR, Munson AE, Germolec DR, Walker VR, et al. Octamethylcyclotetrasiloxane exhibits estrogenic activity in mice via ERα. Toxicol Appl Pharmacol 2003;192:254–61.

[66] Stanczyk FZ, Archer DF, Bhavnani BR. Ethinyl estradiol and 17β-estradiol in combined oral contraceptives: pharmacokinetics, pharmacodynamics and risk assessment. Contraception 2013;87:706–27.

[67] Mattox JH, Shulkman LP. Combined oral hormone replacement therapy formulations. Am J Obstet Gynecol 2001;185:S38–46.

[68] Rhen T, Cidlowski JA. Antiinflammatory action of glucocorticoids—new mechanisms for old drugs. New Engl J Med 2005;353:1711–23.

[69] Lonning PE, editor. Endocrinology and treatment of breast cancer. Clin Endocrinol Metab 2004;18:1–130.

[70] Harris RM, Waring RH. Diethylstilboestrol—a long-term legacy. Maturitas 2012;72:108–12.

[71] Hinz B, Cheremina O, Brune K. Acetaminophen (paracetamol) is a selective cyclooxygenase-2 inhibitor in man. FASEB J 2008;22:383–90.

[72] Mirasol F. Acetaminophen market sees moderate price hike. Chem Mark Rep 1998;254:5.

[73] International Agency for Research on Cancer. Paracetamol—IARC monographs. 1999;73:402.

[74] Kristensen DM, Hass U, Lesné L, Lottrup G, Jacobsen PR, Desdoits-Lethimonier C, et al. Intrauterine exposure to mild analgesics is a risk factor for development of male reproductive disorders in human and rat. Hum Reprod 2011;26:235–44.

[75] Bennett JW, Klich M. Mycotoxins. Clin Microbiol Rev 2003;16:497–516.

[76] Woods HF (chairman). Phytoestrogens and health. Crown copyright, 2003.

How Could Endocrine Disrupters Affect Human Health?

Philippa D. Darbre

Endocrine Disruption and Human Health.
DOI: http://dx.doi.org/10.1016/B978-0-12-801139-3.00002-8

Abstract

This chapter begins with an overview of the extent to which endocrine-disrupting chemicals (EDCs) can enter human tissues from environmental exposure. Retention of EDCs in body tissues may be influenced both by their route of entry and by their resistance to physiological clearance processes. Their endocrine-disrupting activity and biological availability may also be influenced by endogenous metabolic reactions. Measurements using a range of body tissues have demonstrated the ubiquitous distribution of many EDCs across the human population, but the source of the body burden is difficult to establish due to the widespread use of these compounds. The measurement of so many different EDCs in human tissues demonstrates the potential for mixtures of EDCs at low doses to interfere in the long term on hormone regulation with adverse consequences for human health. Many different nonlinear, nonmonotonic dose-responses to EDCs have been demonstrated, and effects at high doses may not always be predictive of effects at low doses. The effects of EDCs vary in different tissues and between individuals, but timing is also important. Critical windows of susceptibility to EDC exposure exist during pre-natal life and early childhood, and some exposures to EDCs in utero can produce long-lasting effects into adult life and on future generations.

2.1 INTRODUCTION

The realization that so many environmental chemicals can exert their effects through disrupting hormone action brings a whole new dimension to toxicology. This is because the action of endocrine-disrupting chemicals (EDCs), through hijacking biological mechanisms (notably by binding to hormone receptors or influencing activity of enzymes involved with hormone synthesis, bioavailability or degradation, as discussed in Chapter 1), enables responses to occur at much lower concentrations than would be expected for classically nonspecific toxicity. Since multiple chemicals can act through the same biological target, this allows for even smaller doses of each chemical to then be added together to generate the final end-point response. Furthermore, the responses will be specifically targeted, and for example, receptor-mediated mechanisms allow responses to be targeted directly to the nucleus, with resulting effects on patterns of gene expression. In addition, timing, duration, and pattern of exposure may be as important as the dose itself, and dose-responses may not even be linear, but instead show a range of nonmonotonic patterns. This means that adverse effects cannot be predicted alone from a single dose of one chemical. A major further concern coming to the forefront of research on endocrine disruption is that some effects may be long-lasting and can even be passed to future generations without any further exposure being necessary. These issues will be outlined in this chapter and discussed in more detail in Chapters 3–15.

Responses to EDCs may range from specific cellular events (such as alteration to the expression of a gene) to altered physiological responses affecting the whole body (see Chapters 3–15). Hormones of the endocrine system are ultimately responsible not only for regulating major physiological processes of development and reproduction, but also for maintenance of all the tissues and organs of the body and for enabling adaptations to environmental changes. Although estrogens are responsible for ensuring female reproduction, their influence extends beyond reproductive tissues into bone, brain, liver, and the cardiovascular system. Thyroid hormones affect all tissues through their role in regulating metabolism. Glucocorticoids have very wide-ranging actions on all tissues through their roles in regulating body fluid homeostasis and glucose metabolism, and in mediating stress responses and inflammation. This is why EDCs are now being found to influence so

> - Female reproductive disorders
>   - Early puberty
>   - Disorders of the uterus
>   - Disorders of the ovaries
>   - Benign breast disease
> - Male reproductive disorders
>   - Urogenital tract malformations
>   - Reduced sperm count and sperm quality
>   - Gynecomastia
> - Thyroid dysfunction
> - Adrenal dysfunction
> - Disorders of the immune system
> - Obesity, metabolic syndrome, and diabetes
> - Cancer of endocrine responsive tissues
> - Cardiovascular disease
> - Bone disorders
> - Developmental disorders
>   - Neurodevelopment (behavioral abnormalities, Alzheimer's disease, Parkinson's disease)

FIGURE 2.1   Human endocrine disorders that have been reported to be affected by EDCs.

many endocrine-sensitive processes (Figure 2.1) [1]. Not only can they interfere in female (Chapter 8) and male (Chapter 9) reproductive processes, but also in thyroid function (Chapter 11), adrenal function (Chapter 12), and immune function (Chapter 14). They can also interfere with metabolism, with resulting effects on obesity and diabetes (Chapters 13 and 15), and with regulation of cell growth, with resulting implications for cancer (Chapter 10). Their effects on developmental processes, including neurodevelopment, have implications for many of the neurological conditions in later life, such as behavioral abnormalities, Alzheimer's disease, and Parkinson's disease (Chapter 13).

2.2 ENTRY INTO HUMAN TISSUES

If EDCs are suspected to exert a functional role in the human body, then the first considerations must be of the extent to which they can enter human tissues from environmental exposure. Entry into the human body may occur through inhalation or oral or dermal routes, and Figure 2.2 outlines some of the main sources of exposure for these different routes. However, none of the sources are mutually exclusive. For example, exposure to pesticides and herbicides may be primarily through inhalation from agricultural spraying, outside spraying in urban gardens or from indoor spraying, but residues may also enter through the oral route from residues in water and food or through the dermal route from inadvertant contamination of the skin. While chemicals impregnated into clothing or soft furnishings would be expected to come into contact mainly with skin, many have also been detected in indoor air, which enables inhalation. Many pharmaceuticals are taken orally, but increasing numbers are now applied in patches to the skin, including nicotine and oral contraception patches.

The route of entry is a major factor in the resulting body uptake. In general, inhalation and oral entry of chemicals will result in greater uptake than dermal application. However,

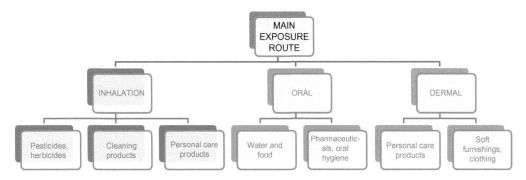

FIGURE 2.2   Examples of human exposure routes for EDCs.

for dermal application, this difference is offset by the near-continuous presence of chemicals in cosmetics, which are not washed off but remain on the skin for long periods, allowing low-level absorption of chemicals over the long term. Furthermore, the shaving of skin prior to cosmetic application can create nicks in the skin that allow greater entry of chemicals into underlying layers of the dermis than would occur in intact skin. The route of entry also influences the metabolic detoxification of EDCs. Since oral and inhaled chemicals will be absorbed into the bloodstream, they will pass through the liver, where they will be subject to metabolic detoxification mechanisms. However, dermally absorbed chemicals will be taken up locally, so they will bypass the liver's metabolism and be subject to metabolic enzymes only locally, in the tissue into which they are absorbed.

The extent to which EDCs are then retained in tissues will depend on the ability of the metabolism to remove them through detoxification reactions catalyzed by the cytochrome P450 enzymes and conjugation systems. Some EDCs, such as phytoestrogens, can be consumed in large amounts in plant material via the diet, but they are removed from the body within hours [2]. However, other EDCs, particularly persistent organic pollutants (POPs), may be taken into the body in only small amounts, but through their resistance to clearance, they may be retained for long periods in body tissues and bioaccumulate over the years, particularly in fatty tissues of the body [3–5].

2.3 CAN EDCs BE ABSORBED FROM DERMAL APPLICATION?

While it is generally accepted that compounds taken in by inhalation or the oral route would enter the human body, there has been more controversy concerning the ability of dermally applied chemicals to be absorbed. Publication in 2004 of measurements of intact paraben esters in human breast tissue [6] sparked debate concerning the wider ability of chemicals applied in lotions to the skin to be absorbed into human tissues [7] (see Chapter 19). Studies from Denmark, however, confirmed the ability of EDCs in cosmetics to be absorbed systemically from dermal application of cosmetic cream in human subjects. Janjua and colleagues demonstrated the systemic absorption of dermally applied butylparaben, diethylphthalate, and dibutylphthalate in 26 healthy male volunteers with levels measurable in blood as little as 1 h after dermal application [8] and in urine after 8–12h [9]. They also measured the rate of absorption of three dermally applied sunscreens [benzo-phenone-3, 3-(4-methylbenzilidene) camphor, and octylmethoxycinnamate] in 32 healthy human volunteers (15 men and 17 women). None of the sunscreens were detectable before the first application but after dermal application, all three were detectable in plasma after 2h and in urine after 24h [10].

2.4 TISSUE MEASUREMENTS

Measurement of body burdens of EDCs requires collection of human tissue samples of which blood (serum), urine, and milk are the most accessible. Serum samples from adults provide a snapshot of circulating EDC levels, and since all organs are infused with blood, this provides a measure of overall body burden. However, levels of nonpersistent EDCs can decrease rapidly after cessation of exposure [8,10], so blood levels can fluctuate according to exposure levels at the time of sampling. Cord blood samples have provided a measure of placental transfer from mother to child [11]. Urine samples are more easily obtained because sampling is noninvasive, so this offers the option of large numbers of measurements with statistical power, but with the proviso that levels of EDCs in the urine will reflect body clearance more than homeostatic body burden. This is especially pertinent for EDCs that are persistent and lipophilic, and therefore not easily cleared from the body, because these would be present in urine at only small concentrations while accumulating over the years in fatty tissues. The use of human milk samples has been instrumental in assessing how maternal body burdens of EDCs influence levels of EDCs are passed to the baby in breast milk. The high fat content of human milk provides an ideal medium for removal of lipophilic EDCs from the mother's breast tissues with a resulting loading passed to the baby [1,12–15]. Far fewer measurements have been made using specific body tissues for obvious reasons of difficulty in obtaining samples, but it remains crucial to obtain measurements of EDCs in relevant organs where the health problems originate even if sample sizes are small. For example, it has been known for many years that relative levels of different polychlorinated biphenyl (PCB) congeners may vary between maternal blood and breast milk [16], and therefore measurements in blood cannot always be assumed to reflect levels in the human breast.

Over the past 20 years, biomonitoring of levels of EDCs has been steadily increasing following both government investment and technical advances. The National Health and Nutrition Examination Survey (NHANES), established in the United States, has provided the most extensive survey of EDCs across the U.S. population, and is unique in that it links the blood and urine specimens with interviews and physical examinations. This national survey has demonstrated that many of the EDCs listed in Chapter 1 are found ubiquitously in the U.S. population, demonstrating the widespread contamination of the population with these compounds. Figure 2.3 shows arithmetic mean serum concentrations of one polybrominated diphenyl ether (PBDE) congener (A), one PCB congener (B), and a breakdown product of the persistent insecticide dichlorodiphenyltrichloroethane (DDT) (C) in three separate sampling periods: 2003–2004, 2005–2006, and 2007–2008 of the NHANES study [17]. DDT and PCBs have been banned in the United States for over 30 years, but the PBDE congener has only more recently ceased production. It is evident that the population

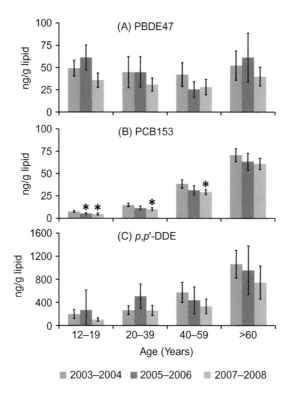

FIGURE 2.3   Arithmetic mean concentrations (ng/g lipid) across four age groupings for three POPs in serum samples of the U.S. population using three separate NHANES sampling periods. (A) 2,2′,4,4′-tetrabromodiphenyl ether (BDE-47); (B) 2,2′,4,4′,5,5′-hexachlorobiphenyl (PCB-153); (C) 2,2-bis(4-chlorophenyl)-1,1-dichloroethene (*p,p*′-DDE). Error bars indicate 95% confidence intervals (95% CI). Significantly different 95% CI of the arithmetic mean compared with NHANES 2003–2004 is indicated with an asterisk. *Source: Reproduced with permission from Sjordin et al. [17].*

is ubiquitously contaminated, even with compounds banned decades previously, and that contamination increases with age. However, there were significant reductions in the PCB congener (B) across three of the age groups with time, suggesting that discontinuation of these chemicals is resulting in a reduction in body burdens. Phthalate esters are another class of industrial chemicals that are widely used in consumer products and to which the human population is exposed (see Chapter 1). Figure 2.4 shows urinary levels of four monoester phthalate metabolites, as measured in the NHANES samples of 1999–2000 [18]. Detectable levels of the metabolites MEP, MBP, MBzP, and MEHP were found in more than 75% of the samples, suggesting widespread exposure of the U.S. population to diethyl phthalate, dibutyl phthalate or diisobutyl phthalate, benzylbutyl phthalate, and di-(2-ethylhexyl) phthalate (DEHP), respectively [18]. Table 2.1 lists some other EDCs that have been measured in human urine samples of the general U.S. population in the NHANES studies. Benzophenone-3 [used as an ultraviolet (UV) filter] [19], bisphenol A (used in plastics) [20], 4-tertiary-octylphenol (used to make resins and surfactants) [20], triclosan (used as an antimicrobial agent) [21], and parabens (used as preservatives) [22] were all measured

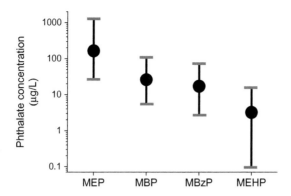

FIGURE 2.4 Levels of four phthalate metabolites in the urine of the U.S. population. Data taken from the NHANES study (1999–2000), as published by Silva and colleagues in 2004 [18]. Monoethyl phthalate (MEP), monobutyl phthalate (MBP), monobenzyl phthalate (MBzP), and mono-(2-ethylhexyl) phthalate (MEHP). Black dots show median values. The upper and lower red lines show the 90th and 10th percentiles, respectively. $N = 2540$, participants greater than or equal to 6 years of age.

ubiquitously in the urine samples (Table 2.1). The phytoestrogens genistein and daidzein (found in soybeans) were also measured ubiquitously, as was their metabolite equol [23] (Table 2.1). Enterlactone and enterodiol, the metabolites of lignans, were also measured ubiquitously [23] (Table 2.1).

Assessing the source of body burdens of EDCs can be very difficult due to the widespread use of so many of the compounds. For example, while parabens have been used extensively as preservatives in cosmetics applied to the skin, they are also used in preservation of food and pharmaceutical products (oral entry) [24] and of paper products [25], and their widespread use has led to their presence in indoor air [26], enabling inhalation. Parabens were first measured in human breast tissue in 2004 [6] but have since been measured in human urine, blood, milk, and placenta [27]. One or more parabens is measurable in 96% of human urine samples across the U.S. population in the NHANES samples of 2005–2006 [22,28] and in 158 of 160 breast tissue samples from the United Kingdom [29], but the source is impossible to identify due to the numerous consumer products to which parabens are added.

2.4.1 Biomarkers

Interpretation of the presence of EDCs in human tissues has been a subject of much controversy. Just the measurement of an EDC in human tissue cannot be taken to imply that there will be adverse functional consequences, but on the other hand, there could be. If EDCs were not present in human tissues, there would be no issue. However, since so many EDCs have been measured in human tissues, research needs to address what implications for human health exist, and under what circumstances. A next step in understanding whether the EDCs have any functional consequences in the tissues in which they are measured would be to develop biomarkers. The ability of EDCs to induce vitellogenin, an exclusively female protein, in male fish provides a very clear biomarker of exposure of the fish to EDCs in the aquatic environment in which they have been living [30]. Development of clear biomarkers for EDCs

TABLE 2.1   EDCs Measured in Human Urine Under the NHANES Using Urine Samples from the U.S. General Population of Those Greater Than or Equal to 6 Years of Age

Compound	NHANES	Sample number	% Population in which detected	Concentration in human urine (Median) (μg/L)	Reference
EDCs IN CONSUMER PRODUCTS					
Benzophenone-3	2003–2004	2517	96.80%	18.0	[19]
Bisphenol A	2003–2004	2517	92.60%	2.7	[20]
4-tertiary-octylphenol	2003–2004	2517	57.40%	0.3	[20]
Triclosan	2003–2004	2517	74.60%	13.0	[21]
Methylparaben	2005–2006	2548	99.10%	63.5	[22]
Propylparaben	2005–2006	2548	92.70%	8.7	[22]
Butylparaben	2005–2006	2548	47%	<LOD	[22]
Ethylparaben	2005–2006	2548	42.40%	<LOD	[22]
PHYTOESTROGENS					
Genistein	1999–2000	2557	93.2%	27.3	[23]
Daidzein	1999–2000	2554	98.5%	69.8	[23]
Equol	1999–2000	2182	73.9%	8.0	[23]
Enterolactone	1999–2000	2548	98.2%	315.0	[23]
Enterodiol	1999–2000	2527	92.2%	34.0	[23]

Total EDC levels in the urine sample.

in human tissues would be very beneficial in identifying functional consequences of the presence of the EDCs. Such biomarkers could be molecular (demonstrating some specific change to expression of one or more genes), histological (changes to tissue architecture), or physiological (specific changes to body function clearly linked to EDC exposure).

2.5 ROLE OF METABOLISM IN BIOLOGICAL ACTIVITY OF EDCs

2.5.1 Metabolism May Alter the Endocrine-Disrupting Properties of an EDC

On occasion, normal metabolism can produce harmful compounds, and therefore, the body has evolved a range of metabolic capabilities that can detoxify such compounds using cytochrome P450 enzymes. These enzymes can also help to rid the body of unwanted toxic foreign compounds, including pharmaceuticals and environmental chemicals, but in so doing, they can sometimes inadvertently turn a harmless parent foreign compound into a compound with unwanted activity. In this way, some environmental compounds that of themselves possess only weak or no endocrine-disrupting properties can be converted into compounds with greater endocrine-disrupting activity. Environmental contamination of animal tissues with DDT includes not only the parent compound, but a mixture of related compounds generated from breakdown and metabolism, and o,p'-DDT has been reported to possess more potent estrogenic activity than the parent DDT compound [31,32]. Hydroxylation of organochlorine compounds is particularly pertinent because the introduction of hydroxyl groupings onto ring structures can generate phenolic groupings, which especially in the para position, can facilitate binding into the ligand binding domain of the estrogen receptor (ER) (see Chapter 3). Some PCB congeners bind only weakly to ERs and their more potent estrogenic activity in vitro and in vivo has been related to metabolic conversion to more reactive intermediates through the hydroxylation [33,34] or generation of catechol metabolites [35].

On the other hand, some foreign compounds may have their endocrine-disrupting activity reduced by endogenous metabolic reactions. For example, the estrogenic activity of the alkyl esters of p-hydroxybenzoic acid (parabens) increases with the linear length of the alkyl chain from methylparaben to n-butylparaben [36] and with branching in the alkyl chain from n-butylparaben to isobutylparaben [37], but all the parabens are subject to endogenous esterase activity, which converts them into the common metabolite p-hydroxybenzoic acid with lower estrogenic activity [38]. The presence of intact paraben esters in human tissues is indicative; therefore, they have escaped metabolism by esterases [7,29].

2.5.2 EDCs May Alter Endogenous Enzyme Activities

EDCs can also act though interfering with activities of different metabolic enzymes. Some EDCs can alter the activity of enzymes involved in steroid hormone biosynthesis or degradation. This has resulting consequences to the levels of hormones secreted, thereby perturbing the homeostatic balance between the concentrations of different hormones, with inevitable physiological consequences. Several pesticides (p,p'-DDT, methoxychlor, lindance, dieldrin, and tributyltin), herbicides (atrazine), fungicides (vinclozolin and prochloraz), bisphenol A, phthalates, octylphenol, and some PCBs may all modulate hormone synthesis by this mechanism [39] (see Chapter 3).

Phytoestrogens have been shown to have diverse actions on a range of enzymes [2], including the inhibition of protein tyrosine kinases [40], inhibition of enzymes involved in regulating cell cycle progression [41], inhibition of DNA topoisomerase [42,43], and inhibition of enzymes regulating angiogenesis [44,45].

2.6 BIOLOGICAL AVAILABILITY

Since steroid hormones are hydrophobic molecules that are only somewhat soluble in water, they are found in biological fluids and transported in the bloodstream either in a conjugated form, where they are linked to a hydrophilic moiety (usually as sulfate or glucuronide derivatives), or bound to carrier proteins. The unbound, unconjugated or "free" fraction is only a small proportion of the total (usually 1–2%) and is considered to represent the biologically available hormone that is free to enter cells.

2.6.1 Binding to Serum Proteins

Androgens and estrogens are bound mainly to steroid hormone binding globulin (SHBG) and, to a lesser extent, serum albumin. Corticosteroid-binding globulin (CBG) is the main carrier protein for glucocorticoids. About 20% of progesterone is carried by CBG, and the remainder by serum albumin. Since the binding globulin inhibits the activity of the hormones, bioavailability of the steroid molecules is influenced by the level of the binding globulin and by the relative binding affinity of competing hormones. Many EDCs also compete for binding to these carrier proteins in the bloodstream and thus can alter the levels of unbound bioavailable steroid [46]. Some phytoestrogens can alter levels of SHBG [47].

2.6.2 Modification by Conjugation

Conjugation of steroids is used to increase their hydrophilicity and is a major step in steroid catabolism and excretion. Two major forms of conjugate are used: glucuronides and sulfates. Glucuronidation involves the addition of a glucuronic acid to a hydroxyl group of the steroid using glucuronyl transferase. Sulfation involves the addition of sulfate onto a hydroxyl group of the steroid using sulfotransferases, and sulfatases can act to remove the sulfate group. EDCs can also be conjugated using these enzymes in order to enhance their hydrophilicity for excretion, but the extent of their conjugation can vary in different tissues. For example, it has been reported that more than 90% of parabens found in human urine are in conjugated form [28,48], but in human milk, the parabens are largely in unconjugated form [49,50]. This would suggest that while parabens can be conjugated for excretion in the urine, they are predominantly in a biologically available form in the human breast.

Although in general, it has been assumed that conjugation would negate any biological activity, experimental results have not always confirmed this. For the phytoestrogens genistein, daidzein, and equol, some estrogenic activity was retained in several of the sulfated forms, and sulfation of daidzein at the 7-position actually increased estrogenic activity [51].

2.7 DOSE-RESPONSE CONSIDERATIONS

Classical toxicology is based on the premise that "the dose makes the poison," a concept first introduced by the Swiss chemist Paracelsus (1493–1541), who is sometimes referred to as "the father of toxicology." This framework holds much truth because some toxic substances can be harmless in low doses and some harmless substances can become toxic at high doses. However, EDCs have challenged these basic concepts of toxicology because their ability to act through receptor-mediated mechanisms allows them to act at very low doses and often in a nonlinear manner. The dose-response curves can take many different forms, but one of the simplest is sigmoidal. The classical example of a biological sigmoid response curve is for oxygen binding to hemoglobin in the blood, where the response is sigmoidal because the binding is cooperative in that the first oxygen binds less easily than subsequent oxygens. However, hormones also act with a sigmoidal curve because hormone receptors are limited in number in a cell and therefore there comes a point where no matter how much more hormone is present, the response cannot be increased—this effect is called "saturation" because every receptor has 1 molecule of hormone bound to it. Likewise,

EDCs can also act with sigmoidal or other shaped dose-response curves. Furthermore, for some EDCs, effects at low doses may not be predictive of effects at high doses, with mechanisms of action being even quite different at low and high doses. The phytoestrogen genistein, for example, can increase the growth of estrogen-responsive cells at low doses by an ER-mediated mechanism; but at high doses, it inhibits cell growth by a different mechanism that does not involve ER [52]. Many different types of nonlinear, nonmonotonic responses to EDCs have now been demonstrated [53] and are discussed in detail in Chapter 7.

2.7.1 Receptor Binding Affinity Versus Response Efficacy

For receptor-mediated mechanisms of action, another dose-response consideration is that a low binding affinity of an EDC to a hormone receptor may not always equate to a weak efficacy for the end-point response (termed *potency*). Receptor-mediated mechanisms of ligand activity depend on two fundamental events: ligand affinity and ligand efficacy [54]. Most EDCs have been labeled "weak" on the basis that they bind with lower affinity to the hormone receptor than the endogenous hormone. However, not all EDCs are weak in their actions (efficacy) if sufficient concentrations are present. Ligand affinity for the receptor can be measured using in vitro techniques such as ligand binding assays (see Chapters 3–6), where the weaker the ligand binding affinity for the receptor, the higher the concentration of ligand needed to saturate the receptor or to compete off a radiolabeled ligand. Ligand efficacy refers to the ability of the ligand to influence receptor-mediated signaling pathways which might have end-point responses such as expression of a gene or proliferation of responsive cells. If the relative binding affinity to the receptor is low, then higher concentrations are needed for the end-point response, but this cannot be taken to imply that the end-point response (efficacy) is weak or partial. Taking parabens as an example, displacement of radiolabeled estradiol in competitive ER binding assays requires higher concentrations of parabens than physiological estrogens [55], demonstrating that parabens have lower relative binding affinity to ER (Figure 2.5A). Furthermore, relative binding affinity decreases with the shortening of the linear length of the alkyl chain from *n*-butylparaben to methylparaben, and higher concentrations are needed to displace radiolabeled estradiol from the receptor (Figure 2.5A) [55]. However, this does not result in reduced efficacy if sufficient concentration of paraben is present. Indeed, in whole-cell assays, with sufficient concentration, parabens give responses in terms of increased proliferation of human breast cancer cells of the same magnitude as 17β-estradiol (Figure 2.5B) [36]. Parabens are not partial agonists, as might be implied by the term "weak"; rather, they give full agonist responses in whole cells. When questioning effects of their presence in human tissues, the question, therefore, is how much is present in the human tissue, not whether they have a low relative binding affinity for ER.

2.7.2 Effect of Length of Time on Response

Much is now discussed concerning the possibility that EDCs may be able to act at low doses in the long term. This is an important environmental consideration because the ubiquitous measurement of EDCs in human blood or urine (see Section 2.4) implies that they are present in the long term in the human body, and this is out of line with most laboratory

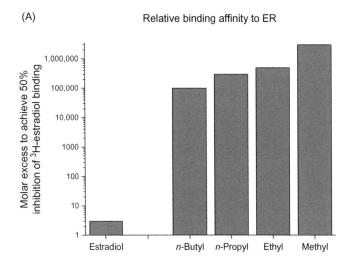

(A)

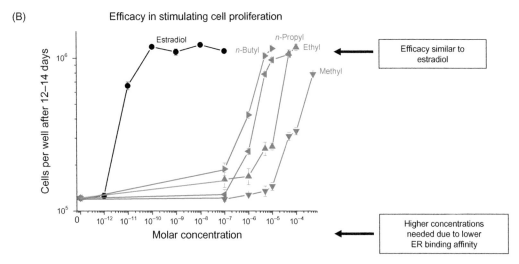

(B)

FIGURE 2.5 Comparison for four parabens of their relative binding affinities to ER (A) compared to their relative efficacies in stimulating the proliferation of MCF7 human breast cancer cells in culture (B). Methylparaben (Methyl), ethylparaben (ethyl), *n*-propylparaben (*n*-Propyl), *n*-butylparaben (*n*-Butyl). Relative binding affinity (A) is shown as the molar concentration needed to displace 50% ³H-estradiol from ER in a competitive binding assay. Relative efficacy (B) is shown as the molar concentration needed to stimulate proliferation of MCF7 human breast cancer cells after 14 days. *Source: Data taken for (A) from Ref. [55] and (B) from Ref. [36].*

studies, which are conducted over a short time scale (such as only a few days). The principle that partial agonist effects can be enhanced over a longer time period has been shown in the case of the estrogen agonist properties of triclosan [56]. Other studies have demonstrated that proliferation of estrogen-responsive human breast cancer cells in culture can be observed with reduced concentrations of parabens if the assay time is lengthened [57].

2.8 EFFECT OF EXPOSURE TO MIXTURES OF CHEMICALS

The ability of multiple EDCs to act by a common mechanism, such as through binding to a specific hormone receptor, suggests that an end-point response might be achievable by mixing several chemicals. Such additive effects would enable individual chemicals to act in combination at lower doses than would be needed for each chemical alone. The ubiquitous measurement of so many EDCs in human blood or urine (see Section 2.4) demonstrates that the human body is not exposed to one chemical at a time, but rather to multiple chemicals in complex mixtures that have entered the human body according to individual lifestyles. Therefore the concept of mixtures of chemicals generating end-point responses is plausible. Laboratory studies have shown that combining estrogen-mimicking chemicals can produce responses in circumstances where no response would have been measurable for each chemical alone in the so-called something from nothing response [58–60]. The additive effects of chemicals have also been demonstrated in animal models, where mixtures of estrogenic chemicals induced vitellogenin (a female protein) in male fish in an additive manner [61].

One long-standing issue has been whether there might be synergistic rather than additive effects, especially if multiple EDCs were to act through complementary as well as common mechanisms. A paper was published in the journal *Science* in 1996 describing synergistic effects between low concentrations of EDCs [62]. The results of synergism were challenged as not reproducible [63], however, and the original paper was retracted [64]. This high-profile retraction, which was associated with a verdict of scientific misconduct by the U.S. Office of Research Integrity, inserted a large element of fear into the scientific community concerning any suggestion of synergy, but 10 years later, some reports again suggested that synergy might be observed between EDCs in amphibians [65].

A further implication of chemical mixtures is that if EDCs act by a common mechanism of action, then different combinations of EDCs could give the same response. This poses a challenge for epidemiological studies, which classically have relied on the presence of a specific chemical as evidence of cause and effect. A new paradigm is now needed to enable the analysis of different mixtures of chemicals to be assessed for a common end-point. This is supported by measurements of 19 individual POPs where different levels of each POP were measured in different people, but overall, 1 or more POPs were measurable at a high level [66]. Analogous results have been reported for parabens, in that five paraben esters were measured in 158 of 160 human breast tissue samples from women with primary breast cancers, but samples with high levels of one ester did not necessarily have high levels of another ester [29]. Further analysis of functionality showed that levels of parabens were at sufficient concentrations in some of these breast tissue samples to enable adverse cellular responses in vitro, but it was different combinations of esters that enabled the end-point response [57].

2.9 EFFECT OF TIMING OF EXPOSURE

Timing of exposure may also affect the action of EDCs and is another important determinant of response. Many of the hormones of the body are released in a cyclical manner,

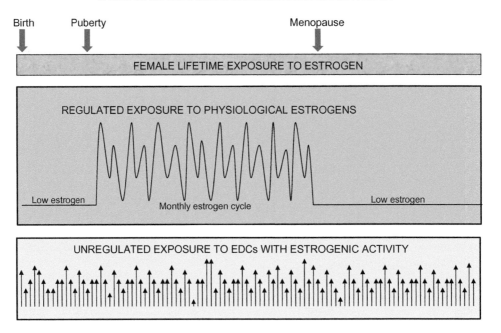

FIGURE 2.6   The importance of timing in the exposure of the human breast to environmental chemicals with estrogenic activity. Levels of physiological estrogens are highest between puberty and menopause, and levels fluctuate during the monthly menstrual cycle. Exposure to environmental estrogens can occur at any stage of life and is not in synchrony with physiological regulation.

and circadian rhythms are an important homeostatic mechanism. EDCs do not enter the body in any physiologically regulated manner and thus may have an impact by disrupting normal cyclical hormonal patterns. For example, the female is exposed to the highest levels of estrogen only between puberty and menopause; furthermore, the levels of estrogen fluctuate during the normal monthly menstrual cycle, as illustrated in the cartoon in Figure 2.6. However, exposure to EDCs with estrogen-disrupting activity is not regulated in synchrony with physiological estrogen exposure. Some EDCs, particularly the POPs, may enter continuously in small amounts over a lifetime, but they bioaccumulate such that there may be increasing loads in body fat with age. Other EDCs, such as phytoestrogens, may be only short-lived in the body, so their presence would depend on whether the exposure was intermittent or continuous. However, overall body burden would be the sum of all the thousands of individual compounds, and this would not parallel physiological regulation.

2.9.1 Critical Windows of Susceptibility

Although EDCs may enter the human body throughout life, there are some specific stages when the human body is particularly susceptible to EDCs. One critical window of susceptibility is the prenatal period, which has been highlighted by the developmental disorders caused by exposure of the human embryo/fetus to diethylstilbestrol (DES) in utero and has been confirmed through a range of studies using animal models [67] (see Chapters 8–10,13). Growth and differentiation during embryonic and fetal life is tightly regulated by the endocrine system, and small changes to hormone levels through interference from EDCs have the potential to alter developmental programming, leading to alterations to tissue and organ development that would become permanent. Disruption at this critical window, therefore, can result in developmental alterations that will persist into adult life, with various consequences to adult health (see Chapter 13). Furthermore, the greater sensitivity of the developing embryo/fetus to hormones compared to adult tissues enables lower doses of chemicals to produce effects at this sensitive life stage than would be needed to influence adult health. Although in utero is a sensitive life stage, the developing young child also remains sensitive to endocrine disruption through exposure to EDCs in the milk of early life and exposures to EDCs in the home environment (Chapter 13).

2.9.2 Latency Periods

Many effects of EDCs are not realized at the time of exposure, and many consequences may become visible only after a period of time has elapsed. This time interval between exposure and response is termed a *latency period.* Most effects of EDC exposure in utero will have a latency period, and the length of time may differ according to the end-point response. For example, hypospadias and cryptorchidism may be visible early after birth in baby boys, while fertility problems would not be evident until after puberty, and any resulting cancers may take decades to develop (see Chapter 9).

In considerations of female breast cancer, for which the major risk factor is estrogen exposure, it is relevant to note that the breast may be especially susceptible to carcinogenesis in early life [68], when endogenous estrogen levels are low; on the other hand, the majority of the symptoms of breast cancer arise in postmenopausal women [69], again when endogenous estrogen levels are low. This demonstrates a long latency period and is not consistent with physiological estrogens being the sole driving force (see Chapter 10).

2.10 TRANSGENERATIONAL EFFECTS

Exposure to several EDCs prior to birth is now known not only to produce long-lasting effects into adult life, but also effects that are passed to future generations without needing any further exposure. Such transgenerational effects were first reported for the pesticide vincolzolin, which, when administered to developing rodents, produced adverse effects on the developing testis, and the adverse effects were passed on for three generations [70]. It seems likely that the mechanism is epigenetic, involving alterations to the genome that do not change nucleotide sequences but rather influence patterns of gene expression through modifications such as DNA methylation or histone modification (see Chapter 13).

2.11 EDCs DO NOT HAVE THE SAME EFFECT IN ALL TISSUES

In assessing the outcome of exposure to EDCs, it must be taken into account that there will be differences in responses in different tissues. For example, if an EDC acts by binding to ERs, it will not affect cells that have no ERs, but even estrogen-responsive tissues can vary in their responses to estrogen. This may, in part, relate to the relative level of the two types of ER, ERα and ERβ, which can mediate differing responses (see Chapter 3) [71]. However, it has long been known that the breast and uterus can give opposing responses to estrogen; in particular, the use of tamoxifen as an antiestrogen to inhibit ER-mediated proliferation of breast cancer cells can result in unwanted agonist responses in the uterus [72]. This has led to the development of selective ER modulators, which have more specific effects on the required target tissue [73], but such tissue-specific effects imply that any EDC also can be expected to have different effects on different tissues.

2.12 EDCs DO NOT HAVE THE SAME EFFECTS IN EVERY INDIVIDUAL: THE INTERACTION OF GENETICS WITH ENVIRONMENT

Just as EDCs do not have the same effect on every tissue of the body, the effects of EDCs vary between individual people. For example, as described in Chapters 8–10, not every woman who was prescribed DES during pregnancy developed reproductive abnormalities or endocrine cancers, although many have; and not every child exposed in utero to DES has associated health problems, although again, many have [67]. Resulting consequences will depend on a complex array of interactions between the individual genetic background and the lifestyle factors and choices of that individual. Genetic factors play a major role in regulating susceptibility to disease, but the speed of increase in many endocrine-related disorders and diseases over recent decades rules out genetic factors as a sole determinant. Incorporating an understanding of the mechanisms underlying susceptibility to disease now requires a paradigm shift to accepting that EDCs may compromise human health, even if they do not do so for every person. Sickle cell anemia, a single gene disorder, is caused by production of a hemoglobin with an abnormal structure (HbS), and production of HbS rather than the normal HbA can be predicted from inheritance of two mutated beta globin (β^S) alleles. People who inherit two β^S alleles will make HbS rather than HbA and will have sickle cell anemia. However, susceptibility to disease is only partly determined by genetics; although, for example, loss of function of *BRCA1* or *BRCA2* genes can compromise the ability of such people to repair DNA, increasing their susceptibility to development of cancer, it does not mean that every person will definitely go on to develop cancer [74]. At present, the genetic and environmental determinants of EDC action are only beginning to be uncovered, and it is a daunting task to define these complex interactions for so many thousands of chemicals that act not only alone, but together in complex mixtures.

References

[1] Bergman A, Heindel JJ, Jobling S, Kidd KA, Zoeller RT, editors. The state of the science of endocrine-disrupting chemicals—2012. United Nations Environment Programme (UNEP) and World Health Organisation (WHO); 2013. <http://unep.org/pdf/9789241505031_eng.pdf>.

[2] Woods HF (chairman). Phytoestrogens and health. Crown copyright 2003. <http://cot.food.gov.uk/sites/default/files/cot/phytoreport0503.pdf>.

[3] World Health Organisation. DDT and its derivatives. Environmental Health Criteria 1979; Number 9.

[4] World Health Organisation. Polychlorinated biphenyls and terphenyls. Environmental Health Criteria 1992; Number 140.

[5] World Health Organisation. Polychlorinated dibenzo-p-dioxins and dibenzofurans. Environmental Health Criteria 1989; Number 88.

[6] Darbre PD, Aljarrah A, Miller WR, Coldham NG, Sauer MJ, Pope GS. Concentrations of parabens in human breast tumours. J Appl Toxicol 2004;24:5–13.

[7] Darbre PD, Harvey PW. Paraben esters: review of recent studies of endocrine toxicity, absorption, esterase and human exposure, and discussion of potential human health risks. J Appl Toxicol 2008;28:561–78.

[8] Janjua NR, Mortensen GK, Andersson AM, Kongshoj B, Skakkebaek NE, Wulf HC. Systemic uptake of diethyl phthalate, dibutyl phthalate, and butyl paraben following whole-body topical application and reproductive and thyroid hormone levels in humans. Environ Sci Technol 2007;41:5564–70.

[9] Janjua NR, Frederiksen H, Skakkebaek NE, Wulff HC, Andersson AM. Urinary excretion of phthalates and paraben after repeated whole-body topical application in humans. Int J Androl 2008;31:118–30.

[10] Janjua NR, Kongshoj B, Andersson AM, Wulf HC. Sunscreens in human plasma and urine after repeated whole-body topical application. JEADV 2008;22:456–61.

[11] Needham LL, Grandjean P, Heinzow B, Jørgensen PJ, Nielsen F, Sjödin A, et al. Partition of environmental chemicals between maternal and fetal blood. Environ Sci Technol 2011;45:1121–6.

[12] Solomon GM, Weiss PM. Chemical contaminants in breast milk: time trends and regional variability. Environ Health Perspect 2002;110:A339–47.

[13] LaKind JS, Amina Wilkins A, Berlin CM. Environmental chemicals in human milk: a review of levels, infant exposures and health, and guidance for future research. Toxicol Appl Pharmacol 2004;198:184–208.

[14] Fuerst P. Dioxins, polychlorinated biphenyls and other organohalogen compounds in human milk. Mol Nutr Food Res 2006;50:922–33.

[15] Tanabe S, Kunisue T. Persistent organic pollutants in human breast milk from Asian countries. Environ Pollut 2006;146:400–13.

[16] Darbre PD. Environmental contaminants in milk: the problem of organochlorine xenobiotics. Biochem Soc Trans 1998;26:106–12.

[17] Sjödin A, Jones RS, Caudill SP, Wong LY, Turner WE, Calafat AM. Polybrominated diphenyl ethers, polychlorinated biphenyls, and persistent pesticides in serum from the National Health and Nutrition Examination Survey: 2003–2008. Environ Sci Technol 2014;48:753–60.

[18] Silva MJ, Barr DB, Reidy JA, Malek NA, Hodge CC, Caudill SP, et al. Urinary levels of seven phthalate metabolites in the U.S. population from the National Health and Nutrition Examination Survey (NHANES) 1999–2000. Environ Health Perspect 2004;112:331–8.

[19] Calafat AM, Wong LY, Ye X, Reidy JA, Needham LL. Concentrations of the sunscreen agent benzophenone-3 in residents of the United States: National Health and Nutrition Examination Survey 2003–2004. Environ Health Perspect 2008;116:893–7.

[20] Calafat AM, Ye X, Wong LY, Reidy JA, Needham LL. Exposure of the U.S. population to bisphenol A and 4-tertiary-octylphenol: 2003–2004. Environ Health Perspect 2008;116:39–44.

[21] Calafat AM, Ye X, Wong LY, Reidy JA, Needham LL. Urinary concentrations of triclosan in the U.S. population: 2003–2004. Environ Health Perspect 2008;116:303–7.

[22] Calafat AM, Ye X, Wong LY, Bishop AM, Needham LL. Urinary concentrations of four parabens in the U.S. population: NHANES 2005–2006. Environ Health Perspect 2010;118:679–85.

[23] Valentin-Blasini L, Sadowski MA, Walden D, Caltabiano L, Needham LL, Barr DB. Urinary phytoestrogen concentrations in the U.S. population (1999–2000). J Expo Anal Environ Epidemiol 2005;15:509–23.

[24] Andersen FA. Final amended report on the safety assessment of methylparaben, ethylparaben, propylparaben, isopropylparaben, butylparaben, isobutylpraben and benzylparaben as used in cosmetic products. Int J Toxicol 2008;27(Suppl. 4):1–82.

[25] Liao C, Kannan K. Concentrations and composition profiles of parabens in currency bills and paper products including sanitary wipes. Sci Total Environ 2014;475:8–15.

[26] Canosa P, Rodriguez I, Rubi E, Cela R. Determination of parabens and triclosan in indoor dust using matrix solid-phase dispersion and gas chromatography with tandem mass spectrometry. Anal Chem 2007;79:1675–81.

[27] Darbre PD, Harvey PW. Parabens can enable hallmarks and characteristics of cancer in human breast epithelial cells: a review of the literature with reference to new exposure data and regulatory status. J Appl Toxicol 2014;34:925–38.

[28] Ye X, Bishop AM, Reidy JA, Needham LL, Calafat AM. Parabens as urinary biomarkers of exposure in humans. Environ Health Perspect 2006;114:1843–6.

[29] Barr L, Metaxas G, Harbach CAJ, Savoy LA, Darbre PD. Measurement of paraben concentrations in human breast tissue at serial locations across the breast from axilla to sternum. J Appl Toxicol 2012;32:219–32.

[30] Jobling S, Nolan M, Tyler CR, Brighty G, Sumpter JP. Widespread sexual disruption in wild fish. Environ Sci Technol 1998;32:2498–506.

[31] Bitman J, Cecil HC, Harris SJ, Fries GF. Estrogenic activity of o,p⊠-DDT in the mammalian uterus and avian oviduct. Science 1968;162:371–2.

[32] Welch RM, Levin W, Conney AH. Estrogenic action of DDT and its analogs. Toxicol Appl Pharmacol 1969;14:358–67.

[33] Nesaretnam K, Corcoran D, Dils RR, Darbre P. 3,4,3′,4′-Tetrachlorobiphenyl acts as an estrogen *in vitro* and *in vivo*. Mol Endocrinol 1996;10:923–36.

[34] Meerts IATM, Hoving S, van den Berg JHJ, Weijers BM, Swarts HJ, van der Beek EM, et al. Effects of *in utero* exposure to 4-hydroxy-2,3,3′,4′,5-pentachlorobiphenyl (4-OHCB107) on developmental landmarks, steroid hormone levels, and female estrous cyclicity in rats. Toxicol Sci 2004;82:259–67.

[35] Garner CE, Jefferson WN, Burka LT, Matthews HB, Newbold RR. *In vitro* estrogenicity of the catechol metabolites of selected polychlorinated biphenyls. Toxicol Appl Pharmacol 1999;154:188–97.

[36] Byford JR, Shaw LE, Drew MG, Pope GS, Sauer MJ, Darbre PD. Oestrogenic activity of parabens in MCF7 human breast cancer cells. J Steroid Biochem Mol Biol 2002;80:49–60.

[37] Darbre PD, Byford JR, Shaw LE, Horton RA, Pope GS, Sauer MJ. Oestrogenic activity of isobutylparaben *in vitro* and *in vivo*. J Appl Toxicol 2002;22:219–26.

[38] Pugazhendhi D, Pope GS, Darbre PD. Oestrogenic activity of *p*-hydroxybenzoic acid (common metabolite of paraben esters) and methylparaben in human breast cancer cell lines. J Appl Toxicol 2005;25:301–9.

[39] Whitehead SA, Rice S. Endocrine-disrupting chemicals as modulators of sex steroid synthesis. Best Pract Res Clin Endocrinol Metab 2006;20:45–61.

[40] Akiyama T, Ishida J, Nakagawa S, Ogawara H, Watanabe S, Itoh N, et al. Genistein, a specific inhibitor of tyrosine-specific protein kinases. J Biol Chem 1987;25:5592–5.

[41] Cappelletti V, Fioravanti L, Miodini P, Di Fronzo G. Genistein blocks breast cancer cells in the G2M phase of the cell cycle. J Cell Biochem 2000;79:594–600.

[42] Kondo K, Tsuneizumi K, Watanabe T, Oishi M. Induction of *in vitro* differentiation of mouse embryonal carcinoma (F9) cells by inhibitors of topoisomerases. Cancer Res 1991;51:5398–404.

[43] Boos G, Stopper H. Genotoxicity of several clinically used topoisomerase II inhibitors. Toxicol Lett 2000;27:7–16.

[44] Sarkar FH. Mechanisms of cancer chemoprevention by soy isoflavone genistein. Cancer Metastasis Rev 2002;21:265–80.

[45] Pepper MS, Hazel SJ, Humpel M, Schleuning WD. 8-Prenylnaringenin, a novel phytoestrogen, inhibits angiogenesis *in vitro* and *in vivo*. J Cell Physiol 2004;199:98–107.

[46] Dechaud H, Ravard C, Claustrat F, de la Perriere AB, Pugeat M. Xenoestrogen interaction with human sex hormone-binding globulin (hSHBG). Steroids 1999;64:328–34.

[47] Pino AM, Valladares LE, Palma MA, Mancilla AM, Yanez M, Albala C. Dietary isoflavones affect sex-hormone-binding globulin levels in postmenopausal women. J Clin Endocrinol Metab 2000;85:2797–800.

[48] Dewalque L, Pirard C, Dubois N, Charlier C. Simultaneous determination of some phthalate metabolites, parabens and benzophenone-3 in urine by ultra high pressure liquid chromatography tandem mass spectrometry. J Chromatogr B 2014;949–950:37–47.

[49] Ye X, Bishop AM, Needham LL, Calafat AM. Automated on-line column-switching HPLC-MS/MS method with peak focusing for measuring parabens, triclosan, and other environmental phenols in human milk. Anal Chim Acta 2008;622:150–6.

[50] Schlumpf M, Kypke K, Wittassek M, Angerer J, Mascher H, Mascher D, et al. Exposure patterns of UV filters, fragrances, parabens, phthalates, organochlorpesticides, PBDEs and PCBs in human milk: correlation of UV filters with use of cosmetics. Chemosphere 2010;81:1171–83.

[51] Pugazhendhi D, Watson KA, Mills S, Botting N, Pope GS, Darbre PD. Effect of sulphation on the oestrogen agonist activity of the phytoestrogens genistein and daidzein in MCF-7 human breast cancer cells. J Endocrinol 2008;197:503–15.

[52] Matsumura A, Ghosh A, Pope GS, Darbre PD. Comparative study of oestrogenic properties of eight phytoes-trogens in MCF7 human breast cancer cells. J Steroid Biochem Mol Biol 2005;94:431–43.

[53] Vandenberg LN, Colborn T, Hayes TB, Heindel JJ, Jacobs Jr. DR, Lee DH, et al. Hormones and endocrine-disrupting chemicals: low-dose effects and nonmonotonic dose responses. Endocr Rev 2012;33:378–455.

[54] Strange PG. Agonist binding, agonist affinity and agonist efficacy at G protein-coupled receptors. Br J Pharmacol 2008;153:1353–63.

[55] Darbre PD. Environmental oestrogens, cosmetics and breast cancer. Best Pract Res Clin Endocrinol Metab 2006;20:121–43.

[56] Gee RH, Charles A, Taylor N, Darbre PD. Oestrogenic and androgenic activity of triclosan in breast cancer cells. J Appl Toxicol 2008;28:78–91.

[57] Charles AK, Darbre PD. Combinations of parabens at concentrations measured in human breast tissue can increase proliferation of MCF-7 human breast cancer cells. J Appl Toxicol 2013;33:390–8.

[58] Rajapakse N, Silva E, Kortenkamp A. Combining xenoestrogens at levels below individual no-observed-effect concentrations dramatically enhances steroid hormone action. Environ Health Perspect 2002;110:917–21.

[59] Silva E, Rajapakse N, Kortenkamp A. Something from "nothing"—eight weak estrogenic chemicals combined at concentrations below NOECs produce significant mixture effects. Environ Sci Technol 2002;36:1751–6.

[60] Kortenkamp A. Ten years of mixing cocktails: a review of combination effects of endocrine-disrupting chemi-cals. Environ Health Perspect 2007;115(Suppl. 1):98–105.

[61] Brian JV, Harris CA, Scholze M, Backhaus T, Booy P, Lamoree M, et al. Accurate prediction of the response of freshwater fish to a mixture of estrogenic chemicals. Environ Health Perspect 2005;113:721–8.

[62] Arnold SF, Klotz DM, Collins BM, Vonier PM, Guillette LJ, McLachlan JA. Synergistic activation of estrogen receptor with combinations of environmental chemicals. Science 1996;272:1489–92.

[63] Ramamoorthy K, Wang F, Chen IC, Norris JD, McDonnell DP, Leonard LS, et al. Estrogenic activity of a dieldrin/toxaphene mixture in the mouse uterus, MCF-7 human breast cancer cells, and yeast-based estrogen receptor assays: no apparent synergism. Endocrinology 1997;138:1520–7.

[64] McLachlan JA. Synergistic effect of environmental estrogens: report withdrawn. Science 1997;277:462–3.

[65] Hayes TB, Case P, Chui S, Chung D, Haeffele C, Haston K, et al. Pesticide mixtures, endocrine disruption, and amphibian declines: are we underestimating the impact? Environ Health Perspect 2006;114(S-1):40–50.

[66] Porta M, Pumarega J, Gasull M. Number of persistent organic pollutants detected at high concentrations in a general population. Environ Int 2012;44:106–111. [EPub ahead of print].

[67] Harris RM, Waring RH. Diethylstilboestrol—a long-term legacy. Maturitas 2012;72:108–12.

[68] Russo J, Russo IH. Biology of disease. Biological and molecular bases of mammary carcinogenesis. Lab Invest 1987;57:112–37.

[69] Key TJ, Verkasalo PK, Banks E. Epidemiology of breast cancer. Lancet Oncol 2001;2:133–40.

[70] Skinner MK, Manikkam M, Guerrero-Bosagna C. Epigenetic transgenerational actions of endocrine disruptors. Reprod Toxicol 2011;31:337–43.

[71] Pugazhendhi D, Darbre PD. Differential effects of overexpression of ERα and ERβ in MCF10A immortalized, non-transformed human breast epithelial cells. Horm Mol Biol Clin Investig 2010;1:117–26.

[72] Lonning PE. Endocrinology and treatment of breast cancer. Clin Endocrinol Metab 2004;18:1–130.

[73] Riggs BL, Hartmann LC. Selective estrogen receptor modulators—mechanisms of action and application to clinical practice. N Engl J Med 2003;348:618–29.

[74] Roy R, Chun J, Powell SN. BRCA1 and BRCA2: different roles in a common pathway of genome protection. Nat Rev Cancer 2012;12:68–78.

MECHANISMS AND ASSAY SYSTEMS

Disrupters of Estrogen Action and Synthesis

Philippa D. Darbre

Endocrine Disruption and Human Health.
DOI: http://dx.doi.org/10.1016/B978-0-12-801139-3.00003-X

49

Abstract

This chapter gives an overview of the mechanisms of estrogen action and describes assay strategies to determine how and where environmental chemicals might mimic or interfere in these processes. At a molecular level, environmental compounds may compete with estrogen for binding to intracellular estrogen receptors (ERs), leading to effects on gene expression (genomic action). Some chemicals may interfere either with the effects of cell membrane ERs on signal transduction pathways or the interaction of estrogens with G-protein coupled receptors (GPERs) (nongenomic action). Some chemicals may act by altering the biosynthesis or bioavailability of endogenous estrogens. At a cellular level, environmental chemicals may increase proliferation of cell lines dependent on estrogen for their growth. The most used animal model is the increase in uterine weight in the immature rodent (uterotrophic assay). Estrogenic compounds have been identified as entering the human body from a wide range of environmental sources, including diet, pharmaceuticals, domestic consumer products, and personal care products.

3.1 PHYSIOLOGICAL ACTIONS OF ESTROGEN AND IMPLICATIONS OF DISRUPTION

Estrogens are a group of steroid hormones that regulate reproductive function and secondary sex characteristics in the female, including breast development. They are secreted primarily from the ovary in a cyclical manner during the estrus cycle to prepare a favorable uterine environment for fertilization, implantation of a fertilized egg, and maintenance of the early embryo. However, they also can be produced by the adrenal cortex, placenta, and adipose cells. After menopause, estrogen production from the ovary ceases, and lower levels of estrogen are made mainly from adrenal and adipose tissue. Side effects of the drop in estrogen levels after menopause serve as a reminder of the many other functions of estrogens in the female body, notably in calcium homeostasis, leading to the demineralization of bone and fractures. However, estrogens also influence other physiological functions in the brain, liver, and cardiovascular system. Therefore, environmental chemicals capable of interfering with the actions of physiological estrogens have the potential to have wide-reaching effects on the female body (see Chapter 8).

Although referred to as the female sex hormones, estrogens are synthesized from androgen precursors and secreted in low levels from the testes. Low levels of estrogens, therefore, play important physiological roles not only in the female, but in the male as well. Exposure of the male to high levels of estrogens or environmental chemicals with estrogenic properties also may potentially have major implications for the health of men (see Chapter 9).

3.2 MOLECULAR ACTIONS OF ESTROGEN AND MECHANISMS OF DISRUPTION

Estrogens act by an endocrine mechanism whereby they are secreted by one organ, carried in the blood to influence target cells in distant organs. Like all steroid hormones, estrogens diffuse readily across the lipid bilayer of the cell membrane and therefore do not need any transport proteins to enter cells. At the target cells, estrogens act through interaction with intracellular protein receptors that were first identified in the 1950s and 1960s [1,2].

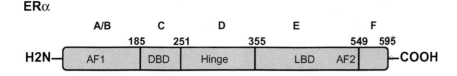

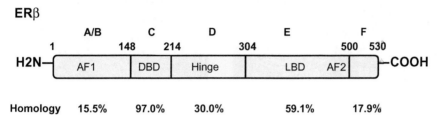

FIGURE 3.1 Functional domains of the human ERs, ERα and ERβ. C region contains the DBD; E region contains the LBD; A/B and E/F regions contain the AF1 and AF2 sites for coregulator binding. Homology between the two receptors in each of the domains is indicated [5].

In 1985, the cDNA for the human estrogen receptor (ER) was cloned [3], but it was renamed ERα after the cloning in 1996 of a second cDNA from a separate human ER gene ERβ [4]. It is, therefore, now recognized that there are two forms of human ER, ERα and ERβ, which are products of different genes encoded on separate chromosomes but share considerable structural homology (Figure 3.1). The receptor protein is organized into four main domains: (1) an N-terminal A/B region containing the ligand-independent activation function AF-1; (2) a DNA-binding domain (DBD) composed of two zinc fingers; (3) a hinge region containing the nuclear localization signal; and (4) an E/F region containing the ligand-binding domain (LBD) and the ligand-dependent transactivation function AF-2. Homology between the ERs is especially evident in the DBD (Figure 3.1) [5].

A common feature of the action of compounds with estrogenic activity is their reversible and saturable binding to cellular ER, and the kinetics of this binding determines their estrogenic potency. Structural studies have shown that both ERα [6] and ERβ [7] bind a single estrogenic molecule to a specific pocket within the LBD. The crystal structure of human ERα has shown that 17β-estradiol is positioned into the LBD by hydrogen bonding of its 3- and 17-hydroxyl groups to specific amino acid side chains and by hydrophobic bonding (van der Waals forces) of the remainder of the steroid ring system to other amino acid side chains (Figure 3.2) [6]. Since the size of the ligand-binding pocket is approximately twice the size of the estradiol molecule, a range of other compounds can also be accommodated, especially given specific structural features of a *para*-hydroxyphenyl grouping present either intrinsically or following metabolic conversion [8]. Figure 3.2 shows how even the long side chain of the antiestrogen raloxifene can be accommodated within the LBD [6]. Figure 3.3 gives examples of a range of very different structures that have been shown capable of binding to the ER. Most contain a *para*-hydroxy

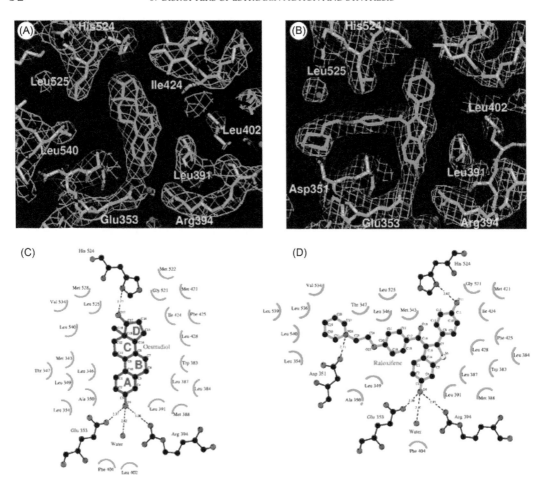

FIGURE 3.2   Binding of 17β-estradiol (A and C) and raloxifene (B and D) to the LBD of human ERα. (A and C) Electron density maps; (C and D) schematic diagram of the interactions. Direct hydrogen bonds are shown by red balls with interconnecting dotted lines. *Source: Reproduced with permission [6].*

group that could form interactions within the LBD similarly to the estradiol molecule. It remains unclear as to whether the chloro-group allows hydrogen bonding in the LBD or whether it is converted to a hydroxyl grouping by metabolic activity within the cells. Most environmental estrogenic chemicals have been organic molecules, but some metal ions (metalloestrogens) also have been shown to be capable of displacing estradiol from binding to ER [9].

Binding of ligand to ER results in conformational change to the ER protein and activation of the receptor. A main mechanism of ER action is as a ligand-activated transcription factor (genomic action), although in recent years, ERs have been shown to act also through the interaction with signal transduction pathways from cell surface receptors and estrogen to act through binding to a distinct G-protein coupled receptor (GPER) (nongenomic actions).

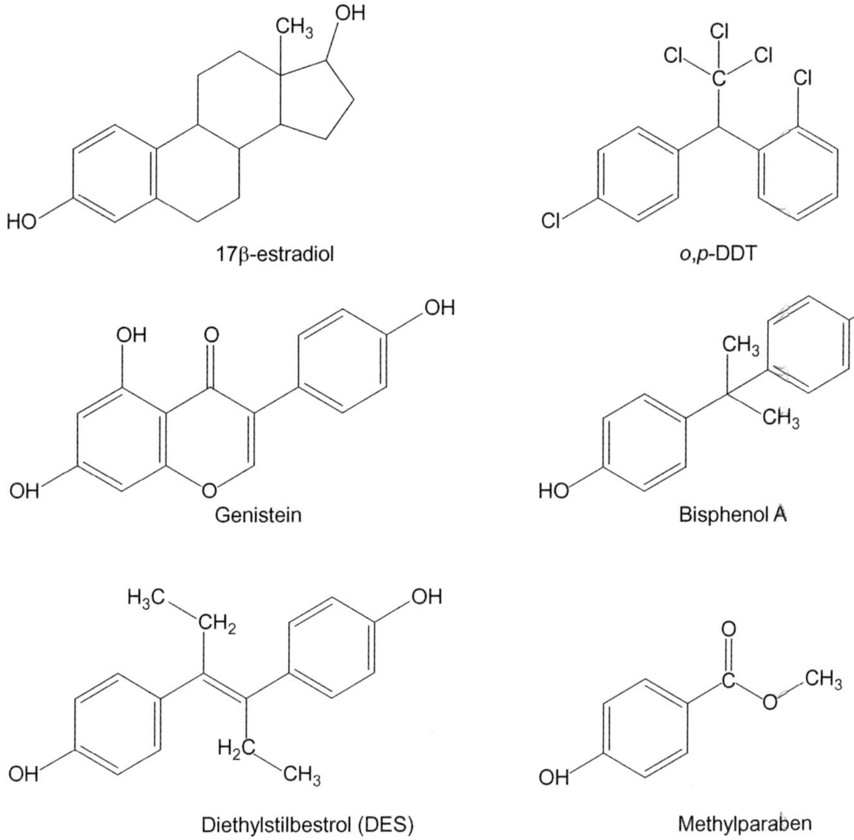

FIGURE 3.3   Chemical structures of different compounds known to bind to human ERs.

3.2.1 Direct Genomic Action

In the direct genomic mechanism, binding of estrogen to ER results in a conformational change to the receptor protein, leading to the dimerization of estrogen-ER complexes, which can then bind to DNA to alter patterns of gene expression (Figure 3.4) [10–13]. Binding of estrogen to the ER causes receptor phosphorylation and the release of associated chaperone proteins, which prevent the ER from binding to DNA in the absence of ligand. The estrogen–ER complexes are then able to dimerize and move into the nucleus, where they bind to specific nucleotide sequences in the DNA termed *estrogen response elements (EREs)*. EREs are found in the vicinity of estrogen-regulated genes and function as enhancer elements to alter levels of gene expression. The consensus ERE sequence is a short palindromic sequence of 12 specific nucleotides spaced by any 3 nucleotides in the middle and defined from 5′ to 3′ as AGGTCA (nnn)TGACCT. When bound to DNA, the ER dimers associate with other coactivator and corepressor proteins to form a complex with RNA polymerase, which transactivates gene expression. Although classically studied estrogen-responsive genes such as the genes for trefoil

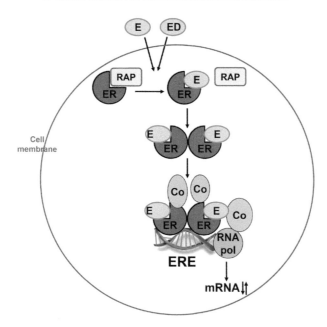

FIGURE 3.4   Direct genomic action of estrogen. Estrogen (E) binds to intracellular ER, resulting in the release of receptor-associated proteins (RAPs), dimerization and binding to estrogen response elements (EREs) in the DNA. Transactivation of gene expression involves binding of coregulators (Co) and RNA polymerase (RNApol) resulting in alteration to the level of hundreds of mRNAs. Endocrine disruptors (EDs) may interfere in this pathway by binding to intracellular ER and setting off a similar sequence of events but with altered consequences to mRNA levels.

growth factor *pS2* [14], progesterone receptor (PR) [15], and cathepsin D [16] are all upregulated by estrogen, global gene expression studies show that not all estrogen-responsive genes are upregulated by the presence of estrogen. In MCF-7 human breast cancer cells, about 70% of genes, which are altered in their expression level, are downregulated following exposure to 17β-estradiol [17]. Microarray studies have also shown that 17β-estradiol can give different profiles of gene expression through the two receptors ERα and ERβ [18].

3.2.2 Indirect Genomic Action

In addition to direct binding of the ER to DNA, ERs can regulate gene expression through interactions with other protein transcription factors. This was first identified from studies showing an interaction of ERβ with the transcription factors Fos and Jun at AP1 response elements (Figure 3.5) [19]. Interactions of ERβ with specificity protein-1 (Sp1) are associated with decreased ligand-dependent gene expression [20,21], but the association of ER with nuclear factor-κB mediates an estradiol-dependent inhibition of gene expression [22].

Interference has also been noted between ER and other transcriptional regulators when the response elements are juxtapositioned in the DNA. This was first shown through identifying interference in the genomic action of ER by binding of an arylhydrocarbon receptor (AhR) with its nuclear translocator (Arnt) to its juxtapositioned dioxin response element in the DNA (Figure 3.6) [23].

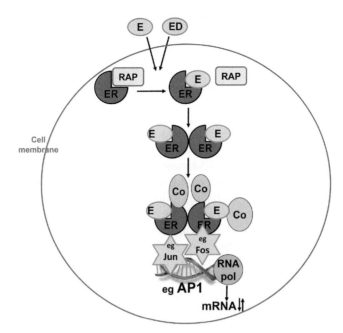

FIGURE 3.5 Indirect genomic action of estrogen. Estrogen (E) binds to intracellular ER resulting in the release of RAPs, dimerization, and binding to other transcription factors such as Jun-Fos. Dimers of Jun-Fos bind to AP-1 response elements in the DNA, and interaction of the ER alters transcription from regulated genes. EDs may interfere in this pathway by binding to intracellular ER and setting off a similar sequence of events, but with altered consequences to mRNA levels.

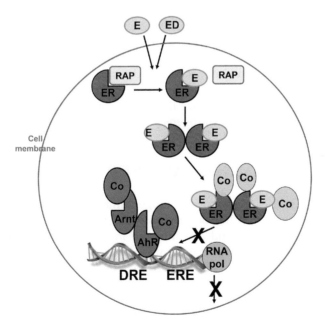

FIGURE 3.6 Indirect genomic action of estrogen. Estrogen (E) binds to intracellular ER, resulting in the release of RAPs, dimerization, and attempts to bind to EREs in the DNA. Juxtapositioned response elements, such as dioxin response elements in the DNA that bind the AhR and its nuclear translocator (Arnt), can influence the ability of estrogen-ER complexes to bind to an ERE [23].

3.2.3 Nongenomic Action

It has been known for a long time that estrogens can also exert rapid actions in cells that are too fast for a mechanism dependent on transcriptional regulation [24], and over the past 15 years, reports have documented that such responses are mediated in cultured cells through alteration to cell-signaling phosphorylation cascades [13,25,26]. The estrogen–ER complex is able to interact at the cell surface with tyrosine kinase receptors to influence mitogen-activated protein kinase and phosphatidyl-inositol-3-kinase signaling pathways [26]. In cultured breast cancer cells, membrane-mediated ERα signaling results in an increase in proliferation [27,28], whereas membrane-mediated ERβ signaling reduces estrogen-stimulated proliferation [28]. Secretion of prolactin is thought to be mediated by ERα bound to the plasma membrane [29]. Some xenoestrogens, which behave as weak agonists in increasing uterine weight in vivo, are strong agonists of membrane-bound receptors [30,31].

In recent years, another G-protein-coupled ER (GPR30, GPER) has been identified and effects of estrogen can be mediated through interaction with GPER [26,32]. It is a 7-trans-membrane spanning protein that has been localized in the nucleus and endoplasmic reticulum, as well as the cell membrane. The full significance of GPER in estrogen action remains to be identified, but the herbicide atrazine is a xenoestrogen that does not bind to ERα or ERβ and seems to act through GPER [33].

3.3 SYNTHESIS OF ENDOGENOUS ESTROGENS AND DISRUPTION OF NECESSARY ENZYMATIC ACTIVITIES

As for all steroid hormones, estrogens are synthesized from cholesterol as the common precursor. In the theca interna of the ovary, cholesterol is converted to androstenedione and testosterone. These can then cross into the surrounding granulosa cells, where aromatase enzymes convert androstenedione into estrone and testosterone into estradiol (Figure 3.7). Some xenoestrogens have been shown to alter the level of cellular aromatase expression, while others have been shown to influence the activity of aromatase, which then interferes with the biosynthesis of endogenous estrogens [34].

3.4 ASSAY SYSTEMS

Due to the release into the environment of large numbers of chemicals with the potential for disrupting estrogen action, it has become essential to develop assay systems to determine not only whether a compound can interfere in estrogen action, but also how and where in the pathways of estrogen action it might act. No single assay system could be expected to provide information on all the necessary end points of disruption of estrogen action and so in general, a range of assays both in vitro and in vivo are necessary. Each has its advantages and disadvantages.

Starting from a minimalist approach, a diagrammatic plan is given in Figure 3.8 for approaching the testing for estrogenic properties of an environmental chemical. Any compound capable of mimicking estrogen action by genomic routes could be expected first to bind to ERs and then

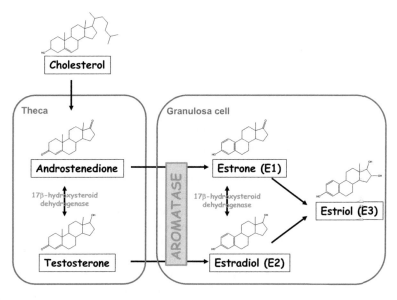

FIGURE 3.7   Biosynthesis of estrogens in the ovary. The precursors are formed in the theca interna and aromatized in the granulosa cells.

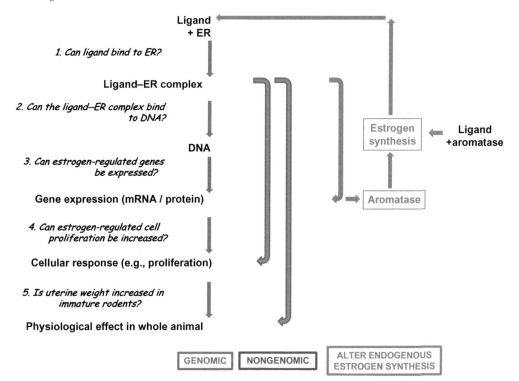

FIGURE 3.8   Schematic diagram illustrating mechanisms by which an environmental chemical might mimic or interfere in estrogen action.

to influence expression of one or more estrogen-regulated genes. On a cellular level, the compound must be able to enter the cell and to influence a cellular function, and a sensitive assay for this has been to determine proliferation of cells dependent on estrogen for their growth. Finally, at a physiological level, the compound must be able to enter a whole animal, reach a target organ, and give a physiological response. The classical gold-standard whole animal assay has become a measured increase in uterine weight in the immature rodent (uterotrophic assay), largely because it is a quantitative assay. The vaginal cornification assay for detecting changes in vaginial epithelium is also used but it is largely qualitative. The in vivo whole animal assay allows for effects to be measured from different routes of administration and gives due allowance to different rates of absorption, metabolism, and clearance in different rodent species.

In vitro assays offer the advantage of simplicity and reproducibility, but they have their limitations in the use of single cell types in isolation and in the artificial environment created by the use of plastic surfaces for the cells to adhere to and by the use of artificial culture media. Some models for culturing cells on different matrices and for co-culturing different cell types have been developed in recent years that have improved the ability to predict the influence of the complex interactions between different cell types within tissues in vivo. The rodent uterotropic assay has become a much used and reliable in vivo assay for compound estrogenicity, but it has limitations when extrapolating to different species (especially when the end point is human health) and different tissues (responses to estrogen can often be opposing in breast compared to uterus, for example).

The estrogenic properties of a compound can be assayed by adding the compound to an assay either on its own or in the presence of the endogenous hormone 17β-estradiol. Both approaches have environmental relevance, because in the human, estrogen levels may be high at specific times of the menstrual cycle, lower at other cycle times, and even lower prior to puberty or after menopause. In general, a chemical with estrogenic activity could be expected to give an agonist response when administered alone. However, if it binds with a lower binding affinity to the ERs than endogenous estrogens, it might be expected to give an antagonist response in the presence of estradiol. All assay systems are designed to detect agonist activity, but not all of them can detect antagonist activity.

In this chapter, typical results of these assays are illustrated using the alkyl esters of *p*-hydroxybenzoic acid (parabens). Parabens are used as antimicrobial preservatives in a wide range of personal care products, foods, and pharmaceuticals to which the human population is exposed. The most commonly used esters are methylparaben, ethylparaben, *n*-propylparaben, *n*-butylparaben, and isobutylparaben. The chemical structure of methylparaben is shown in Figure 3.3: the other parabens differ only in the alkyl grouping. Intact parabens have been measured widely in human body tissues, including in 99% of human urine samples in the United States [35]. All commonly used paraben esters have been shown to bind to human ER and to possess estrogenic activities [36], which makes them a good case study for illustrating results of an environmental compound with estrogenic activity in these assays.

3.4.1 Can a Compound Bind to ER?—ER-Binding Assays in a Cell-Free System

The ability of a compound to bind to ER is usually assayed by a competitive binding assay [37]. This entails incubation of a source of receptor (either a cell lysate containing ER or recombinant ER) with a known amount of ^{3}H-labeled 17β-estradiol in the presence of a range of concentrations of the test compound. After incubation, the unbound [^{3}H]-17βestradiol is removed by adsorption to charcoal, and the bound [^{3}H]-17βestradiol is measured by liquid scintillation counting. A graph can then be plotted of the % [^{3}H]-17βestradiol bound at different molar excesses of the test compound. Compounds requiring a greater molar excess to displace the [^{3}H]-17βestradiol bind more weakly to the ER and have a lower relative binding affinity. The sensitivity for these assays is best achieved through use of a radiolabel. Although it would be ideal to directly measure the binding of each compound with a radiolabel attached, the cost of making the radiolabeled compounds is prohibitively expensive, which is why most assays are carried out measuring the ability of each compound to displace [^{3}H]-17βestradiol, in what is then termed a *competitive binding assay*. The results are usually expressed as the molar concentration of a compound required to displace 50% of the radiolabeled estradiol (IC$_{50}$), or as the ratio of the IC$_{50}$ values for the test compound and estradiol (relative binding affinity).

Many hundreds of compounds have now been shown to displace radiolabeled estradiol from ER in a competitive binding assay, and a paper by Blair and colleagues gives the relative binding affinities for 188 compounds to rat uterine ER [38]. Most environmental compounds tested bind with a lower affinity to receptors than endogenous estrogens. Figure 3.9 shows the results of a competitive binding assay using five paraben esters. Competitive binding of [^{3}H]-17βestradiol to the ER of the MCF-7 human breast cancer cell cytosol could be displaced by decreasing molar excess as the linear length of the alkyl chain increased. This demonstrates that the binding of paraben esters to ER is in the order of *n*-butylparaben > *n*-propylparaben > ethylparaben > methylparaben [39].

Studies comparing the binding of different environmental compounds to ERα and ERβ have shown that while 17β-estradiol binds with a similar affinity to both receptor types, other compounds may bind differently to the two receptors [41]. Since ERβ is widely distributed at low levels across many human tissues, while ERα is more selectively expressed at higher levels within reproductive tissues (especially the breast and uterus) [5], compounds binding with higher affinity to ERβ have the potential to influence a wider range of tissues, and it has been noted that plant phytoestrogens tend to fall within this latter category [41].

With so much experimental information on the affinity with which different chemical structures can bind to human ER, and with the crystal structures of human ERα [6] and ERβ [7] resolved, computer models can now also be designed to allow in silico prediction of ER binding [39].

3.4.2 Can Binding of a Compound to ER Regulate Estrogen-Responsive Gene Expression in Cells In Vitro?

If the ligand can bind to the ER, then the next question is whether the ligand-ER complexes formed are sufficiently functional to enable the transactivation of gene expression. This can be tested in cells containing ER, either using estrogen-regulated, artificial reporter genes introduced into the cells or assaying endogenous genes within the cells that are known to be estrogen-regulated. Human breast cancer cell lines such as MCF-7, T-47-D, or ZR-75-1 have been used extensively because they not only already contain ER, but the cells are estrogen-responsive for gene expression and cell proliferation. However, it is also possible to transfect an ER gene into cells lacking endogenous ER, and this can have the advantage of enabling the selective transfection of ERα or ERβ individually into cells.

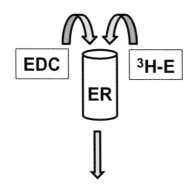

Measure %–³H-estradiol bound to ER

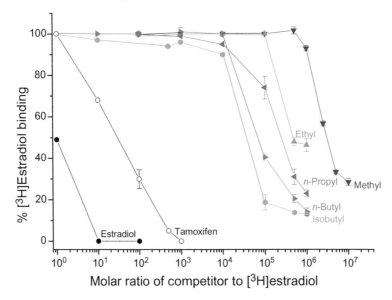

FIGURE 3.9 Competitive binding of parabens to ER from MCF-7 human breast cancer cells. In single-point competitive binding assays, 1.6nM [³H]estradiol was incubated with the indicated molar excess of unlabeled 17β-estradiol, methylparaben, ethylparaben, n-propylparaben, n-butylparaben, or isobutylparaben. *Source: Data are collated from two publications [39,40].*

3.4.2.1 Reporter Gene Assays

A reporter gene [42] is usually constructed within a plasmid such that an ERE sequence is cloned upstream of sequences for the promoter region, the coding region for the reporter gene, and termination signals. This ensures estrogen-regulated expression of messenger RNA (mRNA) and protein for the reporter gene. Reporter genes are chosen on the basis of being easy to assay, and some of the most widely used reporter genes are those coding for the firefly luciferase (*LUC*) gene [43], the bacterial chloramphenicol acetyl transferase (*CAT*) gene [44], the bacterial β-galactosidase (β-GAL) (*LacZ*) gene [45], and the jellyfish green fluorescent protein (GFP) gene [46]. The LUC gene codes for an enzyme that uses the substrate luciferin to generate a flash of light and assay of expression of this enzyme can be carried out by adding luciferin to lysed cells and detecting the flash of light on a luminometer. Commercial companies have developed both expression plasmids into which an ERE can be inserted and kits for assay that stabilize the light signal over several minutes, enabling assays to be performed reproducibly without the need for expensive injection-system luminometers, which were once needed to detect the millisecond flash of light. CAT gene expression can be assayed by incubating lysed cells with ^{14}C-acetylCoA and chloramphenicol, extracting the ^{14}C-acetyl-chloramphenicol into an organic solvent, and counting in a liquid scintillation counter [39]. Expression of the β-GAL gene can be measured by a simple spectrophotometric method through incubating cell lysate with the substrate X-gal (5-bromo-4-chloro-3-indolyl-β-D-galactopyranoside), which is then cleaved by the enzyme to form an intense blue product, and commercial kits are available for this assay. The GFP gene can be measured even more directly using a fluorescence microscope; the advantage of this approach is that any variation in expression between cells can be easily assayed using automated fluorescence-activated cell sorting analysis.

The reporter gene can be introduced (transfected) into the cells by either transient transfection or stable transfection. In transient transfection, the plasmid containing the reporter gene is added to the cells at the time of the assay and expression of the gene can be assayed for a period of 48–72h before any integration of the plasmid into the host genome. This empirical assay enables the assessment of reporter gene expression from effectively naked DNA on the transfected plasmid. However, it does require large amounts of plasmid DNA, and not all cells will take up the plasmid and express the gene. Furthermore, efficiency of transfection may vary in different cultures, so there is a need to control for the relative percentage of transfected cells in each assay. This is usually done by cotransfecting a second reporter gene on a constitutive promoter, and for this purpose, Renilla luciferase is useful because the vector is commercially available and the Renilla luciferase activity can be assayed alongside the firefly luciferase activity using commercial kits.

Stable transfection of the reporter gene entails selecting clones of cells that stably express the reporter gene. This is usually done by cotransfection with a second resistance gene such as the Neo gene, which confers resistance to G418 sulfate. Then G418 sulfate-resistant clones of cells need to be selected for their estrogen-regulated expression of the reporter gene. Having a stably transfected cell line negates the need for large amounts of plasmid for every experiment and the need to control for transfection efficiency, and usually provides a more sensitive assay because all cells express the reporter gene. However, the gene is now stably integrated into the host genome in the form of chromatin and so could be viewed as a more complex assay requiring the ligand–ER complex to regulate a gene integrated as chromatin and where the position of integration can affect expression.

Reporter gene assays have been carried out in a variety of cell types containing ER, either endogenously or with prior transfection of ERα/ERβ into the cells. For specific human health considerations, it is most relevant to use human cells from the target organ of interest. For example, effects of estrogenic compounds measured in human breast tissue are best assessed using primary cultures or cell lines of human breast epithelial cells (immortalized or transformed). However, for more generic questions of whether compounds possess estrogenic properties and for wide screening of large numbers of compounds, yeast cells have been used widely with much success. Although yeast cells are not intrinsically estrogen-responsive, transfection of an ER gene along with an estrogen-responsive reporter gene seem to be all that is needed for the yeast cells to give estrogen-regulated expression of the reporter gene; and colorimetric end-point reporter assays have provided very useful screening tools for identifying the estrogenic activity of compounds. The main disadvantage of yeast cell-based assays is that most seem only able to detect agonist activity of a compound and, for some ill-understood reason (which presumably relates to coactivator or corepressor deficiencies), do not enable antagonist responses.

Figure 3.10 shows the ability of isobutylparaben to regulate the expression of a stably transfected, estrogen-responsive *ERE-CAT* reporter gene in MCF-7 human breast cancer

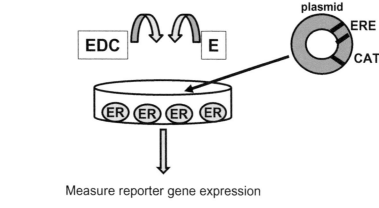

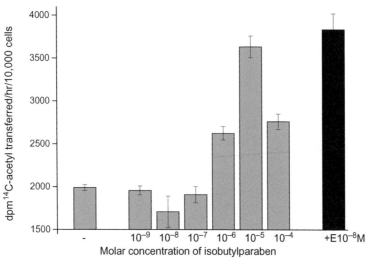

FIGURE 3.10 Regulation of a stably transfected *ERE-CAT* reporter gene by isobutylparaben in MCF-7 human breast cancer cells. CAT gene expression is shown at the indicated concentrations of isobutylparaben or 17β-estradiol and have been published [40].

cells [40]. *CAT* gene expression was measured as the disintegrations per minute (dpm) of ^{14}C-acetyl transferred onto chloramphenicol per hour per 10,000 cells.

3.4.2.2 Endogenous Gene Assays

The assay of endogenous estrogen-regulated genes usually uses human breast cancer cell lines where the genes for trefoil growth factor (*pS2*) [14], PR [15], and cathepsin D [16] have been long recognized as regulated by estrogen. The most widely used and simplest assay is to measure mRNA production by real-time reverse transcriptase polymerase chain reaction (RTPCR), although previous reliance on northern blotting remains valid for these highly expressed mRNAs. At a protein level, immunoassays or western immunoblotting can also be used to measure the levels of these gene products.

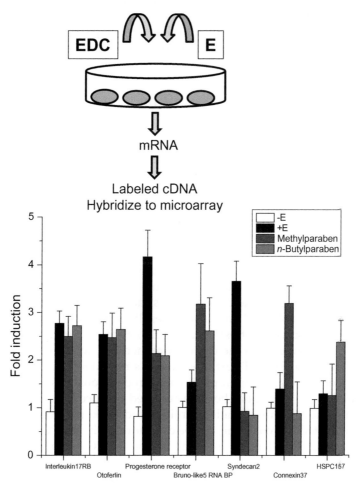

FIGURE 3.11 Microarray analysis reveals some similarities and some differences in the regulation of individual genes by 17β-estradiol (black), methylparaben (blue), and *n*-butylparaben (red) in MCF-7 human breast cancer cells. *Source: Results are as published [47].*

Following the development of microarray technology, it is now possible to assay not only the expression of single genes, but also the profile of expression of thousands of genes using expression microarrays. This allows investigation into the similarity of global gene expression profiles produced by exposure to different xenoestrogens. While some estrogen-regulated genes may be expressed similarly by different xenoestrogens, global gene expression profiles published to date have never been identical with different compounds. Figure 3.11 shows patterns of expression of genes regulated in similar and dissimilar ways by 17β-estradiol and two parabens as selected from the microarray analysis of 19,881 genes in MCF-7 human breast cancer cells [47]. Interleukin 17 receptor B and otoferlin are examples of genes upregulated to a similar extent by 17β-estradiol and both parabens. However, PR gene expression was upregulated to a greater extent by 17β-estradiol than by either of the parabens, and expression of the Bruno-like5 RNA BP gene was upregulated to a greater extent by the parabens than by 17β-estradiol. Expression of the syndecan 2 gene was only upregulated by 17β-estradiol and not by the parabens, yet expression of the connexin37 gene was only upregulated by methylparaben and expression of the HSPC157 gene more by *n*-butylparaben [47].

3.4.3 Can Binding of the Compound to ER Increase Proliferation of Estrogen-Responsive Cells In Vitro?

Although a xenoestrogen may increase expression of estrogen-regulated genes, a further question is whether the whole profile of gene expression produced by exposure to a xenoestrogen can then lead to a cellular response. For this, proliferation of estrogen-responsive human breast cancer cell lines has been used as an end-point assay. ZR-75-1 and some sublines of MCF-7 cells are dependent on estrogen for their growth [48], and the use of MCF-7 cells in the E-SCREEN is a widely validated assay [49]. Lines of MCF-7 and T-47-D cells, which are responsive to estrogen for their proliferation but which still proliferate in the absence of estrogen, can still give valid assays, but they provide less useful models in that the proliferative difference is smaller and it is less easy to assess small changes [48].

For human breast cancer cells to maintain dependence on estrogen for their proliferation, the stock cells need to be kept in the presence of estradiol, insulin, or both: long-term maintenance in the absence of estradiol and insulin results in the loss of proliferative dependence on estrogen [50]. For assay of estrogen regulation of cell proliferation, all sources of estrogen need to be removed from the cell culture medium, which necessitates using both a phenol-red-free medium [51] and dextran-charcoal-stripped serum [52]. The presence of a co-purifying estrogenic contaminant in phenol red preparations was identified in 1985, and the use of phenol-red-free media has become accepted practice [51]. Since serum from any source will contain endogenous steroids, steroids need to be removed from the serum by incubation with activated charcoal. This can be done for 30 min at 56°C to heat-inactivate the serum at the same time [52]; alternatively, it can be done at 4°C overnight if heat inactivation is not needed.

Figure 3.12 shows the effect of five parabens on the proliferation of MCF-7 human breast cancer cells [39,40]. All parabens had the same efficacy as estradiol in stimulating cell proliferation over a 14-day period. However, higher concentrations were needed for maximal

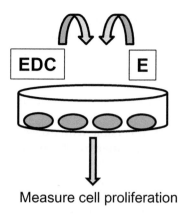

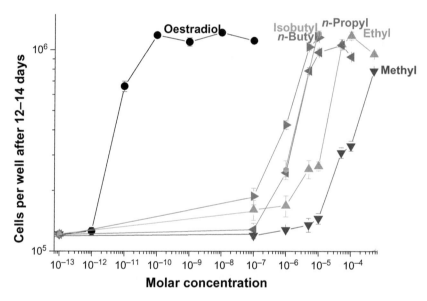

FIGURE 3.12   Effects of the indicated concentrations of parabens on the proliferation of MCF-7 human breast cancer cells in monolayer culture over 12–14 days. Higher concentrations were needed for parabens compared to 17β-estradiol (which is in line with their lower binding affinities to ER), but overall, the efficacies of methylparaben, ethylparaben, n-propylparaben, n-butylparaben, and isobutylparaben were similar to 17β-estradiol when sufficient concentrations were present. *Source: Data are amalgamated from two publications [39,40].*

agonist response for the parabens than for estradiol, which agrees with their lower relative binding affinities to ER [39,40].

   The ability to increase the proliferation of estrogen-responsive human breast cancer cells, especially the MCF-7 cell line, has become a well-validated assay for estrogenic activity of a compound. However, since regulation of proliferation can involve many cross-interacting pathways, it is necessary to also identify whether any alteration to proliferation is ER-mediated or not. The accepted way of achieving this is to carry out proliferation assays with or without the presence of an antiestrogen such as tamoxifen or fulvestrant. Any ER-mediated actions of the compound would be blocked by the presence of the antiestrogen, which would compete for binding to the ER [39]. Any proliferative effects mediated through GPER or other receptor systems would not be blocked by the antiestrogen.

This assay system can identify antagonist as well as agonist responses. However, any antagonist response must be distinguished from nonspecific inhibitory responses or toxicity by demonstrating that the antagonism is reversible with excess estrogen.

Interestingly, this assay system is also sensitive to additive effects. If estrogenic chemicals are combined at concentrations where each individually has a submaximal effect, then the combination can increase the proliferative response above that observed for any of the individual components. This is particularly striking when chemicals are combined at or below their no-observed-effect concentration (NOEC) and has been demonstrated for parabens when combined at NOEC values [53].

3.4.4 Can the Compound Increase Uterine Weight in the Immature Rodent In Vivo?

Any chemical classed as estrogenic also must be able to give rise to a physiological response in a whole animal. This more complex in vivo assay requires the compound to be absorbed from the site of application and then transported to the target organ without being metabolized and cleared from the body before any response is detectable. The gold-standard assay used for measuring estrogenic activity in an animal model has caused an increase in uterine weight in the immature rodent (the uterotrophic assay) [54,55]. The compound can be administered by a variety of routes, including oral, subcutaneous, and dermal. In order to avoid the animal from ingesting any dermally applied compounds, they are usually applied to dorsal skin. Compounds are administered once daily for three days to mice or rats just prior to the onset of puberty. On the fourth day, animals are sacrificed to enable the uterus to be dissected. Increase in uterine weight in the immature rodent is visible by eye. Much of the increase is due to uptake of water, although there is also an increase in cell proliferation. For this reason, two measures of uterine weight are useful: increase in wet weight is used as a measure of the overall tissue weight due to the water uptake but increase in dry weight is used as a measure of the increase in cellular tissue content. The mechanism of increase in the uterine weight remains incompletely understood, but ERα is present in uterine tissue and is thought to drive the uterotrophic response since the uterus of the ERα knockout mouse does not respond to estrogen administration [56].

Although most assays use immature rodents, it is also possible to use ovariectomized rodents, where the source of endogenous estrogen synthesis from the ovary has been stopped. Such animals also give a uterotrophic response to compounds with estrogenic activity, but it has been suggested recently that the overall response is less sensitive [57]. Sensitivity of the assay has also been shown to vary when using different species of rats or mice, so overall conclusions of negative effects in a uterotrophic assay may need to be concluded on the basis of more than one type of rodent [57]. Figure 3.13 shows the results of increase in wet uterine weight in immature mice following exposure to isobutylparaben as compared with estradiol [40].

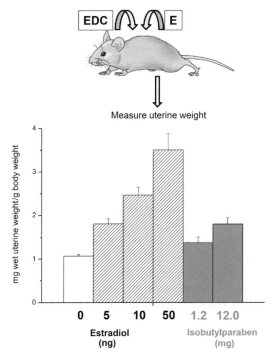

FIGURE 3.13 Effect of subcutaneous administration of isobutylparaben on uterine weight in immature CD1 mice. Mice were treated once daily for three days with the indicated doses of 17β-estradiol or isobutylparaben. *Source: Results are as published [40].*

3.4.5 Can the Compound Interfere with Biosynthesis of Estrogens?

Estrogens are derived from androstenedione and testosterone by the enzyme aromatase, which is a member of the cytochrome P450 family of enzymes (19A1) (Figure 3.7). Some environmental compounds can alter the biosynthesis of endogenous estrogens within the cells, either through binding to ERs and altering the expression of aromatase or through binding directly to aromatase to alter its enzymatic activity (Figure 3.8) [34]. It is possible to assay the effects of compounds on the production of aromatase mRNA by RTPCR, on aromatase protein by Western immunoblotting, or on aromatase activity by measuring estrogen production. Estrogen production is assayed either using antibodies to estradiol in an immunoassay or incubating cytosol with ^{3}H-androstenedione and measuring the release of ^{3}H$_2$O. Any increase in estrogen biosynthesis could act to increase proliferation in cell lines such as MCF-7, which require estrogen for their growth, and this action would be blocked with antioestrogen. In order to distinguish this type of mechanism, it is necessary to assay the cell proliferation in the presence and absence of an aromatase inhibitor, such as letrozole, as well as an antioestrogen.

While some estrogen is synthesized in epithelial cells, it is often synthesized in larger amounts from surrounding stromal fibroblasts [58]. If compounds act to influence estrogen synthesis by stromal cells but it is the epithelial cells that possess the ERs to respond, then paracrine interactions within a tissue also have to be taken into consideration in the assays. This necessitates the use of co-culture systems to identify both increased synthesis and response. A range of co-culture systems are now commercially available that enable epithelial and fibroblast cells to be cultured together but separate them by a membrane so that end points can be measured individually in each cell type.

3.4.6 Bioavailability of Estrogens

As for all steroid hormones, estrogens are lipophilic and so are bound to proteins, steroid hormone-binding globulin (SHBG), or albumin when they are carried in the blood. It is generally agreed that only the free (unbound) estrogen is able to diffuse into the target cell to bring about a response. Therefore, if xenoestrogens can bind to SHBG, then they could cause a net release of additional free estrogen that is biologically available for the tissues to respond to. On the other hand, by binding to SHBG, xenoestrogens might be rendered themselves as not biologically available. The ability of compounds to compete with ^{3}H-estradiol for binding to SHBG can be assayed by radioimmunoassay.

Water solubility of estrogens is increased by conjugation mainly as sulfates or glucuronides for the purposes of excretion. Although it is generally assumed that conjugates of estrogens and xenoestrogens would lack estrogenic activity, some sulfate conjugates of phytoestrogens have been shown to retain estrogenic activity [59]. Furthermore, some phytoestrogens and xenoestrogens have been shown to interfere with sulfotransferase enzymes (SULT isoforms), which carry out the processes of sulfonation [60]. Such effects can be assayed by measuring altered levels of estrogen sulfates and the effects of environmental compounds on the production or activity of the enzymes themselves.

3.5 ENVIRONMENTAL ESTROGENS

Many hundreds of environmental compounds now have been shown to possess the ability to mimic or interfere in estrogen action using assay systems as described in this chapter, and such compounds have been termed *environmental estrogens*. Table 3.1 gives examples of environmental estrogens to which the human population is exposed and which are known to enter human tissues. Of these, some are taken in by informed choice (e.g., in contraceptives and hormone replacement therapy), but by far the greater number enter the human body inadvertently through inhalation or oral and dermal routes following environmental contamination of diet, from use of consumer products in the domestic environment, or from the application of personal care products to human skin [61–63].

Ethinylestradiol is a synthetic estrogen with similar activity to 17β-estradiol [64] and used as a component of oral contraceptives and hormone replacement therapy, although it is also used in some anti-aging cosmetic products. Phytoestrogens are natural components of plants that possess estrogenic activity and are ingested in the diet through consumption of plant materials [65]. Different phytoestrogens possess wide-ranging estrogenic potencies [66]. Many organochlorine compounds have been widely used as pesticides, but the estrogenic activities of compounds such as dichlorodiphenyltrichloroethane (DDT), dieldrin, and

TABLE 3.1 Examples of Environmental Chemicals That Can Bind to ERs and Give Estrogenic Responses, and to Which the Human Population Is Exposed

Use in the environment	Example compounds	Source of human exposure	Evidence for estrogenic activity of example compounds
Pharmaceuticals	Ethinylestradiol	Contraceptive pill, hormone replacement therapy, cosmetics	[64]
Natural component of plants	Genistein, daidzein	Edible plant material (diet)	[65,66]
Pesticides/herbicides	DDT, dieldrin, endosulfan	Animal fat (diet)	[64,67]
Electrical industry	Polychlorinated biphenyls	Animal fat (diet)	[64,68,69]
By-product of incineration	Polychlorinated dioxins	Inhaled; animal fat in diet	[70]
Flame retardant in soft furnishings	Polybrominated organics	Domestic environment	[71]
Plastics, epoxy resins	Bisphenol A	Storage of food and beverages (diet); domestic environment	[72,73]
Plastics	Phthalate esters	Domestic consumer products	[74,75]
Detergent	Alkyl phenols	Domestic environment	[76,77]
Preservative	Parabens	Cosmetics, food, pharmaceuticals	[36]
Antiseptic, preservative	Triclosan	Personal care products, domestic consumer products	[78]
Absorb UV light	Benzophenones	Suncare products, other cosmetics, clothing	[79]
Fragrance	Butylphenylmethylpropional, benzyl salicylate, musks	Personal care products, domestic consumer products	[80,81]

endosulfan [64,67] were identified only after long-term environmental usage had occurred already. Due to their lipophilicity, these compounds remain persistent in the environment and bioaccumulate in fatty tissues of animals. Such compounds, therefore, are ingested in animal fat in the diet, and since they are not easily cleared from the body, they tend to build up in adipose tissue with age. The polychlorinated biphenyls are another group of persistent organochlorine compounds used widely in the electrical industry, and again, their estrogenic properties [64,68,69] were revealed only long after widespread contamination of the environment and transfer into animal fat in the human diet. Polychlorinated dioxins are mainly generated as by-products of incineration, but they also have become widespread in the environment and present in animal fat in the diet. They possess estrogen antagonist properties and weak agonist activity [70]. Many compounds in a range of consumer products used in the domestic environment have now been shown to possess estrogenic activity as well. This includes polybrominated organics used as flame retardants in soft furnishings

[71], components of plastics [72–75], and alkyl phenols used in detergents [76,77]. Finally, it is now recognized that many chemical constituents of personal care products also possess estrogenic activity and are entering human tissues. This includes parabens [36] and triclosan, [78] used as antimicrobial preservatives; benzophenones, used to absorb ultraviolet (UV) light [79]; and many components of fragrance, including polycyclic musks and nitromusks [80], butylphenylmethylpropional (Lilial), and benzyl salicylate [81]. Some applications, such as triclosan in toothpaste, result in entry to the human body by the oral route, and others used in aerosols may result in inhalation, but the majority of excipients of personal care products enter through the skin from dermal exposure (see Chapter 19).

References

[1] Toft D, Gorski J. A receptor molecule for estrogens: isolation from the rat uterus and preliminary characterization. Proc Natl Acad Sci USA 1966;55:1574–81.
[2] Jensen EV, DeSombre ER. Estrogen-receptor interaction. Science 1973;182:126–34.
[3] Walter P, Green S, Greene G, Krust A, Bornert JM, Jeltsch JM, et al. Cloning of the human estrogen receptor cDNA. Proc Natl Acad Sci USA 1985;82:7889–93.
[4] Mosselman S, Polman J, Dijkema R. ER beta: identification and characterization of a novel human estrogen receptor. FEBS Lett 1996;392:49–53.
[5] Gustafsson JA. Estrogen receptor β—a new dimension in estrogen mechanism of action. J Endocrinol 1999;163:379–83.
[6] Brzozowski AM, Pike AC, Dauter Z, Hubbard RE, Bonn T, Engström O, et al. Molecular basis of agonism and antagonism in the oestrogen receptor. Nature 1997;389:753–8.
[7] Pike AC, Brzozowski AM, Hubbard RE, Bonn T, Thorsell AG, Engström O, et al. Structure of the ligand-binding domain of oestrogen receptor beta in the presence of a partial agonist and a full antagonist. EMBO J 1999;18:4608–18.
[8] Pike ACW. Lessons learnt from structural studies of the oestrogen receptor. Best Pract Res Clin Endocrinol Metab 2006;20:1–14.
[9] Darbre PD. Metalloestrogens: an emerging class of inorganic xenoestrogens with potential to add to the oestrogenic burden of the human breast. J Appl Toxicol 2006;26:191–7.
[10] Oettel M, Schillinger E, editors. Estrogens and antiestrogens I. Berlin, Germany: Springer Verlag; 1999.
[11] Nilsson S, Mäkelä S, Treuter E, Tujague M, Thomsen J, Andersson G, et al. Mechanisms of estrogen action. Physiol Rev 2001;81:1535–65.
[12] Cheskis BJ, Greger JG, Nagpal S, Freedman LP. Signaling by estrogens. J Cell Physiol 2007;213:610–7.
[13] Acconcia F, Marino M. The effects of 17β-estradiol in cancer are mediated by estrogen receptor signaling at the plasma membrane. Front Physiol 2011;2:1–8.
[14] Masiakowski P, Breathnach R, Bloch J, Gannon F, Krust A, Chambon P. Cloning of cDNA sequences of hormone-regulated genes from the MCF-7 human breast cancer cell line. Nucleic Acids Res 1982;10:7895–903.
[15] Kastner P, Krust A, Turcotte B, Stropp U, Tora L, Gronemeyer H, et al. Two distinct estrogen-regulated promoters generate transcripts encoding the two functionally different human progesterone receptor forms A and B. EMBO J 1990;9:1603–14.
[16] Krishnan V, Wang X, Safe S. Estrogen receptor-Sp1 complexes mediate estrogen-induced cathepsin D gene expression in MCF-7 human breast cancer cells. J Biol Chem 1994;269:15912–15917.
[17] Frasor J, Danes JM, Komm B, Chang KCN, Lyttle CR, Katzenellenbogen BS. Profiling of estrogen up- and down-regulated gene expression in human breast cancer cells: insights into gene networks and pathways underlying estrogenic control of proliferation and cell phenotype. Endocrinology 2003;144:4562–74.
[18] Tee MK, Rogatsky I, Tzagarakis-Foster C, Cvoro A, An J, Christy RJ, et al. Estradiol and selective estrogen receptor modulators differentially regulate target genes with estrogen receptors α and β. Mol Biol Cell 2004;15:1262–72.
[19] Webb P, Nguyen P, Valentine C, Lopez GN, Kwok GR, McInerney E, et al. The estrogen receptor enhances AP1 activity by two distinct mechanisms with different requirements for receptor transactivation functions. Mol Endocrinol 1999;13:1672–85.

[20] Safe S. Transcriptional activation of genes by 17beta-estradiol through estrogen receptor-Sp1 interactions. Vitam Horm 2001;62:231–52.

[21] Pearce ST, Jordan VC. The biological role of estrogen receptors alpha and beta in cancer. Crit Rev Oncol Hematol 2004;50:3–22.

[22] Ascenzi P, Bocedi A, Marino M. Structure–function relationship of estrogen receptor α and β: impact on human health. Mol Aspect Med 2006;27:299–402.

[23] Klinge CM, Bowers JL, Kulakosky PC, Kamboj KK, Swanson HI. The aryl hydrocarbon receptor (AHR)/AHR nuclear translocator (ARNT) heterodimer interacts with naturally occurring estrogen response elements. Mol Cell Endocrinol 1999;157:105–19.

[24] Selye H. Correlations between the chemical structure and the pharmacological actions of the steroids. Endocrinol 1942;30:437–53.

[25] Powell CE, Soto AM, Sonnenschein C. Identification and characterisation of membrane estrogen receptor from MCF7 estrogen-target cells. J Steroid Biochem Mol Biol 2001;77:97–108.

[26] Soltysik K, Czekaj P. Membrane estrogen receptors—is it an alternative way of estrogen action? J Physiol Pharmacol 2013;64:129–42.

[27] Acconia F, Totta P, Ogawa S, Cardillo I, Inoue S, Leone S, et al. Survival versus apoptotic 17β-estradiol effect: role of ERα and Erβ activated non-genomic signaling. J Cell Physiol 2005;203:193–201.

[28] Marino M, Ascenzi P. Membrane association of estrogen receptor α and β influences 17β-oestradiol-mediated cancer cell proliferation. Steroids 2008;73:853–8.

[29] Norfleet AM, Clarke CH, Gametchu B, Watson CS. Antibodies to the estrogen receptor-alpha modulate rapid prolactin release from rat pituitary tumor cells through plasma membrane estrogen receptors. FEBS J 2004;14:157–65.

[30] Bulayeva NN, Watson CS. Xenoestrogen-induced ERK-1 and ERK-2 activation via multiple membrane-initiated signalling pathways. Environ Health Perspect 2004;112:1481–7.

[31] Watson CS, Bulayeva NN, Wozniak AL, Finnerty CC. Signalling from the membrane via membrane estrogen receptor-alpha: estrogens, xenoestrogens and phytoestrogens. Steroids 2005;70:364–71.

[32] Lappano R, De Marco P, De Francesco EM, Chimento A, Pezzi V, Magglioni M. Cross-talk between GPER and growth factor signalling. J Steroid Biochem Mol Biol 2013;137:50–6.

[33] Albanito L, Lappano R, Madeo A, Chimento A, Prossnitz ER, Cappello AR, et al. G-protein-coupled receptor 30 and estrogen receptor-alpha are involved in the proliferative effects induced by atrazine in ovarian cancer cells. Environ Health Perspect 2008;116:1648–55.

[34] Whitehead SA, Rice S. Endocrine-disrupting chemicals as modulators of sex steroid synthesis. Best Pract Res Clin Endocrinol Metab 2006;20:45–61.

[35] Calafat AM, Ye X, Wong LY, Bishop AM, Needham LL. Urinary concentrations of four parabens in the U.S. Population: NHANES 2005–2006. Environ Health Perspect 2010;118:679–85.

[36] Darbre PD, Harvey PW. Paraben esters: review of recent studies of endocrine toxicity, absorption, esterase and human exposure, and discussion of potential human health risks. J Appl Toxicol 2008;28:561–78.

[37] Leake RE, Habib F. Steroid hormone receptors: assay and characterisation Steroid hormones: a practical approach. Oxford: IRL Press; 1987. pp. 67–97.

[38] Blair RM, Fang H, Branham WS, Hass BS, Dial SL, Moland CL, et al. The estrogen receptor binding affinities of 188 natural and xenochemicals: structural diversity of ligands. Toxicol Sci 2000;54:138–53.

[39] Byford JR, Shaw LE, Drew MG, Pope GS, Sauer MJ, Darbre PD. Oestrogenic activity of parabens in MCF7 human breast cancer cells. J Steroid Biochem Mol Biol 2002;80:49–60.

[40] Darbre PD, Byford JR, Shaw LE, Horton RA, Pope GS, Sauer MJ. Oestrogenic activity of isobutylparaben *in vitro* and *in vivo*. J Appl Toxicol 2002;22:219–26.

[41] Kuiper GG, Carlsson B, Grandien K, Enmark E, Haggblad J, Nilsson S, et al. Comparison of the ligand binding specificity and transcript tissue distribution of estrogen receptors alpha and beta. Endocrinology 1997;138:863–70.

[42] Harvey EN, Snell PA. The analysis of bioluminescences of short duration, recorded with photoelectric cell and string galvanometer. J Gen Physiol 1931;14:529–45.

[43] Arnone MI, Dmochowski IJ, Gache C. Using reporter genes to study cis-regulatory elements. Methods Cell Biol 2004;74:621–52.

[44] Luckow B, Schutz G. CAT constructions with multiple unique restriction sites for the functional analysis of eukaryotic promoters and regulatory elements. Nucleic Acids Res 1987;15:5490.

[45] Patton WF. Detection technologies in proteome analysis. J Chromatogr B 2002;771:3–31.

[46] Inouye S, Tsuji FI. Expression of the gene and fluorescence characteristics of the recombinant protein. FEBS Lett 1994;341:277–80.

[47] Pugazhendhi D, Sadler AJ, Darbre PD. Comparison of the global gene expression profiles produced by methylparaben, n-butylparaben and 17β-oestradiol in MCF7 human breast cancer cells. J Appl Toxicol 2007;27:67–77.

[48] Darbre PD, Daly RJ. Effects of oestrogen on human breast cancer cells in culture. Proc R Soc Edinb 1989;95B:119–32.

[49] Soto AM, Maffini MV, Schaeberie CM, Sonnenschein C. Strengths and weaknesses of in vitro assays for estrogenic and endrogenic activity. Best Pract Res Clin Endocrinol Metab 2006;20:15–33.

[50] Shaw LE, Sadler AJ, Pugazhendhi D, Darbre PD. Changes in oestrogen receptor-α and -β during progression to acquired resistance to tamoxifen and fulvestrant (Faslodex, ICI 182,780) in MCF7 human breast cancer cells. J Steroid Biochem Mol Biol 2006;99:19–32.

[51] Berthois Y, Katzenellenbogen JA, Katzenellenbogen BS. Phenol red in tissue culture media is a weak estrogen: implications concerning the study of estrogen-responsive cells in culture. Proc Natl Acad Sci USA 1986;83:2496–500.

[52] Darbre P, Yates J, Curtis SA, King RJB. Effect of estradiol on human breast cancer cells in culture. Cancer Res 1983;43:349–54.

[53] Charles AK, Darbre PD. Combinations of parabens at concentrations measured in human breast tissue can increase proliferation of MCF-7 human breast cancer cells. J Appl Toxicol 2013;33:390–8.

[54] Clode SA. Assessment of in vivo assays for endocrine disruption. Best Pract Res Clin Endocrinol Metab 2006;20:35–43.

[55] Marty MS, O'Connor JC. Key learnings from the endocrine disruptor screening program (EDSP) Tier 1 rodent uterotrophic and Hershberger assays. Birth Defects Res (Part B) 2014;101:63–70.

[56] Dupont S, Krust A, Gansmuller A, Dierich A, Chambon P, Mark M. Effect of single and compound knockouts of estrogen receptors alpha (ERalpha) and beta (ERbeta) on mouse reproductive phenotypes. Development 2000;127:4277–91.

[57] Lemini C, Jaimez R, Avila ME, Franco Y, Larrea F, Lemus AE. In vivo and in vitro estrogen bioactivities of alkyl parabens. Toxicol Ind Health 2003;19:69–79.

[58] Miki Y, Ono K, Hata S, Suzuki T, Kumamoto H, Sasano H. The advantages of co-culture over mono cell culture in simulating in vivo environment. J Steroid Biochem Mol Biol 2012;131:68–75.

[59] Pugazhendhi D, Watson KA, Mills S, Botting N, Pope GS, Darbre PD. Effect of sulphation on the oestrogen agonist activity of the phytoestrogens genistein and daidzein in MCF-7 human breast cancer cells. J Endocrinol 2008;197:503–15.

[60] Waring RH, Ayers S, Gescher AJ, Glatt HR, Meinl W, Jarratt P, et al. Phytoestrogens and xenoestrogens: the contribution of diet and environment to endocrine disruption. J Steroid Biochem Mol Biol 2008;108:213–20.

[61] Darbre PD. Environmental oestrogens, cosmetics and breast cancer. Best Pract Res Clin Endocrinol Metab 2006;20:121–43.

[62] Darbre PD, Charles AK. Environmental oestrogens and breast cancer: evidence for a combined involvement of dietary, household and cosmetic xenoestrogens. Anticancer Res 2010;30:815–28.

[63] Darbre PD, Fernandez MF. Environmental oestrogens and breast cancer: long-term low-dose effects of mixtures of varied chemical combinations. J Epidemiol Community Health 2013;67:203–5.

[64] Soto AM, Sonnenschein C, Chung KL, Fernandez MF, Olea N, Serrano FO. The E-SCREEN assay as a tool to identify estrogens: an update on estrogenic environmental pollutants. Environ Health Perspect 1995;103(Suppl. 7): 113–22.

[65] Woods HF. Phytoestrogens and health. London: Food Standards Agency Publication; 2003. Crown Copyright, <http://cot.food.gov.uk/pdfs/phytoreport0503>.

[66] Matsumura A, Ghosh A, Pope GS, Darbre PD. Comparative study of oestrogenic properties of eight phytoestrogens in MCF7 human breast cancer cells. J Steroid Biochem Mol Biol 2005;94:431–43.

[67] Soto AM, Chung KL, Sonnenschein C. The pesticides endosulfan, toxaphene, and dieldrin have estrogenic effects on human estrogen-sensitive cells. Environ Health Perspect 1994;102:380–3.

[68] Nesaretnam K, Corcoran D, Dils RR, Darbre P. 3,4,3′,4′-Tetrachlorobiphenyl acts as an estrogen in vitro and in vivo. Mol Endocrinol 1996;10:923–36.

[69] Nesaretnam K, Darbre P. 3,5,3′,5′-Tetrachlorobiphenyl is a weak oestrogen agonist *in vitro* and *in vivo*. J Steroid Biochem Mol Biol 1997;62:409–18.

[70] Safe S, Wormke M. Inhibitory aryl hydrocarbon receptor—estrogen receptor α cross-talk and mechanisms of action. Chem Res Toxicol 2003;16:807–16.

[71] Feliciano MM, Bigsby RM. The polybrominated diphenyl ether mixture DE-71 is mildly estrogenic. Environ Health Perspect 2008;116:605–11.

[72] Jorgensen ECB, Long M, Hofmeister MV, Vinggaard AM. Endocrine-disrupting potential of bisphenol A, bisphenol A dimethacrylate, 4-*n*-nonylphenol, and 4-*n*-octylphenol *in vitro*: new data and a brief review. Environ Health Perspect 2007;115:69–76.

[73] Rubin BS. Bisphenol A: an endocrine disruptor with widespread exposure and multiple effects. J Steroid Biochem Mol Biol 2011;127:27–34.

[74] Jobling S, Reynolds T, White R, Parker MG, Sumpter JP. A variety of environmentally persistent chemicals, including some phthalate plasticizers, are weakly estrogenic. Environ Health Perspect 1995;103:582–7.

[75] Harris CA, Henttu P, Parker MG, Sumpter JP. The estrogenic activity of phthalate esters *in vitro*. Environ Health Perspect 1997;105:802–11.

[76] White R, Jobling S, Hoare SA, Sumpter JP, Parker MG. Environmentally persistent alkylphenolic compounds are estrogenic. Endocrinology 1994;135:175–82.

[77] Laws SC, Carey SA, Ferrell JM, Bodman GJ, Cooper RL. Estrogenic activity of octylphenol, nonylphenol, bisphenol A and methoxychlor in rats. Toxicol Sci 2000;54:154–67.

[78] Gee RH, Charles A, Taylor N, Darbre PD. Oestrogenic and androgenic activity of triclosan in breast cancer cells. J Appl Toxicol 2008;28:78–91.

[79] Schlumpf M, Cotton B, Conscience M, Haller V, Steinmann B, Lichtensteiger W. *In vitro* and *in vivo* estrogenicity of UV screens. Environ Health Perspect 2001;109:239–44.

[80] Gomez E, Pillon A, Fenet H, Rosain D, Duchesne MJ, Nicholas JC, et al. Estrogenic activity of cosmetic components in reporter cell lines: parabens, UV screens, and musks. J Toxicol Environ Health Part A 2005;68:239–51.

[81] Charles AK, Darbre PD. Oestrogenic activity of benzylsalicylate, benzylbenzoate and butylphenylmethylpropional (Lilial) in MCF7 human breast cancer cells *in vitro*. J Appl Toxicol 2009;29:422–34.

4

Disruptors of Androgen Action and Synthesis

J. Thomas Sanderson

Abstract

Various environmental chemicals have been found to exert antiandrogenic effects in exposed animals and there is a concern that such compounds may also result in adverse effects in humans. Attempts to elucidate potential mechanisms of antiandrogenic action require knowledge of the functions of androgens in the body and the various ways in which environmental chemicals may disrupt these functions. Environmental antiandrogens may compete with the endogenous androgens testosterone and dihydrotestosterone (DHT) for the androgen receptor (AR), thus blocking its intracellular signaling pathway, which is responsible for the majority of androgenic functions. Other disruptions of androgen function may be caused by inhibition of androgen biosynthesis via catalytic inhibition of key steroidogenic enzymes. Two important enzymes that can be targets for environmental chemicals are cytochrome P450 17-mediated steroid

Endocrine Disruption and Human Health.
DOI: http://dx.doi.org/10.1016/B978-0-12-801139-3.00004-1

17α-hydroxylase/17,20-lyase and steroid 5α-reductase activity, which are responsible for the production of the precursor C19-steroids dehydroepiandrosterone (DHEA) and androstenedione, and the conversion of testosterone to its more potent androgenic metabolite DHT, respectively. Various environmental chemicals, most notably pesticides, such as the DDT metabolite p,p-DDE, and fungicides, such as vinclozolin, procymidone, and prochloraz, have been identified to act via several of these antiandrogenic mechanisms to cause reproductive malformations in male rats exposed either in utero or in adult life. In addition to in vivo models to screen for proandrogenic or antiandrogenic compounds (rodent Hershberger assay), several in vitro cell bioassays have been developed for the rapid, mechanism-based screening of disruptors of androgen action either at the level of AR signaling (LNCaP human prostate cancer cells or various reporter-gene systems) or at the level of steroidogenesis (H295R human adrenocortical carcinoma cells). Interestingly, very few if any environmental chemicals have been found to act as androgen mimics, in contrast to the many compounds found to act as estrogens in the environment. The consequences of human exposure to environmental levels of antiandrogens remains unclear.

4.1 PHYSIOLOGICAL ACTIONS OF ANDROGENS

Androgens perform key roles during embryogenesis, postnatal development, and in adulthood [1]. Although considered the male sex hormone, androgens also are produced in women and have important effects in both sexes. During male fetal development, androgens are produced as early as 8 weeks of gestation once embryonic stromal cells derived from the gonadal ridge of the mesenchyme start to differentiate into Leydig cells. At this time, androgens play a key role in the development of the prostate, scrotum, and penis, as well as in the ultimate decent of the testes between 7 months of fetal development and birth. Once a male reaches puberty, testicular androgen production by luteinizing hormone (LH) receptor-expressing Leydig cells increases under the influence of increased pituitary secretion of LH. The increased testosterone levels support the formation of functional seminiferous tubules and differentiation of germ cells into sperm. Pituitary follicle-stimulating hormone (FSH) secretion also increases, which, in cooperation with androgens, acts on the FSH receptor-expressing Sertoli cells to support sperm production. During this time, the actions of androgens become evident in males in the form of increased development of muscle mass and inhibition of fat deposition, among various other secondary sex characteristics, such as the growth of facial and body hair. In the adult male, androgens are responsible for maintaining libido, muscle mass, erythropoiesis, bone mineral density, prostate function, and spermatogenesis. In the adult brain, androgens reduce the frequency of pulsatile LH secretion by the pituitary in a negative feedback loop to control testicular androgen production. The role of testosterone, the main circulating androgen in males, is not always straightforward, as some of its actions are due to its potent androgenic metabolite dihydrotestosterone (DHT) in tissues that express steroid 5α-reductase (SRD5A), such as prostate, skin, and epididymis, or even due to estradiol in tissues where aromatase is expressed, such as bone, epididymis, and brain.

4.2 ANDROGEN BIOSYNTHESIS AND METABOLISM

Androgens in humans are synthesized de novo from cholesterol in several steroidogenic tissues, such as the testes in males, the ovaries in females, and the adrenal cortex in

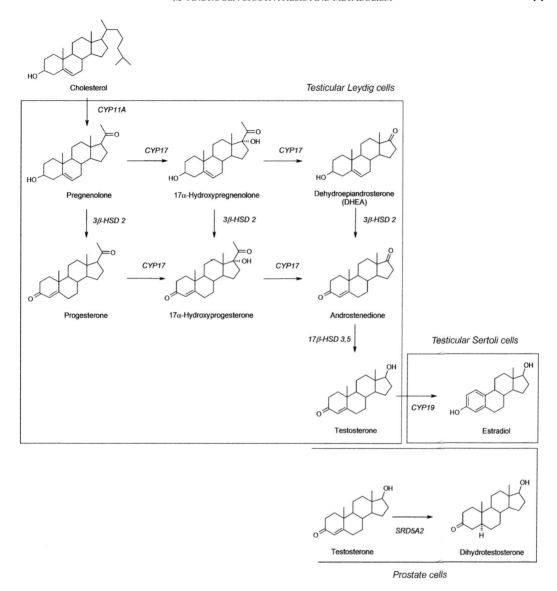

FIGURE 4.1   Biosynthesis de novo of androgens from cholesterol in steroidogenic tissues such as the testes. Testosterone is converted to the potent androgenic metabolite DHT in various peripheral tissues, as illustrated here in the prostate.

both sexes [2]. Androgen biosynthesis (Figure 4.1) begins with the conversion of cholesterol to pregnenolone by cytochrome P45011A (CYP11A, cholesterol side-chain cleavage) and subsequent conversion to progesterone by 3β-hydroxysteroid dehydrogenase type 2 (HSD3B2). Both pregnenolone and progesterone are substrates for CYP17, which exhibits dual steroid 17α-hydroxylase/17,20-lyase activity, producing the 17α-hydroxylated metabolites of pregnenolone and progesterone, which are subsequently converted into dehydroepiandrosterone (DHEA) and androstenedione, respectively [3]. In humans, the 17,20-lyase activity of CYP17 depends on the availability of cofactor cytochrome b5 [3] and appears to have a preference for the conversion of 17α-hydroxypregnenolone to DHEA exhibiting a K_m value 30 times lower than that for 17α-hydroxyprogesterone [4]. DHEA can undergo conversion to androstenedione by HSD3B2. The weakly androgenic 17-keto-steroid androstenedione is converted to the active 17-hydroxy-form of testosterone by 17β-hydroxysteroid dehydrogenase type 3 (HSD17B3) in testes and by aldo-keto reductase 1C3 (AKR1C3) in other peripheral tissues [5], including the ovaries in females [6]. Depending on the tissue, testosterone may subsequently be converted to its highly potent androgenic metabolite DHT by SRD5A1/2.

The biologically active androgens DHT and testosterone are deactivated mainly in the liver, but also to a lesser extent in nonhepatic tissues, such as prostate and skin. Biological deactivation of androgens may occur via oxidation or reduction reactions and subsequent conjugation pathways, after which the metabolites are excreted via the kidneys. Testosterone is reduced by hepatic AKR1D1 (steroid 5β-reductase) to biologically inactive 17β-hydroxy-5β-androstane-3-one, but also undergoes hepatic oxidation by cytochrome P450 enzymes to produce various hydroxylated metabolites (predominantly 6β-hydroxytestosterone by CYP3A4/5), which are conjugated with sulfate by hepatic sulfotransferases (predominantly by hepatic SULT2A1) [7] or with glucuronide by glucuronyl transferases (preferentially by hepatic UGT2B7, 15, and 17) [8,9]. DHT is catabolized by hepatic AKR1C4 [10] to produce the metabolite 5α-androstane-3α-17β-diol, which undergoes subsequent sulfate or glucuronide conjugation and renal excretion.

4.3 ANDROGEN RECEPTOR

4.3.1 Genomic Mechanisms of Androgen Action

The androgen receptor (AR) gene (official nomenclature *NR3C4*) is located on chromosome Xq11-12 and contains eight exons coding for a protein of about 110 kDa with about 919 amino acids dependent on the number of polyglutamine and polyglycine repeats. Similar to other nuclear receptors, the AR contains an N-terminal domain, DNA-binding domain (DBD), a hinge region, and a ligand-binding domain, with each domain having specific functions (Figure 4.2) [11,12]. The AR acts as a transcription factor and mediates the genomic actions of testosterone and DHT (Figure 4.3). Unligated AR is present in the cytoplasm in a complex with heat shock proteins (HSPs). Once bound to androgen, the AR dissociates from its HSPs and undergoes dimerization, phosphorylation, and

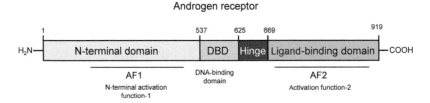

FIGURE 4.2   Structural and functional domains of the AR. *Source: Adapted from Ref. [12].*

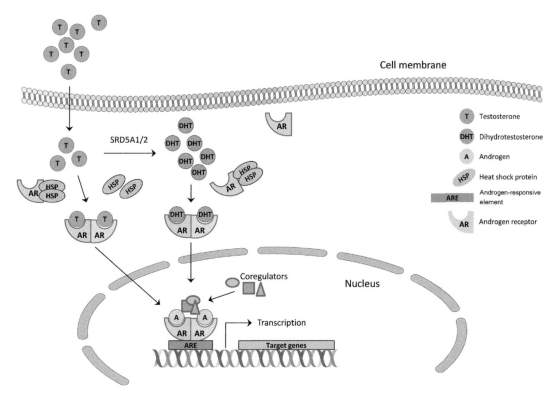

FIGURE 4.3 Classic genomic mechanism of the action of androgens. Circulating testosterone (T) enters the target cell, where it either binds directly to the AR or is converted by the enzyme steroid 5α-reductase (SRD5A1/2) to DHT, which binds with greater affinity to AR.

translocation to the nucleus of the target cell. Here, it recognizes and binds androgen-responsive elements (AREs) on the DNA and then recruits other transcriptional coregulators (e.g., coactivators and corepressors) to initiate or repress gene transcription. The types of genes that are activated or repressed are highly cell-specific and are commonly involved in cell proliferation, communication, differentiation, and prostate cancer progression [13]. In males, AR is expressed strongly in the prostate, epididymis, skeletal muscle, liver, adrenal, and central nervous system. In females, AR expression is lower, but it is most prominent in the mammary gland, uterus, vulvar epithelium, vaginal mucosa, and ovarian follicles. In the female brain, as in males, the AR is important to mediating the effects of androgens on libido and sexual behavior.

4.3.2 Nongenomic Actions of Androgens and the AR

The AR is capable of exerting effects within the cell without interacting with DNA, and these nongenomic pathways of signal transduction are characterized by direct AR-protein interactions, resulting in rapid cellular responses. Usually the activation of nongenomic pathways requires ARs to be ligand-bound, although constitutive ligand-independent activation may occur in diseases such as prostate cancer. Often these pathways involve the activation of specific kinases, such as Akt, protein kinase A, mitogen-activated protein kinases (ERK1/2), and protein kinase C [14,15], resulting in the phosphorylation and activation or inactivation of proteins involved in the cell cycle. Another frequently observed nongenomic action of androgen-bound AR is a rapid increase in intracellular calcium levels in certain cell types, such as Sertoli cells [16], T cells [17], cardiomyocytes, and hippocampal neurons [18]. Increasing evidence suggests that these responses are mediated by a membrane-bound form of AR (mAR) that may be activated extracellularly by androgens.

One of the implications of the existence of nongenomic pathways of androgen-mediated AR action is that even short-term changes in hormone levels, possibly caused by an acute temporary exposure to an endocrine-disrupting chemical (EDC), may result in altered cellular responses critical to human health [14].

4.4 ROLE OF ANDROGENS AND THE AR IN HUMAN DISEASES

Defects in the AR gene and subsequent loss of functional protein may result in human disorders such as androgen insensitivity syndrome, which is characterized by hypospadias, infertility, and gynecomastia in males. On the other hand, overexpression of functional AR and increased synthesis of androgens are implicated in prostate cancer growth and progression. In early-stage, androgen-dependent prostate cancer, androgens stimulate cell proliferation and increase the expression of various prostate-specific proteins such as prostate-specific antigen (PSA), which is commonly used as a marker of benign prostate hyperplasia or prostate cancer. In prostate cancer, ligand-bound AR is also involved in the posttranslational (nongenomic) induction of the key proliferative protein cyclin D1 [19] and the genomic downregulation of E-cadherin [20], which functions as a cell adhesion protein that allows cell–cell communication and is generally involved in maintaining cell and tissue structure. Loss of E-cadherin and other cadherins may promote cell migration and invasion and thus cancer progression and metastasis [20]. The main driver of androgen-dependent prostate cancer cell proliferation and progression is DHT, which is formed locally in high concentrations by conversion of testosterone due to the overexpression of steroid 5α-reductase (SRD5A1), whereas in normal prostate epithelium and in benign prostate hyperplasia, the SRD5A2 form is predominant [21–23]. Other key mechanisms involved in AR-mediated prostate cancer progression include (1) overexpression of AR [24], (2) increased constitutive ligand-independent activation of AR, (3) decreased degradation of AR, (4) increased intracellular synthesis of androgens, and (5) mutations in AR causing a broadening of ligand-binding selectivity [25,26]. Each of these mechanisms has complex causes that are far from well understood. AR overexpression occurs in 80% of prostate cancer patients that no longer respond to antiandrogen treatment through a process of gene amplification in response to androgen-deprivation therapy [27–29].

In females, it is thought that overexposure to androgens during fetal development and throughout adult life is an important factor in the development of polycystic ovary syndrome (PCOS). The occurrence of PCOS has been associated with increased androgen synthesis by the ovarian theca cells due to increased expression of GATA6, which is known to increase the transcription of the key androgen biosynthetic enzyme CYP17 [30].

4.5 ANTIANDROGENS

Antiandrogens are useful in the treatment of prostate cancer, benign prostate hyperplasia, precocious puberty, and male pattern baldness, as well as hirsutism in females and acne in both sexes. Antiandrogens used for therapeutic purposes (Table 4.1) are either AR

TABLE 4.1 Steroidal and Nonsteroidal Antiandrogens Designed to Block the AR or Inhibit Androgen Biosynthesis in the Treatment of Androgen-Dependent Prostate Cancer

Antiandrogen	Structure	Classification	Mechanism(s) of antiandrogenicity and other endocrine activities
Cyproterone acetate		Steroidal antiandrogen	Competitive AR antagonist [31] Partial AR agonist in the absence of endogenous androgens Progesterone receptor agonist [31] Inhibitor of steroidogenesis (reduced corticosteroid and androgen biosynthesis by inhibiting CYP21 and CYP17, respectively) [31] Antigonadotropic [31]
Hydroxyflutamide		Nonsteroidal antiandrogen	AR antagonist and active metabolite of flutamide [32]
Bicalutamide		Nonsteroidal antiandrogen	AR antagonist and a more potent derivative of hydroxyflutamide [33]
Finasteride		Steroid 5α-reductase inhibitor	Inhibits the catalytic activity of, preferentially, SRD5A2 preventing the conversion of testosterone to DHT in benign prostate hyperplastic tissue [34,35]
Dutasteride		Steroid 5α-reductase inhibitor	Inhibits the catalytic activity of SRD5A1 and SRD5A2 preventing the conversion of testosterone to DHT [36]
Abiraterone		Inhibitor of 17α-hydroxylase and 17,20-lyase activity	Inhibits both catalytic activities of CYP17, preventing the conversion of pregnenolone and/or progesterone to C19 steroids [37–39]

antagonists, such as the steroidal progesterone derivative cyproterone acetate; nonsteroidal antagonists, such as hydroxyflutamide and bicalutamide; or inhibitors of testosterone or DHT synthesis, such as the steroidal CYP17 inhibitor abiraterone [37] and the SRD5A inhibitors finasteride and dutasteride [34]. Inappropriate exposure to antiandrogens during critical periods of human development such as pregnancy may result in pseudohermaphroditism in male offspring; exposure during puberty will delay male virilization [40]. AR antagonists block the action of endogenous androgens by competing for the AR ligand-binding site. AR agonists, once bound, induce a number of conformational changes that protect ARs against protein degradation and allow them to accumulate in the cytoplasm [41], homodimerize, recruit coregulators, and translocate to the nucleus. One mechanism of action of AR antagonists is to prevent this agonist-mediated conformational protection against degradation [42,43], resulting in downregulation of the receptor or an inability of the AR to shed its HSPs, thus preventing homodimerization; or modifying the conformational change such that binding of coregulators is no longer possible or preferential binding of corepressors occurs [44]. A modified conformational change may also result in increased access of the AR to phosphatases that would prevent AR phosphorylation and transactivation [45].

An alternative mechanism of antiandrogenicity is the inhibition of androgen biosynthesis. Finasteride and dutasteride are therapeutic molecules used effectively in the treatment of benign prostate hyperplasia and chemoprevention of prostate cancer, respectively. Dutasteride is a dual SRD5A1/2 inhibitor, whereas finasteride is a relatively selective SRD5A2 inhibitor. Both reduce DHT levels in target tissues by preventing its formation from testosterone, with finasteride being selective for the nonmalignant prostate, as it is the predominant organ to express SRD5A2. Finasteride is less effective in blocking DHT synthesis in prostate cancer tissues, as these tumors overexpress SRD5A1, and the dual inhibitory properties of dutasteride make it a better option. Inhibitors of CYP17 such as abiraterone are particularly effective at lowering androgen (and estrogen levels), as they block the production of all C19 steroids through inhibition of steroid 17,20-lyase activity, but they also prevent the normal biosynthesis of glucocorticoids in adrenal cortex by inhibiting the 17α-hydroxylase activity of the enzyme (Figure 4.1). The inhibition of adrenal 17α-hydroxylase activity results in increased pituitary secretion of adrenocorticotropic hormone (ACTH), which stimulates the synthesis of mineralocorticoids, resulting in hypertension, hypokalemia, and fluid retention [38]. To minimize such side effects, current research is focusing on the development of selective 17,20-lyase inhibitors of CYP17.

4.6 BIOASSAYS FOR THE EVALUATION OF DISRUPTORS OF ANDROGENIC ACTION

There is growing scientific and public concern that chemicals found in the human environment may interfere negatively with the endocrine system, thus resulting in increased (male) infertility, incidences of certain endocrine cancers, advanced onset of puberty, and various other pathologies related to the endocrine system. Chemicals of concern include medications, food additives, commercial/industrial products, pesticides, and other environmental contaminants. Although a large amount of research has focused on the proestrogenic and antiestrogenic effects of chemicals in relation to reproductive toxicity and various endocrine cancers, such as those of the breast and uterus, relatively little is known about the possible pro- or antiandrogenic effects of environmental chemicals in humans. To identify such compounds, various in vivo and in vitro assays of androgen action and synthesis have been developed.

4.6.1 In Vivo Bioassays of Androgenic Action

The Hershberger assay is the classic method of detecting anabolic and androgenic activities of compounds in vivo [46]. It can be designed to identify either AR agonists or antagonists, as well as inhibitors of SRD5A. Male rats are castrated at about 42 days of age, after which they are allowed to recover for at least 7 days before being exposed to the compound or mixture of interest once a day for 10 days by oral gavage or subcutaneous injection [47,48]. Animals are exposed to various doses of the compound of interest, either alone to determine proandrogenic activity or in combination with testosterone to determine antiandrogenic effects. Important controls include castrated rats exposed to the vehicle alone, testosterone alone, and testosterone in combination with an established antiandrogen such as cyproterone acetate, hydroxyflutamide, or bicalutamide. After the exposures, the rats are killed and weighed, and then undergo autopsy to determine the weights of accessory sex organs, including ventral prostate, seminal vesicles, levator ani-bulbocavernosus muscles, glans penis, and Cowper's gland. Other useful measurements include serum testosterone and LH levels, as well as liver, kidney, and adrenal weights, as they may shed light on the mechanisms of pro- or antiandrogenic action or to identify systemic toxicity.

4.6.2 In Vitro Bioassays of Androgenic Action

In vivo screening tools are costly and time-consuming, and the challenge is to be able to evaluate as many of the potentially EDCs that are found in the environment as efficiently as possible. For this reason, a number of in vitro bioassays have been developed for the identification of proandrogenic or antiandrogenic compounds. These include AR-binding assays and reporter-gene assays that measure AR transcriptional activation by transfecting cells with a human AR expression vector and a plasmid containing a luciferase gene with multiple AREs and a strong promoter [49,50]. Whereas AR binding assays have limited value because they do not distinguish between (partial) agonists and antagonists, the reporter-gene assays will be able to identify proandrogenic and antiandrogenic compounds and provide a measure of potency relative to that of a known positive control for agonism (e.g., DHT) or antagonism (e.g., bicalutamide). LNCaP human androgen-dependent prostate cancer cells are also used to screen for compounds that may exhibit proandrogenic or antiandrogenic effects, as these cells have the advantage of responding to (anti)androgenic compounds in a number of AR-dependent ways, including altered cell proliferation, AR nuclear accumulation, and PSA expression [51,52]. LNCaP cells have the additional advantage that they express SRD5A1, allowing the cell line to be used to determine inhibitory or stimulatory effects on *SRD5A1* gene expression and catalytic steroid 5α-reductase activity. On the other hand, LNCaP cells contain a mutated AR with a single point mutation T877A in the ligand-binding domain, which increases its promiscuity for ligands other than androgens, thus allowing other steroid hormones to transactivate the receptor [25]. Whether this translates into an increased promiscuity for antiandrogens that would otherwise not block androgen-mediated transactivation of wild-type AR is not known.

Screening tools for the evaluation of compounds that can interfere with androgen biosynthesis include microsomal preparations of rat or human testes and adrenals [53,54] and various cell-based systems, such as R2C rat Leydig carcinoma cells, human Leydig cells in primary culture, or H295R human adrenocortical carcinoma cells [55–57]. Microsomal fractions of human tissues that express the key androgen biosynthetic enzymes CYP17 and SRD5A1/2 have been particularly useful and important in identifying catalytic inhibitors of steroid 17,20-lyase and 5α-reductase activity, as such inhibitors are effective in the treatment of androgen-dependent prostate cancer [3]. One disadvantage of microsomes is that the effects of compounds on the genetic, posttranscriptional, and posttranslational regulation of steroidogenic enzymes cannot be determined [58]. Simple cell-based assays provide this possibility, as they may retain the regulatory machineries that control steroidogenic enzyme expression, synthesis, and degradation. Cell-based assays can be used to determine the induction or downregulation of androgen biosynthetic enzymes by chemical exposure, as well as to measure the effects of chemicals on catalytic activity and cell viability. The H295R cell line is increasingly used as a bioassay for the screening of disruption of steroidogenesis and has been incorporated into the OECD Guidelines for the Testing of Chemicals [59]. Effects on androgen biosynthesis in H295R cells can be assessed in several ways, including measuring changes in levels of testosterone or DHT and androgen precursors such as androstenedione and DHEA, and by determining the effects on the gene expression of essential androgen biosynthetic enzymes such as CYP17 [60,61], HSD17B3/5, and SRD5A1 [51] using RT-PCR methods or their catalytic activities using selective enzyme substrates [62].

4.7 ENVIRONMENTAL DISRUPTORS OF ANDROGENIC ACTION

In comparison to the large numbers of estrogenic compounds identified in the environment, relatively few chemicals have been found to disrupt androgenic action, and of those identified, their properties have almost invariably been antiandrogenic. A number of antiandrogenic environmental chemicals have been shown to act as antagonists for ARs, such as the dicarboximide fungicides vinclozolin and procymidone [63], and organochlorines such as the 1,1,1-trichloro-2,2-*bis*(p-chlorophenyl)ethane (DDT) metabolite 1,1-dichloro-2,2-*bis* (p-chlorophenyl)ethylene (p,p′-DDE) (Table 4.2).

Vinclozolin has been registered as a fungicide in the United States since 1981 and is used in large quantities on fruit and vegetable crops throughout the world. Humans may be exposed to vinclozolin occupationally (e.g., farm workers), or via water, air, and diet [77,78]. The antiandrogenic actions of vinclozolin have been studied in detail both in vivo and in vitro [79]. Vinclozolin has been reported to directly antagonize the AR by competing with DHT for the ligand-binding site. [69], preventing its activation by endogenous androgens. Exposure of pregnant rats from gestational day 14 to postnatal day 3 to vinclozolin at doses of 100 and 200 mg/kg body weight/day resulted in the demasculinization of male offspring [65], which exhibited vaginal pouches, ectopic testes, atrophy of the seminiferous tubules, and hypospadias. At puberty, the male rats had smaller prostates, fewer seminal vesicles,

TABLE 4.2   Several Environmental Chemicals with Structures and Known Mechanisms of Antiandrogenicity In Vitro and In Vivo

Environmental chemical (CAS number)	Structure	Classification	Mechanism(s) of antiandrogenicity and reported effects
Vinclozolin (50471-44-8)		Dicarboximide fungicide	Competitive AR antagonist in vitro [64] Demasculinization and feminization of male rats exposed in utero [65–67] Altered mammary gland morphology in female rats exposed in utero [68] Increased AR antagonism by metabolite 3′,5′-dichloro-2-hydroxy-2-methylbut-3-enanilide (M2) [63,69] Inhibition of AR-mediated responses in LNCaP cells [51,52]
Prochloraz (67747-09-5)		Imidazole fungicide	AR antagonist in vitro [70] Demasculinization and reproductive malformations in male rats exposed in utero [71] Antiandrogenic effects in prostate and testes in adult rats [70] Inhibition of CYP17 activity in vivo and in vitro [72–74]
Procymidone (32809-16-8)		Dicarboximide fungicide	AR antagonist in vitro [49] and in vivo [75]
p,p′-DDE (72-55-9)		Metabolite of organochlorine pesticide *p,p′*-DDT	AR antagonist in vitro [63,76] Demasculinization of male rats exposed in utero [66]

lower plasma testosterone levels, and lower body weights. In a later study, alterations were observed in androgen-mediated gene expression in the prostates of castrated/testosterone supplemented adult male rats exposed to 200 mg/kg of vinclozolin for 4 days [66]. Female offspring of rats exposed to 1 mg/kg/day of vinclozolin for the duration of pregnancy had altered female mammary glands at postnatal day 35, including an increase in epithelial branching and loss of epithelial cell polarization, although these alterations were less pronounced at postnatal day 50 [68]. These effects of vinclozolin were consistent with altered mammary gland development in female mice lacking AR [80]. Procymidone (Table 4.2), another widely used fungicide of the same chemical class as vinclozolin, exhibits similar reproductive toxicities related to its antiandrogenic effects due to blockade of AR signaling [75]; and the same has been observed for the DDT metabolite *p,p′*-DDE [66,76].

Antiandrogenic effects mediated through interference with steroidogenesis have been attributed to a number of environmental chemicals, including a variety of pesticides and industrial chemicals, as well as certain antifungal medications. Prochloraz (Table 4.2) is an imidazole fungicide that owes its antifungal activity to the inhibition of fungal CYP51A1 [81,82], the enzyme responsible for 14α-demethylation of lanosterol, a conversion required for the biosynthesis of ergosterol, which is an essential component of the fungal cell membrane. However, the inhibitory properties of prochloraz, as for many imidazole and triazole fungicides or antifungal medications, are not particularly selective. Prochloraz is known to inhibit the activity of several cytochrome P450 enzymes in the steroidogenesis pathway such as CYP17 [51,72] and CYP19 [83,84]. In addition, prochloraz, but not other imidazole pesticides [85], binds the AR and blocks its activation [70]. In rats exposed in utero from gestational day 14–18 to various doses of prochloraz (31.5–250 mg/kg/day), the males (but not the females) developed various reproductive malformations, such as reduced anogenital distance and appearance of female-like areolas, vaginal pouches, and hypospadias. Most effects were evident at the two highest doses of 125 and 250 mg/kg/day. Another study showed that prochloraz, in a Hershberger assay, markedly reduced ventral prostate size, seminal vesicle number, and size of bulbourethral gland at all test doses (50–200 mg/kg/day for 7 days). These effects were similar to those caused by exposure to the AR antagonist flutamide (75 mg/kg/day), but prochloraz had additional effects on the thyroid hormone (T_4) and FSH levels which distinguished its mechanism(s) of endocrine disruption from that of flutamide. Prochloraz, therefore, is considered to be an antiandrogenic endocrine disruptor with multiple modes of action [86].

References

[1]   Griffin JE, Wilson JD. Disorders of the testes and the male reproductive tract. In: Larsen PR, Kronenberg HM, Melmed S, Polonsky KS, editors. William's textbook of endocrinology (10th ed.). Philadelphia, PA: Elsevier Health Sciences; 2003. pp. 706–69.
[2]   Hanukoglu I. Steroidogenic enzymes: structure, function, and role in regulation of steroid hormone biosynthesis. J Steroid Biochem Mol Biol 1992;43:779–804.
[3]   Porubek D. CYP17A1: a biochemistry, chemistry, and clinical review. Curr Top Med Chem 2013;13:1364–84.
[4]   Hosaka M, Oshima H, Troen P. Studies of the human testis. XIV. Properties of C17-C20 lyase. Acta Endocrinol (Copenh) 1980;94:389–96.
[5]   Peltoketo H, Luu-The V, Simard J, Adamski J. 17beta-hydroxysteroid dehydrogenase (HSD)/17-ketosteroid reductase (KSR) family; nomenclature and main characteristics of the 17HSD/KSR enzymes. J Mol Endocrinol 1999;23:1–11.
[6]   Nelson VL, Qin KN, Rosenfield RL, Wood JR, Penning TM, Legro RS, et al. The biochemical basis for increased testosterone production in theca cells propagated from patients with polycystic ovary syndrome. J Clin Endocrinol Metab 2001;86:5925–33.
[7]   Strott CA. Sulfonation and molecular action. Endocr Rev 2002;23:703–32.
[8]   Beaulieu M, Levesque E, Hum DW, Belanger A. Isolation and characterization of a novel cDNA encoding a human UDP-glucuronosyltransferase active on C19 steroids. J Biol Chem 1996;271:22855–62.
[9]   Chouinard S, Yueh MF, Tukey RH, Giton F, Fiet J, Pelletier G, et al. Inactivation by UDP-glucuronosyltransferase enzymes: the end of androgen signaling. J Steroid Biochem Mol Biol 2008;109:247–53.
[10] Penning TM, Burczynski ME, Jez JM, Hung CF, Lin HK, Ma H, et al. Human 3alpha-hydroxysteroid dehydrogenase isoforms (AKR1C1-AKR1C4) of the aldo-keto reductase superfamily: functional plasticity and tissue distribution reveals roles in the inactivation and formation of male and female sex hormones. Biochem J 2000;351:67–77.
[11] Gelmann EP. Molecular biology of the androgen receptor. J Clin Oncol 2002;20:3001–15.

[12] Lonergan PE, Tindall DJ. Androgen receptor signaling in prostate cancer development and progression. J Carcinog 2011;10:20.

[13] Bolton EC, So AY, Chaivorapol C, Haqq CM, Li H, Yamamoto KR. Cell- and gene-specific regulation of primary target genes by the androgen receptor. Genes Dev 2007;21:2005–17.

[14] Foradori CD, Weiser MJ, Handa RJ. Non-genomic actions of androgens. Front Neuroendocrinol 2008;29: 169–81.

[15] Bennett NC, Gardiner RA, Hooper JD, Johnson DW, Gobe GC. Molecular cell biology of androgen receptor signalling. Int J Biochem Cell Biol 2010;42:813–27.

[16] Gorczynska E, Handelsman DJ. Androgens rapidly increase the cytosolic calcium concentration in Sertoli cells. Endocrinology 1995;136:2052–9.

[17] Benten WP, Lieberherr M, Sekeris CE, Wunderlich F. Testosterone induces Ca^{2+} influx via non-genomic surface receptors in activated T cells. FEBS Lett 1997;407:211–4.

[18] Foradori CD, Werner SB, Sandau US, Clapp TR, Handa RJ. Activation of the androgen receptor alters the intracellular calcium response to glutamate in primary hippocampal neurons and modulates sarco/endoplasmic reticulum calcium ATPase 2 transcription. Neuroscience 2007;149:155–64.

[19] Xu Y, Chen SY, Ross KN, Balk SP. Androgens induce prostate cancer cell proliferation through mammalian target of rapamycin activation and post-transcriptional increases in cyclin D proteins. Cancer Res 2006;66:7783–92.

[20] Liu YN, Liu Y, Lee HJ, Hsu YH, Chen JH. Activated androgen receptor downregulates E-cadherin gene expression and promotes tumor metastasis. Mol Cell Biol 2008;28:7096–108.

[21] Wako K, Kawasaki T, Yamana K, Suzuki K, Jiang S, Umezu H, et al. Expression of androgen receptor through androgen-converting enzymes is associated with biological aggressiveness in prostate cancer. J Clin Pathol 2008;61:448–54.

[22] Iehle C, Radvanyi F, Gil Diez de Medina S, Ouafik LH, Gerard H, Chopin D, et al. Differences in steroid 5alpha-reductase iso-enzymes expression between normal and pathological human prostate tissue. J Steroid Biochem Mol Biol 1999;68:189–95.

[23] Thomas LN, Lazier CB, Gupta R, Norman RW, Troyer DA, O'Brien SP, et al. Differential alterations in 5alpha-reductase type 1 and type 2 levels during development and progression of prostate cancer. Prostate 2005;63:231–9.

[24] Yang L, Xie S, Jamaluddin MS, Altuwaijri S, Ni J, Kim E, et al. Induction of androgen receptor expression by phosphatidylinositol 3-kinase/Akt downstream substrate, FOXO3a, and their roles in apoptosis of LNCaP prostate cancer cells. J Biol Chem 2005;280:33558–33565.

[25] Veldscholte J, Berrevoets CA, Ris-Stalpers C, Kuiper GG, Jenster G, Trapman J, et al. The androgen receptor in LNCaP cells contains a mutation in the ligand binding domain which affects steroid binding characteristics and response to antiandrogens. J Steroid Biochem Mol Biol 1992;41:665–9.

[26] Tepper CG, Boucher DL, Ryan PE, Ma AH, Xia L, Lee LF, et al. Characterization of a novel androgen receptor mutation in a relapsed CWR22 prostate cancer xenograft and cell line. Cancer Res 2002;62:6606–14.

[27] Koivisto P, Kononen J, Palmberg C, Tammela T, Hyytinen E, Isola J, et al. Androgen receptor gene amplification: a possible molecular mechanism for androgen deprivation therapy failure in prostate cancer. Cancer Res 1997;57:314–9.

[28] Linja MJ, Savinainen KJ, Saramaki OR, Tammela TL, Vessella RL, Visakorpi T. Amplification and overexpression of androgen receptor gene in hormone-refractory prostate cancer. Cancer Res 2001;61:3550–5.

[29] Visakorpi T, Hyytinen E, Koivisto P, Tanner M, Keinanen R, Palmberg C, et al. In vivo amplification of the androgen receptor gene and progression of human prostate cancer. Nat Genet 1995;9:401–6.

[30] Wood JR, Nelson VL, Ho C, Jansen E, Wang CY, Urbanek M, et al. The molecular phenotype of polycystic ovary syndrome (PCOS) theca cells and new candidate PCOS genes defined by microarray analysis. J Biol Chem 2003;278:26380–90.

[31] Neumann F. The antiandrogen cyproterone acetate: discovery, chemistry, basic pharmacology, clinical use and tool in basic research. Exp Clin Endocrinol 1994;102:1–32.

[32] McGinnis MY, Mirth MC. Inhibition of cell nuclear androgen receptor binding and copulation in male rats by an antiandrogen, Sch 16423. Neuroendocrinology 1986;43:63–8.

[33] Furr BJ. The development of Casodex (bicalutamide): preclinical studies. Eur Urol 1996;29(Suppl. 2):83–95.

[34] Nacusi LP, Tindall DJ. Targeting 5alpha-reductase for prostate cancer prevention and treatment. Nat Rev Urol 2011;8:378–84.

[35] Gisleskog PO, Hermann D, Hammarlund-Udenaes M, Karlsson MO. A model for the turnover of dihydrotestosterone in the presence of the irreversible 5 alpha-reductase inhibitors GI198745 and finasteride. Clin Pharmacol Ther 1998;64:636–47.

[36] Clark RV, Hermann DJ, Cunningham GR, Wilson TH, Morrill BB, Hobbs S. Marked suppression of dihydrotestosterone in men with benign prostatic hyperplasia by dutasteride, a dual 5alpha-reductase inhibitor. J Clin Endocrinol Metab 2004;89:2179–84.

[37] Sonpavde G, Attard G, Bellmunt J, Mason MD, Malavaud B, Tombal B, et al. The role of abiraterone acetate in the management of prostate cancer: a critical analysis of the literature. Eur Urol 2011;60:270–8.

[38] Attard G, Reid AH, Auchus RJ, Hughes BA, Cassidy AM, Thompson E, et al. Clinical and biochemical consequences of CYP17A1 inhibition with abiraterone given with and without exogenous glucocorticoids in castrate men with advanced prostate cancer. J Clin Endocrinol Metab 2012;97:507–16.

[39] Duc I, Bonnet P, Duranti V, Cardinali S, Riviere A, De Giovanni A, et al. In vitro and in vivo models for the evaluation of potent inhibitors of male rat 17alpha-hydroxylase/C17,20-lyase. J Steroid Biochem Mol Biol 2003;84:537–42.

[40] Wilson JD. Androgens. Goodman LS, Gilman A, Hardman JG, Gilman AG, Limbird LE, editors. Goodman & Gilman's the pharmacological basis of therapeutics (9th ed.). New York, NY: McGraw-Hill; 1996. pp. 1441–57.

[41] Zhou ZX, Lane MV, Kemppainen JA, French FS, Wilson EM. Specificity of ligand-dependent androgen receptor stabilization: receptor domain interactions influence ligand dissociation and receptor stability. Mol Endocrinol 1995;9:208–18.

[42] Kuil CW, Mulder E. Mechanism of antiandrogen action: conformational changes of the receptor. Mol Cell Endocrinol 1994;102:R1–R5.

[43] Kuil CW, Berrevoets CA, Mulder E. Ligand-induced conformational alterations of the androgen receptor analyzed by limited trypsinization. Studies on the mechanism of antiandrogen action. J Biol Chem 1995;270:27569–76.

[44] Grosse A, Bartsch S, Baniahmad A. Androgen receptor-mediated gene repression. Mol Cell Endocrinol 2012;352:46–56.

[45] Yang CS, Xin HW, Kelley JB, Spencer A, Brautigan DL, Paschal BM. Ligand binding to the androgen receptor induces conformational changes that regulate phosphatase interactions. Mol Cell Biol 2007;27:3390–404.

[46] Hershberger LG, Shipley EG, Meyer RK. Myotrophic activity of 19-nortestosterone and other steroids determined by modified levator ani muscle method. Proc Soc Exp Biol Med 1953;83:175–80.

[47] Marty MS, O'Connor JC. Key learnings from the Endocrine Disruptor Screening Program (EDSP) Tier 1 rodent uterotrophic and Hershberger assays. Birth Defects Res B Dev Reprod Toxicol 2014;101:63–79.

[48] Yamasaki K, Sawaki M, Noda S, Muroi T, Takakura S, Mitoma H, et al. Comparison of the Hershberger assay and androgen receptor binding assay of twelve chemicals. Toxicology 2004;195:177–86.

[49] Vinggaard AM, Joergensen EC, Larsen JC. Rapid and sensitive reporter gene assays for detection of antiandrogenic and estrogenic effects of environmental chemicals. Toxicol Appl Pharmacol 1999;155:150–60.

[50] Sonneveld E, Jansen HJ, Riteco JA, Brouwer A, van der Burg B. Development of androgen- and estrogen-responsive bioassays, members of a panel of human cell line-based highly selective steroid-responsive bioassays. Toxicol Sci 2005;83:136–48.

[51] Robitaille CN, Rivest P, Sanderson JT. Antiandrogenic mechanisms of pesticides in human LNCaP prostate and H295R adrenocortical carcinoma cells. Toxicol Sci 2014. Epub ahead of print (doi: http://dx.doi.org/10.1093/toxsci/kfu212).

[52] Lorenzetti S, Marcoccia D, Narciso L, Mantovani A. Cell viability and PSA secretion assays in LNCaP cells: a tiered in vitro approach to screen chemicals with a prostate-mediated effect on male reproduction within the ReProTect project. Reprod Toxicol 2010;30:25–35.

[53] Ayub M, Levell MJ. Inhibition of rat testicular 17 alpha-hydroxylase and 17,20-lyase activities by anti-androgens (flutamide, hydroxyflutamide, RU23908, cyproterone acetate) in vitro. J Steroid Biochem 1987;28:43–7.

[54] Ayub M, Levell MJ. Inhibition of human adrenal steroidogenic enzymes in vitro by imidazole drugs including ketoconazole. J Steroid Biochem 1989;32:515–24.

[55] Mason JI, Bird IM, Rainey WE. Adrenal androgen biosynthesis with special attention to P450c17. Ann NY Acad Sci 1995;774:47–58.

[56] Rainey WE, Bird IM, Sawetawan C, Hanley NA, McCarthy JL, McGee EA, et al. Regulation of human adrenal carcinoma cell (NCI-H295) production of C19 steroids. J Clin Endocrinol Metab 1993;77:731–7.

[57] Gazdar AF, Oie HK, Shackleton CH, Chen TR, Triche TJ, Myers CE, et al. Establishment and characterization of a human adrenocortical carcinoma cell line that expresses multiple pathways of steroid biosynthesis. Cancer Res 1990;50:5488–96.

[58] Sanderson JT. The steroid hormone biosynthesis pathway as a target for endocrine-disrupting chemicals. Toxicol Sci 2006;94:3–21.

[59] OECD. Test No. 456: H295R steroidogenesis assay, OECD Publishing.

[60] Gracia T, Hilscherova K, Jones PD, Newsted JL, Higley EB, Zhang X, et al. Modulation of steroidogenic gene expression and hormone production of H295R cells by pharmaceuticals and other environmentally active compounds. Toxicol Appl Pharmacol 2007;225:142–53.

[61] Hilscherova K, Jones PD, Gracia T, Newsted JL, Zhang X, Sanderson JT, et al. Assessment of the effects of chemicals on the expression of ten steroidogenic genes in the H295R cell line using real-time PCR. Toxicol Sci 2004;81:78–89.

[62] Canton RF, Sanderson JT, Nijmeijer S, Bergman A, Letcher RJ, van den Berg M. *In vitro* effects of brominated flame retardants and metabolites on CYP17 catalytic activity: a novel mechanism of action? Toxicol Appl Pharmacol 2006;216:274–81.

[63] Vinggaard AM, Niemela J, Wedebye EB, Jensen GE. Screening of 397 chemicals and development of a quantitative structure–activity relationship model for androgen receptor antagonism. Chem Res Toxicol 2008;21:813–23.

[64] Kelce WR, Monosson E, Gamcsik MP, Laws SC, Gray Jr. LE. Environmental hormone disruptors: evidence that vinclozolin developmental toxicity is mediated by antiandrogenic metabolites. Toxicol Appl Pharmacol 1994;126:276–85.

[65] Gray Jr. LE, Ostby JS, Kelce WR. Developmental effects of an environmental antiandrogen: the fungicide vinclozolin alters sex differentiation of the male rat. Toxicol Appl Pharmacol 1994;129:46–52.

[66] Kelce WR, Lambright CR, Gray Jr. LE, Roberts KP. Vinclozolin and p,p′-DDE alter androgen-dependent gene expression: *in vivo* confirmation of an androgen receptor-mediated mechanism. Toxicol Appl Pharmacol 1997;142:192–200.

[67] Gray Jr. LE, Ostby J, Monosson E, Kelce WR. Environmental antiandrogens: low doses of the fungicide vinclozolin alter sexual differentiation of the male rat. Toxicol Ind Health 1999;15:48–64.

[68] El Sheikh Saad H, Toullec A, Vacher S, Pocard M, Bieche I, Perrot-Applanat M. *In utero* and lactational exposure to vinclozolin and genistein induces genomic changes in the rat mammary gland. J Endocrinol 2013;216:245–63.

[69] Wong C, Kelce WR, Sar M, Wilson EM. Androgen receptor antagonist versus agonist activities of the fungicide vinclozolin relative to hydroxyflutamide. J Biol Chem 1995;270:19998–20003.

[70] Vinggaard AM, Nellemann C, Dalgaard M, Jorgensen EB, Andersen HR. Antiandrogenic effects *in vitro* and *in vivo* of the fungicide prochloraz. Toxicol Sci 2002;69:344–53.

[71] Noriega NC, Ostby J, Lambright C, Wilson VS, Gray Jr. LE. Late gestational exposure to the fungicide prochloraz delays the onset of parturition and causes reproductive malformations in male but not female rat offspring. Biol Reprod 2005;72:1324–35.

[72] Blystone CR, Lambright CS, Howdeshell KL, Furr J, Sternberg RM, Butterworth BC, et al. Sensitivity of fetal rat testicular steroidogenesis to maternal prochloraz exposure and the underlying mechanism of inhibition. Toxicol Sci 2007;97:512–9.

[73] Ohlsson A, Ulleras E, Oskarsson A. A biphasic effect of the fungicide prochloraz on aldosterone, but not cortisol, secretion in human adrenal H295R cells—underlying mechanisms. Toxicol Lett 2009;191:174–80.

[74] Nielsen FK, Hansen CH, Fey JA, Hansen M, Jacobsen NW, Halling-Sorensen B, et al. H295R cells as a model for steroidogenic disruption: a broader perspective using simultaneous chemical analysis of 7 key steroid hormones. Toxicol In Vitro 2012;26:343–50.

[75] Ostby J, Kelce WR, Lambright C, Wolf CJ, Mann P, Gray Jr LE. The fungicide procymidone alters sexual differentiation in the male rat by acting as an androgen-receptor antagonist *in vivo* and *in vitro*. Toxicol Ind Health 1999;15:80–93.

[76] Kelce WR, Stone CR, Laws SC, Gray LE, Kemppainen JA, Wilson EM. Persistent DDT metabolite p,p′-DDE is a potent androgen receptor antagonist. Nature 1995;375:581–5.

[77] Leblanc JC, Malmauret L, Guerin T, Bordet F, Boursier B, Verger P. Estimation of the dietary intake of pesticide residues, lead, cadmium, arsenic and radionuclides in France. Food Addit Contam 2000;17:925–32.

[78] Vitelli N, Chiodini A, Colosio C, De Paschale G, Somaruga C, Turci R, et al. Occupational and environmental exposure to anilide and dicarboximide pesticides. G Ital Med Lav Ergon 2007;29:276–7.

[79] Kavlock R, Cummings A. Mode of action: inhibition of androgen receptor function—vinclozolin-induced malformations in reproductive development. Crit Rev Toxicol 2005;35:721–6.

[80] Yeh S, Hu YC, Wang PH, Xie C, Xu Q, Tsai MY, et al. Abnormal mammary gland development and growth retardation in female mice and MCF7 breast cancer cells lacking androgen receptor. J Exp Med 2003;198:1899–908.

[81] Vanden Bossche H, Marichal P, Gorrens J, Bellens D, Verhoeven H, Coene M-C, et al. Interaction of azole derivatives with cytochrome P-450 isozymes in yeast, fungi, plants and mammalian cells. Pestic Sci 1987;21:289–306.

[82] Vanden Bossche H, Koymans L. Cytochromes P450 in fungi. Mycoses 1998;41(Suppl. 1):32–8.

[83] Vinggaard AM, Hnida C, Breinholt V, Larsen JC. Screening of selected pesticides for inhibition of CYP19 aromatase activity *in vitro*. Toxicol In Vitro 2000;14:227–34.

[84] Sanderson JT, Boerma J, Lansbergen GW, van den Berg M. Induction and inhibition of aromatase (CYP19) activity by various classes of pesticides in H295R human adrenocortical carcinoma cells. Toxicol Appl Pharmacol 2002;182:44–54.

[85] Ayub M, Levell MJ. The effect of ketoconazole related imidazole drugs and antiandrogens on [3H] R 1881 binding to the prostatic androgen receptor and [3H]5 alpha-dihydrotestosterone and [3H]cortisol binding to plasma proteins. J Steroid Biochem 1989;33:251–5.

[86] Vinggaard AM, Hass U, Dalgaard M, Andersen HR, Bonefeld-Jorgensen E, Christiansen S, et al. Prochloraz: an imidazole fungicide with multiple mechanisms of action. Int J Androl 2006;29:186–92.

Disrupters of Thyroid Hormone Action and Synthesis

Jenny Odum

Abstract

Thyroid hormones are essential for the development and maintenance of physiological functions in mammals. Their importance is illustrated by the routine screening of newborn babies to ensure that thyroid hormones are within normal limits. The first section describes the thyroid hormones and how blood levels are controlled by the hypothalamic–pituitary–thyroid (HPT) axis. The basic structure of the thyroid and the synthesis of thyroid hormones are then discussed. The actions of the thyroid hormones at target tissues are mediated by the thyroid hormone receptors, and the molecular basis of this is described. The second section

Endocrine Disruption and Human Health.
DOI: http://dx.doi.org/10.1016/B978-0-12-801139-3.00005-3

shows how the complexity of the thyroid hormonal system leads to many ways by which it may be disrupted. Modes of action and the biological consequences of thyroid hormone disrupters on human health are illustrated. Finally, assays for detecting thyroid hormone-disrupting chemicals and the current status of international efforts to develop standardized tests are discussed.

5.1 THE IMPORTANCE OF THE THYROID HORMONAL SYSTEM FOR HUMAN HEALTH

5.1.1 Thyroid Hormones and the Hypothalamic–Pituitary–Thyroid Axis

Thyroid hormones are essential for normal development and the maintenance of physiological functions in mammals. In young or fetal mammals, they also are essential for normal brain development and skeletal development. Cretinism, where affected individuals have severely stunted physical and mental growth, has long been known to be associated with reduced levels of thyroid hormones [1]. It was particularly prevalent in regions of the Alps in the nineteenth century where low levels of dietary iodine resulted in hypothyroidism (low levels of thyroid hormones) and impaired neurological development. Recognition of this link led to the supplementation of diets with iodine, which has solved this problem in these areas [2]. There are also several maternal conditions, such as congenital hypothyroidism, that have led to lowered thyroid hormone levels in offspring, resulting in lowered IQ, delayed language development, and poorer attention and memory skills [3,4]. In many countries, newborn babies are now screened for hypothyroidism by measuring thyroid hormone levels in blood. These measures have largely eliminated cretinism and milder forms of this disease in the developed world [5,6].

Although this book focusses on human health, it is worth noting that the thyroid hormone system plays a key role in the development of all vertebrates in addition to mammals and there is a high level of evolutionary conservation of the thyroid system. An excellent review of the thyroid system that covers both mammalian and nonmammalian systems was published by the Organisation for Economic Cooperation and Development (OECD) in 2006 [7]. Metamorphosis in amphibia depends on thyroid hormones, and virtually every tissue in the body is influenced because thyroid hormones initiate the biochemical and morphological changes in the transition from larva to adult [8,9]. Another example is flatfish, which experience postembryonic remodeling during metamorphosis [10]. They change from a bilaterally symmetrical body to an asymmetric form with gradual translocation of one eye to the opposite side of the head. As with amphibian metamorphosis, all the developmental programs of flatfish metamorphosis are ultimately under the control of thyroid hormones.

Returning to mammalian systems, the two biologically active thyroid hormones are thyroxine (T4) and triiodothyronine (T3) [7]. These are small biphenolic molecules derived from tyrosine and iodinated (Figure 5.1). T4 and T3 are produced in the thyroid gland. In the circulation, the concentrations of T4 are generally higher than those of T3 (10- to 50-fold) [11], but T3 is the more active ligand at the thyroid hormone receptor (TR). T4 is deiodinated to T3 at the site of action [12]. Although some T3 is also produced in the thyroid, the action of peripheral deiodinases is thought to be largely responsible for the levels of T3 in the blood [13].

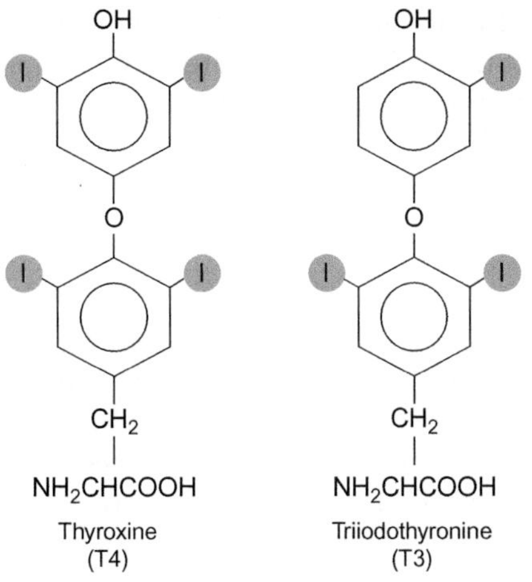

FIGURE 5.1   The structures of T4 and T3, with the positions of iodine highlighted.

As indicated previously, thyroid hormones have many functions. They help to regulate intermediary metabolism, energy intake, and thermogenesis [14,15]. During mammalian development, they are also involved in brain and skeletal development [16,17]. Thyroid hormones, their receptors, retinoids, and receptors (RAR and RXR) together play critical roles in embryonic development and physiology [18]. Thyroid hormones are also involved in the development of sensory organs such as the eye and ear. The development of the inner ear, cochlear, and cone photoreceptors in the eye have been shown to depend upon thyroid hormones [19–21].

Thyroid hormone delivery to target tissues is regulated by a complex series of networks. These control the synthesis of T4 and T3, the concentrations within the blood, generation of the active ligand at the target cell, and removal of thyroid hormones by metabolism within the liver. The hypothalamic–pituitary–thyroid (HPT) axis is central to this regulation and operates a system of feedback control mechanisms, similar to other hormonal systems [22]. Although the HPT axis operates as a loop, it can be envisaged as starting at the hypothalamus, where neurons of the hypothalamic paraventricular nucleus synthesize thyrotropin-releasing hormone (TRH) [23]. This hormone is delivered to the pituitary via the hypothalamic–pituitary-portal vessels, which provides a vascular link between these two organs.

TRH then acts on thyrotroph cells within the anterior pituitary to stimulate the production of thyroid-stimulating hormone (TSH), also known as *thyrotropin* [24]. TSH is carried in the blood to the thyroid gland where it binds to receptors on the surface of the thyroid follicular cells, stimulating adenylate cyclase [25]. The increased cAMP produced by this binding triggers a cascade of events that bring about the synthesis and release of thyroid hormones into the circulation (see discussion later in this chapter).

In the blood, thyroid hormones are carried by specific carrier proteins. In humans, most thyroid hormones (~75%) are carried by thyroid-hormone-binding globulin (TBG), which has high affinity for T4 and a lesser affinity for T3 [26]. A further 15% of thyroid hormones are carried by transthyretin (TTR) and the remainder by serum albumin. In the fetal and early postnatal rat, levels of TBG are high but then decline, becoming almost undetectable in adults [27,28]. The majority of thyroid hormones are carried by serum albumin in adult rats.

At the target tissues, T3 and T4 are actively transported into the cells, where T4 is converted into the more active T3 by deiodinases (Types 1 and 2). Deiodination of T4 by Type 3 results in the production of reverse T3 (rT3), an inactive form of thyroid hormone. T3 and T4 then bind to the TRs within the target cell (see the later discussion).

Once released from the receptors, the thyroid hormones reenter the circulation. Finally, T4 and T3 are removed from the blood in the liver. They are transported into the hepatocytes, where they are metabolized by Phase 2 xenobiotic metabolizing enzymes, UDP-glucuronosyltransferases, and sulfotransferases [29,30]. The conjugated thyroid hormones (largely glucuronide conjugates) are then excreted in the bile [27].

Regulation of the HPT axis is achieved at several points so that concentrations of thyroid hormone can be closely controlled [7]. This is an area where research is uncovering new mechanisms of regulation that may allow fine-tuning of the system at different life stages or within different organs to keep concentrations of thyroid hormone within optimum limits [31].

The thyroid hormones have a negative feedback effect on the release of TSH from the pituitary and the release of TRH from the hypothalamus. TRH has also been shown to regulate the release of TSH [32]. Other factors may regulate the HPT axis as well; for example, fasting has been shown to suppress the TRH neurons, causing reduced levels of T3 and T4 [33,34]. Active concentration of thyroid hormones into target cells may also be a point of control. The local production of T3 from T4 is another mechanism of regulation where the level of deiodination controls subsequent receptor activation [35,36]. Formation of rT3 rather than T3 may be a further way of controlling thyroid hormone action. Figure 5.2 shows some of the better-known points of control of the HPT axis.

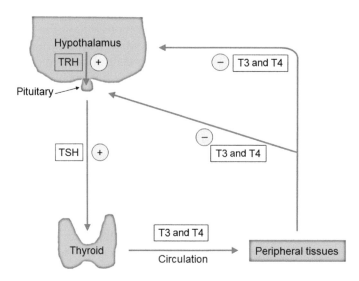

FIGURE 5.2   The HPT axis showing release of the hormones TRH, TSH, T3, and T4 and their actions in feedback control of the axis.

The complexity of the HPT axis and the different ways by which the levels of the thyroid hormones are controlled provide the scope for disruption by endocrine active chemicals. Possible ways by which these chemicals may act, as well as some examples, are given in this chapter and in several other reviews [22,31,37,38]. Most chemicals acting on the thyroid hormonal system ultimately perturb the levels of T4 and T3, which then may result in a change in the level of TSH via the feedback control mechanism. Blood concentrations of T4, T3, and TSH are the most commonly used biomarkers for determining effects on the thyroid system [7,31].

5.1.2 The Basic Structure of the Thyroid

The mammalian thyroid gland comprises two oval lobes on each side of the trachea, joined across the trachea by a thin isthmus. When viewed microscopically, the thyroid is made of spherical follicles surrounded by connective tissue and supported by a rich vascular network. The follicles are generally similar in size, although on a microscope slide, they may appear different because they will be sliced at different points during the cutting of thin sections. The follicles are lined by an epithelium that has a simple cuboidal shape and the center of the follicle is filled with a substance called *colloid*. The colloid contains thyroglobulin, which acts as a reservoir for the thyroid hormones. The structure of the thyroid follicle is integral to the process of the synthesis of the thyroid hormones, as shown in the next section and in Figure 5.3. When the thyroid is actively synthesizing and secreting

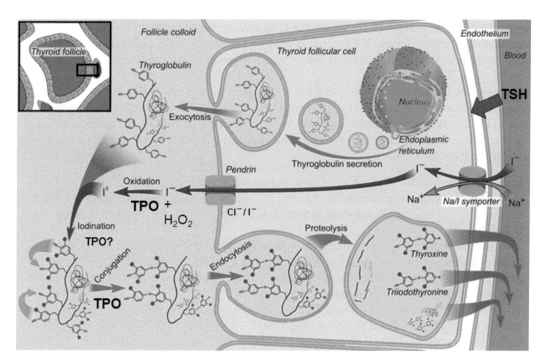

FIGURE 5.3   The production of thyroid hormones within the thyroid follicle. *Source: Figure reproduced with permission from http://creativecommons.org/licenses/by-sa/3.0/.*

thyroid hormones, the structure of the follicle can be seen to change. The epithelial cells become taller and more columnar as they become active. The appearance of the colloid may also change as the processes of synthesis and excretion of the thyroid hormones are stimulated in response to TSH [27]. The microscopic appearance of the thyroid is also a key end point for detecting effects on the thyroid hormonal system. Macroscopically, these effects may lead to changes in the weight of the thyroid [7,39,40].

The parathyroid glands are located on the ventral surface of the thyroid and have a role in the regulation of calcium. The interstitium around the follicles may contain "C" cells that produce calcitonin, which regulates calcium. These will not be discussed further in this chapter, as there are few, if any, chemicals that are known to perturb this system.

5.1.3 Thyroid Hormone Synthesis

Synthesis of the thyroid hormones takes place within the thyroid follicle and is illustrated in Figure 5.3. The protein thyroglobulin is synthesized on ribosomes within the thyroid follicular cells. Thyroglobulin is a large (660-KD) dimeric protein, rich in tyrosine residues [25]. The thyroid hormone precursors are derived from the tyrosine residues on thyroglobulin. Carbohydrate and sugar moieties are added to thyroglobulin within the Golgi complex, and the protein is then exocytosed across the apical membrane into the colloidal space [7].

The thyroid follicular cells absorb iodine from the blood by means of the sodium-iodide symporter (NIS). This transporter protein concentrates iodine 20- to 40-fold within the thyroid, translocating two molecules of Na^+ to one of I^- to achieve the concentration of iodine against a concentration gradient. Iodide is then transported by pendrin (a sodium-independent chloride/iodide transporter), from the follicular cell, across the apical membrane, and into the follicular colloidal space [7].

Synthesis of the thyroid hormones then takes place within the follicular colloidal space. Thyroperoxidase (TPO) is the key enzyme involved in the synthesis of the thyroid hormones [41–43]. It is a membrane-bound protein attached to the apical membrane of the follicular cell and protruding into the colloidal space. It performs three functions in the synthesis of the thyroid hormones:

1. Iodide must be oxidized to a higher state before it can react with the tyrosine residues. Hydrogen peroxide is generated within the follicle by an enzyme system located at the apical surface, close to TPO. Iodide is then oxidized by TPO to its reactive state (I_{3^-}: triiodide ion).
2. The reactive iodide then immediately reacts with tyrosine residues on thyroglobulin to form protein-bound monoiodotyrosine (MIT) and diiodotyrosine (DIT). This step is generally called "the organification of iodine." There is some debate about whether this step is catalyzed by TPO or is nonenzymic.
3. The iodotyrosine residues MIT and DIT are then coupled with an ether bond (–O–) in a reaction catalyzed by TPO. The coupling of MIT + DIT results in T3; the coupling of DIT + DIT results in T4; and the coupling of DIT + MIT results in inactive rT3.

The thyroglobin containing the bound hormone is then endocytosed back into the follicular cell. Fusion of the endosome with a lysome is followed by proteolysis within the cell.

Fusion of the lysome with the basolateral cell membrane results in release of T4 and T3 into the circulation.

This process results in the thyroid having a reservoir of covalently linked thyroid hormone within the colloid that is readily available in case the hypothalamic-pituitary sensing system requires the release of thyroid hormones into the blood. TSH acts on the follicular cells to stimulate the process of release of thyroid hormones.

The response to TSH and the extent to which there is a reservoir of thyroid hormone varies according to species [44]. Humans have a large reservoir of thyroid hormones within their thyroid compared to rats and the appearance of the follicular cells is more quiescent than that of rats [45]. Rats readily respond to chemicals or treatments that affect thyroid hormones by releasing bound hormone and actively synthesizing new thyroid hormone. This results in rats having active thyroids, and hypertrophy (increase in cell size) and hyperplasia (increase in cell number) of follicular cells is often observed in response to treatment. In humans, follicular cell hypertrophy, which allows the release of hormone from thyroglobulin, may be observed in humans, but hyperplasia is rare [27,46].

5.1.4 The Molecular Basis of Thyroid Hormone Action

The actions of the thyroid hormones are largely mediated by the TRs [2,47], which are members of the superfamily of the ligand-dependent transcription factors, similar to the estrogen receptor and the androgen receptor. There are two TR genes, $TR\alpha$ and $TR\beta$, which between them produce four functional TRs (TRα1, TRβ1, TRβ2, and TRβ3). TR1α is a T3-binding splice product; that is, regions of the messenger RNA (mRNA) newly formed from transcription of $TR\alpha$ are excluded from the final processed mRNA to form a spliced product that is translated into a protein. It is predominantly expressed in brain, heart, and skeletal muscle. TRα2 and TRα3 are also splice products, but they do not bind T3 and therefore are not generally considered to be bona fide TRs. The $TR\beta$ gene produces three major T3-binding splice products. TRβ1 is expressed widely; TRβ2 is expressed primarily in the retina, inner ear, and brain; and TRβ3 is expressed in the liver, kidney, and lung [2].

Within the cell, the TRs form heterodimers with the retinoic acid X receptor (RXR). The unliganded complex binds to corepressors such as nuclear receptor corepressor 1 (NCoR) or silencing mediator of retinoic acid and thyroid hormone receptor (SMRT), repressing gene transcription [17,48]. Binding the ligand (T3) causes a conformational change, resulting in disruption of the corepressors, binding and promotion of co-activator binding. This is followed by the recruitment of polymerase III and gene transcription. This process is illustrated in Figure 5.4.

The tissue- and cell-specific actions of TRs are influenced by ligand availability, transport of the thyroid hormones into the cell, expression of the TR isoforms within cell types, the presence of coactivators and repressors, and the sequence and location of the thyroid hormone response elements (TREs). The TRs may also interact with other pathways and signaling systems. This is likely to be especially important for the retinoic acid receptor (RAR), which may heterodimerize with TRs in a similar manner to RXR. Disruption of these processes may have severe consequences in developing animals. Interaction of the TRs with other receptors, such as PPARα and PPARγ in the liver, have also been described. These interactions have effects on fatty acid oxidation and lipid homeostasis [49,50].

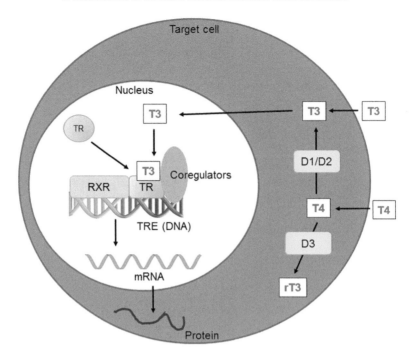

FIGURE 5.4   Action of the thyroid hormones within a target cell. T4 and T3 are transported into the cell, and T4 is deiodinated to T3 by deiodinases 1 and 2 (D1 and D2). T4 may be deiodinated by deiodinase 3 (D3) to the inactive rT3. T3 binds to TR, causing a conformational change that triggers heterodimerization with RXR. Association of co-regulators then occurs, binding to DNA at the TRE and ultimately transcription occurs, followed by translation.

In addition to the classical nuclear TRs, nongenomic actions of thyroid hormones have also been described. Membrane receptors (specific integrin $\alpha v/\beta3$ receptors) acting to transduce signals have been identified in blood vessels and the heart [17].

5.2 DISRUPTION OF THE THYROID HORMONAL SYSTEM

5.2.1 Modes of Action for Thyroid Hormone Disruption

The processes and systems described previously demonstrate the complexity of the thyroid hormonal system and offer many potential sites at which it may be disrupted. There are many examples of exogenous chemical disruption of the thyroid hormonal system, ranging from the simple inorganic anion perchlorate that inhibits NIS to complex halogenated aromatic chemicals such as polychlorinated biphenyls (PCBs) that may act as ligands for TRs. Chemicals may also affect more than one target within this system.

Possible modes through which thyroid-disrupting chemicals may act include:

- Inhibition of iodine uptake by the thyroid (including inhibition of NIS)
- Inhibition of TPO

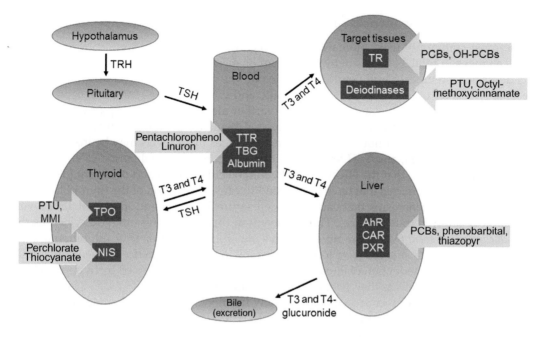

FIGURE 5.5   Possible targets within the thyroid hormonal system and chemicals known to interact with them. PTU and methimazole (MMI) inhibit TPO activity. Perchlorate and thiocyanate anions compete with iodine uptake via NIS. Pentachlorophenol and linuron interfere with the binding of thyroid hormones to blood carrier proteins. PCBs and their hydroxylated metabolites bind to TR. PTU and octyl-methoxycinnamate inhibit deiodinase activity. PCBs, phenobarbital, and thiazopyr bind to some of the hepatic nuclear receptors and cause increased activity of UDP-glucuronosyltransferases.

- Interference with thyroid hormone storage and release from the follicle
- Interference with binding to blood proteins (e.g., TBG, TTR, albumin)
- Inhibition of peripheral deiodinase activity
- Binding to TRs (agonism or antagonism)
- Increased metabolism of thyroid hormones in the liver; for example, via activation of the hepatic receptors aryl hydrocarbon receptor (AhR), constitutive androstane receptor (CAR), and pregnane X receptor (PXR) and subsequent induction of Phase II xenobiotic-metabolizing enzymes
- Decreased metabolism of thyroid hormones in the liver (e.g., inhibition of Phase II xenobiotic-metabolizing enzymes)
- Effects on other receptors that may heterodimerize with PRs or interact via cross talk (e.g., RXR)
- Effects on nongenomic receptors

Examples of chemicals acting on the thyroid hormonal system have been described in reviews by Howdeshell [38], Miller et al. [31], WHO [22], and Zoeller [37]. Figure 5.5 illustrates targets within this system and some examples of chemicals that may act at these targets.

5.2.2 Possible Consequences of Thyroid Hormone Disruption

The most commonly used biomarker for detecting effects on the thyroid hormone system is changes in total T4 levels in blood (serum or plasma). Most of the actions on the targets described previously will result in changes in this marker. However, direct binding to the TRs, effects on other receptors via cross talk, and effects on nongenomic receptors may not affect T4 levels because they act at a point farther along the signaling pathway than T4. Increased blood TSH is also a commonly measured biomarker, although in some instances, chemicals may alter T4 but not affect TSH. Small changes in T4 levels may be insufficient to trigger a change in TSH, and TSH levels may also reset after an initial period of stimulation. It is possible, therefore, that the effect on TSH could be either be missed or absent [39,51].

The majority of chemicals that have been found to cause disruption of the thyroid hormone system do so via mechanisms that cause reduced serum T4 levels and increased TSH levels in laboratory animals (rats or mice). The first event in this sequence is often described as the *molecular initiating event (MIE)*. Examples of MIEs may be inhibition of TPO, inhibition of NIS, or activation of hepatic nuclear receptors. A commonly observed sequence of events in animal studies following the reduction of circulating T4 is increased TSH followed by hypertrophy of the thyroid follicular cells as the system attempts to increase the levels of T4 by releasing more hormone from the colloid store, synthesizing new hormone, or both. If the degree of inhibition of T4 by the thyroid-disrupting chemical is too great and compensation is not achieved by these measures, then hyperplasia of the thyroid follicular cells may occur as a result of prolonged stimulation by TSH in an attempt to raise T4 levels. The combined hypertrophy and hyperplasia then lead to an overall increase in the weight of the thyroid [27,31] (Figure 5.6).

The control mechanisms within the thyroid hormone system may allow it to compensate for chemical perturbation and readjust hormone levels to remain within homeostatic limits. The extent to which it is able to compensate will depend upon factors such as the potency of the initial interaction, the exposure level or dose of the chemical, the duration of exposure, the species under study, and the life stage of that species. The potency of the initial interaction is a combination of the strength of the molecular interaction (e.g., IC_{50}: the concentration causing 50% inhibition of activity) and the magnitude of the effect (e.g., the optimum concentration results in 80% inhibition of TPO activity).

In rats and mice, the most commonly described adverse outcomes resulting from exposure to thyroid-disrupting chemicals that decrease plasma T4, are neurological effects and thyroid tumors. When propylthiouracil (PTU), a pharmaceutical inhibitor of TPO used to treat hyperthyroidism, was administered to pregnant rats, impaired motor activity, learning, memory, and hearing resulted in the offspring [52–54]. Perchlorate, a natural environmental

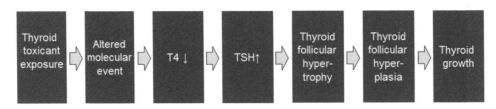

FIGURE 5.6   Typical events in a mode of action following exposure to thyroid-disrupting chemicals.

contaminant and an ingredient of some rocket fuels, caused increased incidences of thyroid follicular tumors in rats and mice after administration in drinking water for two years [55].

The consequences of alterations in the concentrations of thyroid hormones during fetal development have been the subject of much research [18,38]. Although it is well known that severe decreases in serum thyroid hormones cause abnormal brain development in both rats and humans, it is becoming clear that smaller changes may also be associated with neural insufficiency. Small differences (about 25%) in maternal T4 during early pregnancy were associated with reduced IQ scores in children, even though the degree of T4 reduction was not considered to constitute clinical hypothyroidism [56,57]. These types of studies are supported by experimental animal studies where a 28% reduction in T4 in 2-week old pups given low doses of PTU resulted in a marked reduction in cell density of the corpus callosum of the brain [58].

Zoeller and Rovet [18] reviewed the timing of normal brain development in humans and rats and the importance of thyroid hormones (Figure 5.7). The timing of events and their

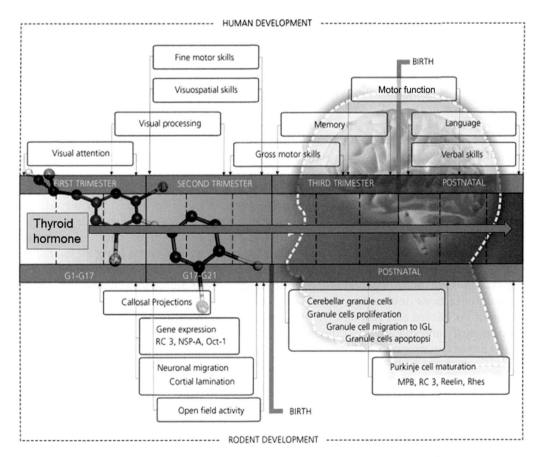

FIGURE 5.7   Scheme illustrating how thyroid hormone insufficiency produces effects in humans (upper panel) and rodents (lower panel). Thyroid hormone insufficiency in the early prenatal, late prenatal, and early postnatal periods causes different effects. *Source: From Zoeller and Rovet [18], with permission.*

dependence on, initially, maternal thyroid hormones and, later, fetal thyroid hormones illustrate the importance of maintaining the thyroid hormone system within tight limits during this time. Disruption of the thyroid hormone system and the potential consequences for neurological effects, therefore, is highly relevant for human health. Effects on other organ systems have also been associated with altered thyroid homeostasis in clinical studies (e.g., the cardiovascular system, cholesterol, and lipids [59]). This is not surprising given the broad spectrum of target organs for thyroid hormones, which is an area of research for chemicals affecting the thyroid.

The appearance of thyroid tumors in rats and mice exposed to thyroid-disrupting chemicals is not generally thought to pose a similar hazard for humans. In rodents, persistent elevation of TSH, as a result of lowered circulating T4, leads to thyroid hypertrophy and hyperplasia as described previously (Figure 5.6). Over a prolonged period of time, the constant stimulation of the follicular cells may lead to neoplasia and the development of thyroid follicular tumors. However, there are important physiological and biochemical differences between the thyroid hormone systems of rodents and humans. The differences in the appearance of the thyroid have been described already, but other factors are also important. In the rat, the reserve capacity of thyroid hormones is smaller than humans, T4 has a much shorter half-life than in humans (12h compared to 5–9 days), and constitutive levels of TSH are about 25-fold higher in rats than in humans. The shorter half-life of T4 is thought to be related to the absence of TBG in adult rats, which leads to a higher turnover rate of thyroid hormones. In adult humans, thyroid hormones are tightly bound to TBG in blood. The consequence of these differences is that the thyroid of rodents is a much more active organ than that of humans. Thyroid tumors are a relatively common finding in rat long-term studies, while the only known human thyroid carcinogen is ionizing radiation. Several analyses have been conducted to investigate the human relevance of rodent thyroid follicular tumors and have concluded that the relevance is low [27,60,61].

Adverse outcome pathways (AOPs) have recently been developed from mode of action approaches to toxicology and follow a series of events from an MIE to a possible adverse outcome [62,63]. AOPs identify key events along a toxicity pathway and can be used to consider a detailed mechanism of action for a specific chemical or generic modes of action for chemicals or classes of chemicals that may act in a similar manner. Identifying all the factors involved and the key events on a pathway is an active area of research. Not all chemicals acting via a specific mode of action will produce all the effects along an AOP and identifying biological interactions or chemical characteristics that determine these will help to make an AOP useful for hazard and risk assessment. An AOP that integrates all the modes of action listed previously and the adverse outcomes of thyroid tumors, neurological dysfunction, or both that have been proposed for thyroid-disrupting chemicals is illustrated in Figure 5.8.

5.2.3 Testing for Thyroid Hormone Disruption

In recent years, the OECD, within its test guideline program, has taken a global lead in developing standardized test guidelines for testing for endocrine disrupting chemicals. The assays are contained within the "OECD Conceptual Framework for the Screening and Testing of Endocrine-Disrupting Chemicals" (CF), which was modified and updated in 2012 [64]. The CF consists of five different levels, where the assays at each level increase in complexity and provide different types of information about the potential of a chemical to cause

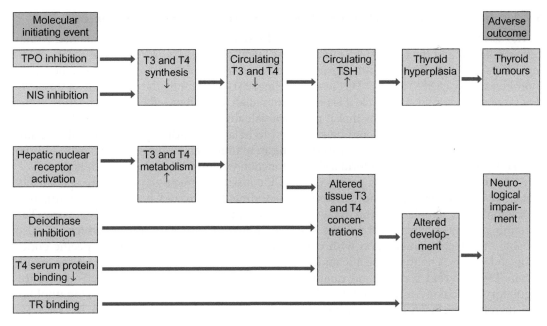

FIGURE 5.8   AOP illustrating disruption of the thyroid hormonal system and the adverse end points of thyroid tumors and neurological impairment. Note that there are other possible outcomes and many more steps along this pathway still to be elucidated. *Source: Adapted from Miller et al. [31].*

endocrine disruption. The CF is intended to provide a guide to the tests available that can provide information for assessment of potential endocrine disrupters and can be viewed as a "toolbox" of tests. It is not, however, a testing strategy whereby testing would progress automatically from Level 1 to Level 5. Assays can be selected at any level from the CF depending upon the testing objective. An OECD document on the standardized test guidelines for evaluating chemicals for endocrine disruption has also recently been published [40]. This provides guidance on how to interpret the outcome of individual tests and how to increase evidence of whether a substance may be an endocrine disrupter. The assays in the CF are currently mostly focused on the estrogen, androgen, and thyroid hormonal pathways; and disruption of steroidogenesis. Other pathways will be included as science and assays evolve.

Unfortunately, the complexity of the thyroid hormonal system has meant that standardization of in vitro assays for interaction with end points within this system has lagged behind those developed for modes of action involving estrogen, androgen, and steroidogenesis disruption. Therefore, at present there are no in vitro thyroid assays within the CF. There are, however, several in vivo assays within Levels 3–5 of the CF that contain end points for detecting effects on the thyroid. The lack of standardized in vitro assays for thyroid end points has increased the efforts within OECD groups and other organizations involved in assay validation, such that the available possible assays have been grouped and listed, and validation activities are now being organized [65,66]. Suitable in vivo and possible in vitro assays are discussed next.

5.2.3.1 *In Vivo Assays for Detecting Thyroid Hormone-Disrupting Chemicals*

The assays capable of detecting effects on the thyroid hormonal system are contained within Levels 3, 4, and 5 of the OECD CF (Table 5.1). At Level 3, the assays of the CF are short screening assays and provide information primarily about selected pathways. The amphibian metamorphosis assay (AMA) [OECD TG (Test Guideline) 231] is currently the only assay at this level that targets the thyroid, and while it is not a mammalian assay, the well-conserved nature of the thyroid hormone system means that it provides valuable information across taxa. A chemical that is positive in the AMA should be suspected to be a thyroid-disrupting chemical in mammals and a possible candidate for further testing in mammalian systems. The *Xenopus* embryo thyroid signaling assay may perform a similar function when and if it passes validation.

At Level 4, the mammalian assays of the CF consist of three assays that are specifically designed to test for endocrine disruption (including the thyroid hormonal system); that is, the male and female pubertal assays and the adult male endocrine screening assay. The remaining assays at this level are the standard regulatory toxicity assays, which are also capable of detecting interaction with endocrine systems but do not contain specific endocrine end points. The three specific endocrine tests all contain end points such as serum T4, serum TSH, thyroid weight, and quantitative histopathology of the thyroid. Some of the regulatory toxicology tests contain end points such as thyroid weight and histopathology and therefore are useful for assessing effects on the thyroid (TG 407, TG 408, TG 415, TG

TABLE 5.1　Assays Within the OECD CF (2012) with End Points for Detecting Disruption of the Thyroid Hormonal System

Level of OECD CF	Standardized test methods suitable for detecting possible thyroid disrupting chemicals in mammals
Level 3 In vivo assays providing data about selected endocrine mechanism(s)/pathway(s)	• Amphibian metamorphosis assay (OECD TG 231) • *Xenopus* embryo thyroid-signaling assay (when and if TG is available)
Level 4 In vivo assays providing data on adverse effects on endocrine relevant end points	• Repeated dose 28-day study (OECD TG 407) • Repeated dose 90-day study (OECD TG 408) • One-generation reproduction toxicity study (OECD TG 415) • Male pubertal assay • Female pubertal assay • Intact adult male endocrine screening assay • Chronic toxicity and carcinogenicity studies (OECD TG 451-3) • Reproductive screening test (OECD TG 421 if enhanced) • Combined 28-day/reproductive screening assay (OECD TG 422 if enhanced) • Developmental neurotoxicity study (OECD TG 426)
Level 5 In vivo assays providing more comprehensive data on adverse effects on endocrine relevant end points over more extensive parts of the life cycle of the organism	• Extended one-generation reproductive toxicity study (OECD TG 443). • Two-generation reproduction toxicity study (OECD TG 416 most recent update)

451-3, TG 421-2, and TG 426) (Table 5.1). Recent updates to TG 407 and proposed updates to TG 421-2 also include serum T4, serum TSH, and quantitative histopathology. TG 453 (carcinogenicity study) will detect the adverse effect of thyroid tumors and TG 426 (developmental neurotoxicity study) will detect some adverse effects on the brain and behavior.

At Level 5, the mammalian assays of the CF consist of extensive reproductive studies (TG 443 and TG 416). The extended one-generation reproductive toxicity study (TG 443) is preferable for detecting endocrine disruption because it provides an evaluation of a number of endocrine end points in the juvenile and adult F1, which are not included in the two-generation study (TG 416). The thyroid end points in the extended one-generation reproductive toxicity study include serum T4, serum TSH, thyroid weight, and quantitative histopathology of the thyroid in both or all generations. In addition, this study includes many end points concerned with development of the brain and behavior. The high statistical sensitivity of this study (in terms of animal numbers), end points and exposure of sensitive life stages should enable the detection of thyroid hormone-disrupting chemicals acting via all possible mechanisms.

5.2.3.2 *In Vitro Assays for Detecting Thyroid Hormone-Disrupting Chemicals*

Potential in vitro assays for detecting thyroid hormone-disrupting chemicals have been divided into several groups (or blocks) depending on which aspects of thyroid regulation they cover. Table 5.2 illustrates the blocks and the model systems that have been suggested

TABLE 5.2   Potential In Vitro Assays for Detecting Thyroid Hormone-Disrupting Chemicals

Block/Target	Model system	Example reference
BLOCK 1: CENTRAL REGULATION VIA THE HTP AXIS		
TRH production (hypothalamus)	Genomic assay indicates TRH production in human glioblastoma-astrocytoma cells	Garcia et al. (2000)
TRH activation (pituitary)	TRH activation assay in human cell line	Millipore commercial kit
TSH receptor activation (thyroid)	TSH-mediated cAMP production in Chinese hamster ovary cells expressing TSH receptor	Santini et al. (2003)
BLOCK 2: THYROID HORMONE SYNTHESIS		
TPO	Inhibition of TPO-mediated oxidation of iodide, guiacol, or Amplex Ultrared in a cell-free assay	Freyberger and Ahr (2006) Paul et al. (2013)
NIS-mediated iodide uptake	Uptake of radioiodide into rat thyroid cell line	Arturi et al. (2002)
BLOCK 3: BINDING AND TRANSPORT OF THYROID HORMONES IN SERUM		
T4 binding proteins, TTR and TBG	Displacement T4 from its binding site on the serum binding proteins TTR or TBG	Aqai et al. (2012)
BLOCK 4: METABOLISM AND EXCRETION OF THYROID HORMONES		
Liver 5′-deiodinase type 1	Inhibition of deiodinase type 1 activity by measuring appearance of ^{125}I-rT3 without and with the chemical	Freyberger and Ahr (2006)

(Continued)

TABLE 5.2   (Continued)

Block/Target	Model system	Example reference
Sulfation	Inhibition or upregulation of cellular sulfotransferases in intact human cell lines expressing enzyme or human recombinant enzyme	Martin et al. (2012)
Glucuronidation	Inhibition or upregulation of cellular UDP-glucuronosyltransferases in intact human cell lines expressing enzyme or human recombinant enzyme	Hamers et al. (2011)
BLOCK 5: DISTRIBUTION OF THYROID HORMONES BY CELLULAR TRANSPORTERS		
TH membrane transporters	T4 transport in cells overexpressing membrane transporters	Westholm et al. (2010)
TH transport across placenta and blood brain barrier	T4 transport in human placenta choriocarcinoma cells or bovine brain cells	Vandenhaute et al. (2011)
BLOCK 6: CELLULAR RESPONSES TO THYROID HORMONES		
Nuclear TR binding	TR competitive binding assay (radioligand)	You et al. (2006)
Nuclear TR activation	TR-mediated agonism and antagonism in reporter gene assay in rat GH3 cell line	Freitas et al. (2011)
Cell-specific responses	Cell proliferation in response to chemical challenge in thyroid hormone-dependent cells (rat pituitary cell line: T-screen)	Kitamura et al. (2005)

Source: Adapted from Refs. [65,66], references are as cited therein.

as possible assays. Many of these assays are fairly well established and are used in research programs and high-throughput screening; examples include TPO inhibition, TTR binding, TBG binding, and TR transactivation. These assays are likely to enter validation programs in the near future so that they can be used in regulatory toxicity testing.

5.3 CONCLUSIONS

The thyroid hormonal system has wide-ranging effects on intermediary metabolism, the cardiovascular system, energy intake, and thermogenesis in mammals. Normal levels of thyroid hormones are also critical for brain and skeletal development in the developing young. Disruption of the thyroid hormonal system may have many consequences for human health and effects monitored to date include lowered IQ. There are several in vivo tests in experimental animals that detect disruption of the thyroid hormonal system, but its complexity and the diversity of potential sites of action mean that validation of in vitro tests has been slow. However, current activities are aiming to address this. The validation of new tests and the development of AOPs for thyroid disruption should facilitate progress in this area of science and risk assessment.

References

[1] Cranefield PF. The discovery of cretinism. Bull Hist Med 1962;36:489–511.

[2] Patel J, Landers K, Li H, Mortimer RH, Richard K. Thyroid hormones and fetal neurological development. J Endocrinol 2011;209:1–8.

[3] Rovet JF. Congenital hypothyroidism: long-term outcome. Thyroid 1999;9:741–8.

[4] Rovet JF. Long-term neuropsychological sequelae of early-treated congenital hypothyroidism: effects in adolescence. Acta Paediatr 1999(Suppl. 88):88–95.

[5] Klein R. History of congenital hypothyroidism. In: Burrow GN, Dussault JH, editors. Neonatal thyroid screening. New York, NY: Raven Press; 1980. pp. 51–9.

[6] Klein R, Mitchell ML. Neonatal screening for hypothyroidism Braverman LE, Utiger RD, editors. The thyroid: a fundamental and clinical text. Philadelphia, PA: Lipponcott-Raven; 1996. pp. 984–8.

[7] OECD. Detailed review paper on thyroid hormone disruption assays. No. 57. OECD Environmental Health and Safety Publications, Series on Testing and Assessment. Available at: <http://www.oecd.org/env/ehs/testing/>; 2006.

[8] Hayes TB. Endocrine disruption in amphibians. In: Sparling DW, Linger G, Bishop CA, editors. Ecotoxicology of amphibians and reptiles. Pensacola, FL: SETAC Press; 2000. pp. 573–93.

[9] Shi YB. Amphibian metamorphosis from morphology to molecular biology. New York, NY: Wiley-Liss Press; 2000.

[10] Schreiber AM. Flatfish: an asymmetric perspective on metamorphosis. Curr Top Dev Biol 2013;103:167–94.

[11] Taurog A, Dorris ML, Doerge DR. Minocycline and the thyroid: antithyroid effects of the drug, and the role of thyroid peroxidase in minocycline-induced black pigmentation of the gland. Thyroid 1996;6:211–9.

[12] St Germain DL, Galton VA. The deiodinase family of selenoproteins. Thyroid 1997;7:655–68.

[13] Chopra IJ. Nature, source and relative significance of circulating thyroid hormones. In: Braverman LE, Utiger RD, editors. The thyroid: a fundamental and clinical text. Philadelphia, PA: Lipponcott-Raven; 1996. pp. 111–24.

[14] Ribeiro MO, Carvalho SD, Schultz JJ, Chiellini G, Scanlan TS, Bianco AC, et al. Thyroid hormone–sympathetic interaction and adaptive thermogenesis are thyroid hormone receptor isoform–specific. J Clin Invest 2001;108:97–105.

[15] Ribeiro MO, Bianco SD, Kaneshige M, Schultz JJ, Cheng SY, Bianco AC, et al. Expression of uncoupling protein 1 in mouse brown adipose tissue is thyroid hormone receptor-beta isoform specific and required for adaptive thermogenesis. Endocrinology 2010;151:432–40.

[16] Sharlin DS, Visser TJ, Forrest D. Developmental and cell-specific expression of thyroid hormone transporters in the mouse cochlea. Endocrinology 2011;152:5053–64.

[17] Brent GA. Mechanisms of thyroid hormone action. J Clin Invest 2012;122:3035–43.

[18] Zoeller RT, Rovet J. Timing of thyroid hormone action in the developing brain: clinical observations and experimental findings. J Neuroendocrinol 2004;16:809–18.

[19] Ng L, Ma M, Curran T, Forrest D. Developmental expression of thyroid hormone receptor beta2 protein in cone photoreceptors in the mouse. Neuroreport 2009;20:627–31.

[20] Gogakos AI, Duncan Bassett JH, Williams GR. Thyroid and bone. Arch Biochem Biophys 2010;503:129–36.

[21] Crofton KM. Developmental disruption of thyroid hormone: correlations with hearing dysfunction in rats. Risk Anal 2004;24:1665–71.

[22] WHO Damstra T, Barlow S, Berman A, Kavlock R, Van der Kraak G, editors. Global assessment of the state-of-the-science of endocrine disruptors. Geneva: World Health Organisation; 2002. p. 180. WHO/PCS/EDC/02.2.

[23] Segerson TP, Kauer J, Wolfe HC, Mobtaker H, Wu P, Jackson IM, et al. Thyroid hormone regulates TRH biosynthesis in the paraventricular nucleus of the rat hypothalamus. Science 1987;238:78–80.

[24] Haisenleder DJ, Ortolano GA, Dalkin AC, Yasin M, Marshall JC. Differential actions of thyrotropin (TSH)-releasing hormone pulses in the expression of prolactin and TSH subunit messenger ribonucleic acid in rat pituitary cells *in vitro*. Endocrinology 1992;130:2917–23.

[25] Taurog A. Thyroid iodine metabolism. In: Braverman LE, Utiger RD, editors. The thyroid: a fundamental and clinical text. Philadelphia, PA: Lipponcott-Raven; 1996.

[26] Schussler GC. The thyroxine-binding proteins. Thyroid 2000;10:141–9.

[27] Hill RN, Crisp TM, Hurley PM, Rosenthal SL, Singh DV. Risk assessment of thyroid follicular cell tumors. Environ Health Perspect 1998;106:447–57.

[28] Vranckx R, Rouaze-Romet M, Savu L, Mechighel P, Maya M, Nunez EA. Regulation of rat thyroxine-binding globulin and transthyretin: studies in thyroidectomized and hypophysectomized rats given tri-iodothyronine or/and growth hormone. J Endocrinol 1994;142:77–84.

[29] Hood A, Klaassen CD. Differential effects of microsomal enzyme inducers on *in vitro* thyroxine (T(4)) and triiodothyronine (T(3)) glucuronidation. Toxicol Sci 2000;55:78–84.

[30] Hood A, Klaassen CD. Effects of microsomal enzyme inducers on outer-ring deiodinase activity toward thyroid hormones in various rat tissues. Toxicol Appl Pharmacol 2000;163:240–8.

[31] Miller MD, Crofton KM, Rice DC, Zoeller RT. Thyroid-disrupting chemicals: interpreting upstream biomarkers of adverse outcomes. Environ Health Perspect 2009;117:1033–41.

[32] Greer MA, Sato N, Wang X, Greer SE, McAdams S. Evidence that the major physiological role of TRH in the hypothalamic paraventricular nuclei may be to regulate the set-point for thyroid hormone negative feedback on the pituitary thyrotroph. Neuroendocrinology 1993;57:569–75.

[33] Legradi G, Emerson CH, Ahima RS, Flier JS, Lechan RM. Leptin prevents fasting-induced suppression of prothyrotropin-releasing hormone messenger ribonucleic acid in neurons of the hypothalamic paraventricular nucleus. Endocrinology 1997;138:2569–76.

[34] Fekete C, Mihaly E, Luo LG, Kelly J, Clausen JT, Mao Q, et al. Association of cocaine- and amphetamine-regulated transcript-immunoreactive elements with thyrotropin-releasing hormone-synthesizing neurons in the hypothalamic paraventricular nucleus and its role in the regulation of the hypothalamic-pituitary-thyroid axis during fasting. J Neurosci 2000;20:9224–34.

[35] Hernandez A, Martinez ME, Liao XH, Van SJ, Refetoff S, Galton VA, et al. Type 3 deiodinase deficiency results in functional abnormalities at multiple levels of the thyroid axis. Endocrinology 2007;148:5680–7.

[36] Ng L, Lyubarsky A, Nikonov SS, Ma M, Srinivas M, Kefas B, et al. Type 3 deiodinase, a thyroid-hormone-inactivating enzyme, controls survival and maturation of cone photoreceptors. J Neurosci 2010;30:3347–57.

[37] Zoeller RT. Environmental chemicals impacting the thyroid: targets and consequences. Thyroid 2007;17:811–7.

[38] Howdeshell KL. A model of the development of the brain as a construct of the thyroid system. Environ Health Perspect 2002;110(Suppl. 3):337–48.

[39] Devito M, Biegel L, Brouwer A, Brown S, Brucker-Davis F, Cheek AO, et al. Screening methods for thyroid hormone disruptors. Environ Health Perspect 1999;107:407–15.

[40] OECD. Guidance document on standardised test guidelines for evaluating chemicals for endocrine disruption. No. 150. OECD Environmental Health and Safety Publications, Series on Testing and Assessment. Available at: <http://www.oecd.org/env/ehs/testing/>; 2012.

[41] Doerge DR. Mechanism-based inhibition of lactoperoxidase by thiocarbamide goitrogens. Identification of turnover and inactivation pathways. Biochemistry 1988;27:3697–700.

[42] Doerge DR, Takazawa RS. Mechanism of thyroid peroxidase inhibition by ethylenethiourea. Chem Res Toxicol 1990;3:98–101.

[43] Doerge DR, Taurog A, Dorris ML. Evidence for a radical mechanism in peroxidase-catalyzed coupling. II. Single turnover experiments with horseradish peroxidase. Arch Biochem Biophys 1994;315:90–9.

[44] Bernier-Valentin F, Kostrouch Z, Rabilloud R, Munari-Silem Y, Rousset B. Coated vesicles from thyroid cells carry iodinated thyroglobulin molecules. First indication for an internalization of the thyroid prohormone via a mechanism of receptor-mediated endocytosis. J Biol Chem 1990;265:17373–80.

[45] McClain RM. Mechanistic considerations for the relevance of animal data on thyroid neoplasia to human risk assessment. Mutat Res 1995;333:131–42.

[46] McClain RM, Rice JM. A mechanistic relationship between thyroid follicular cell tumours and hepatocellular neoplasms in rodents. IARC Sci Publ 1999;147:61–8.

[47] Bernal J. Thyroid hormone receptors in brain development and function. Nat Clin Pract Endocrinol Metab 2007;3:249–59.

[48] Dayan CM, Panicker V. Novel insights into thyroid hormones from the study of common genetic variation. Nat Rev Endocrinol 2009;5:211–8.

[49] Araki O, Ying H, Furuya F, Zhu X, Cheng SY. Thyroid hormone receptor beta mutants: dominant negative regulators of peroxisome proliferator-activated receptor gamma action. Proc Natl Acad Sci USA 2005;102:16251–6.

[50] Liu YY, Heymann RS, Moatamed F, Schultz JJ, Sobel D, Brent GA. A mutant thyroid hormone receptor alpha antagonizes peroxisome proliferator-activated receptor alpha signaling *in vivo* and impairs fatty acid oxidation. Endocrinology 2007;148:1206–17.

[51] Capen CC. Mechanistic data and risk assessment of selected toxic end points of the thyroid gland. Toxicol Pathol 1997;25:39–48.

[52] Axelstad M, Hansen PR, Boberg J, Bonnichsen M, Nellemann C, Lund SP, et al. Developmental neurotoxicity of propylthiouracil (PTU) in rats: relationship between transient hypothyroxinemia during development and long-lasting behavioural and functional changes. Toxicol Appl Pharmacol 2008;232:1–13.

[53] NTP. Two-generation reproduction toxicity study of propylthiouracil (CAS#51-52-5) when administered to Sprague-Dawley rats in the drinking water. Report No. RACB20102; 2003.

[54] Kobayashi K, Tsuji R, Yoshioka T, Kushida M, Yabushita S, Sasaki M, et al. Effects of hypothyroidism induced by perinatal exposure to PTU on rat behavior and synaptic gene expression. Toxicology 2005;212:135–47.

[55] Kessler FJ, Kruskemper HL. Experimental thyroid tumors caused by many years of potassium perchlorate administration. Klin Wochenschr 1966;44:1154–6.

[56] Haddow JE, Palomaki GE, Allan WC, Williams JR, Knight GJ, Gagnon J, et al. Maternal thyroid deficiency during pregnancy and subsequent neuropsychological development of the child. N Engl J Med 1999;341:549–55.

[57] Morreale de EG. Maternal hypothyroxinemia versus hypothyroidism and potential neurodevelopmental. Alterations of her offspring. Ann Endocrinol (Paris) 2003;64:51–2.

[58] Sharlin DS, Tighe D, Gilbert ME, Zoeller RT. The balance between oligodendrocyte and astrocyte production in major white matter tracts is linearly related to serum total thyroxine. Endocrinology 2008;149:2527–36.

[59] Michalopoulou G, Alevizaki M, Piperingos G, Mitsibounas D, Mantzos E, Adamopoulos P, et al. High serum cholesterol levels in persons with 'high-normal' TSH levels: should one extend the definition of subclinical hypothyroidism? Eur J Endocrinol 1998;138:141–5.

[60] Hurley PM. Mode of carcinogenic action of pesticides inducing thyroid follicular cell tumors in rodents. Environ Health Perspect 1998;106:437–45.

[61] Hard GC. Recent developments in the investigation of thyroid regulation and thyroid carcinogenesis. Environ Health Perspect 1998;106:427–36.

[62] Ankley GT, Bennett RS, Erickson RJ, Hoff DJ, Hornung MW, Johnson RD, et al. Adverse outcome pathways: a conceptual framework to support ecotoxicology research and risk assessment. Environ Toxicol Chem 2010;29:730–41.

[63] OECD. Guidance document on developing and assessing adverse outcome pathways. No. 184. OECD Environmental Health and Safety Publications, Series on Testing and Assessment. Available at: <http://www.oecd.org/env/ehs/testing/>; 2013.

[64] OECD. OECD conceptual framework for testing and assessment of endocrine disrupters. OECD Environmental Health and Safety Publications, Series on Testing and Assessment. Available at: <http://www.oecd.org/env/ehs/testing/>; 2012.

[65] OECD. In vitro and ex vivo assays for identification of modulators of thyroid hormone signalling (draft). OECD Environmental Health and Safety Publications, Series on Testing and Assessment. Available at: <http://www.oecd.org/env/ehs/testing/>; 2013.

[66] Murk AJ, Rijntjes E, Blaauboer BJ, Clewell R, Crofton KM, Dingemans MM, et al. Mechanism-based testing strategy using in vitro approaches for identification of thyroid hormone disrupting chemicals. Toxicol In Vitro 2013;27:1320–46.

CHAPTER

6

Disruption of Other Receptor Systems: Progesterone and Glucocorticoid Receptors, Peroxisome Proliferator-Activated Receptors, Pregnane X Receptor, and Aryl Hydrocarbon Receptor

Philippa D. Darbre

OUTLINE

Endocrine Disruption and Human Health.
DOI: http://dx.doi.org/10.1016/B978-0-12-801139-3.00006-5

Abstract

This chapter describes the mechanisms of action of several intracellular ligand-activated transcription factors: progesterone receptor (PR), glucocorticoid receptor (GR), peroxisome proliferator-activated receptors (PPAR), pregnane X receptor (PXR), and aryl hydrocarbon receptor (AhR). Environmental endocrine-disrupting chemicals (EDCs) have been shown to bind to and activate these receptors, giving a range of specific responses that are measurable in assays based both in vitro and in vivo. Disruption of PR may lead to aberrant proliferation and differentiation in reproductive tissues. The wide cellular distribution of GR and its broad range of functions imply that disruption of GR could lead to more general modulation of immune and stress responses, altered glucose metabolism, and loss of maintenance of body fluid homeostasis. Disruption of PPARs can lead to imbalance of lipid homeostasis and regulation of glucose metabolism, and environmental EDCs acting through this route have been shown to cause obesity and have been termed *obesogens*. PXR and AhR can bind a wide range of foreign compounds (xenobiotics) and so act as xenobiotic sensors. Target genes of PXR and AhR include cytochrome P450 enzymes involved in metabolism and clearance of foreign compounds. One main side effect, however, is that some of these cytochrome P450 enzymes also regulate synthesis and breakdown of steroid hormones; therefore, some environmental chemicals may act as EDCs by modulating endogenous steroid hormone levels through PXR- or AhR-mediated mechanisms.

6.1 INTRODUCTION

The majority of studies to date have centered on disruption of estrogen, androgen, or thyroid hormone pathways. This is not for any a priori reason that these receptors are more susceptible to disruption, but rather that the resulting effects on wildlife populations were obvious and the assay systems for these receptors well established. However, it is becoming increasingly evident that environmental chemicals also can disrupt other hormone receptor systems. This includes other members of the steroid receptor superfamily [namely, progesterone receptor (PR) and glucocorticoid receptor (GR)], and more widely, other members of the nuclear receptor superfamily [namely, peroxisome proliferator-activated receptors (PPAR) and pregnane X receptor (PXR)]. The aryl hydrocarbon receptor (AhR) is an orphan receptor with no known endogenous ligand, but the binding of organochlorine compounds such as dioxins can give cellular responses with endocrine outcomes consequent to the altered expression of cytochrome P450 genes. Other endocrine-disrupting chemicals (EDCs) can interfere in prostaglandin synthesis, so they disrupt actions of these essential homeostatic regulators.

6.2 PROGESTERONE RECEPTOR

6.2.1 Mechanisms of Action

The steroid hormone progesterone has its major function in the female in the regulation of ovulation and pregnancy. It acts by binding to intracellular PR, which has a similar domain structure to other steroid hormone receptors in containing a DNA-binding domain (DBD) and a ligand-binding domain (LBD) [1]. In the genomic mechanism, the LBD of the receptor protein interacts with progesterone, causing the release of associated chaperone heat shock proteins, dimerization, binding through the DBD of the receptor to specific progesterone response elements (PREs) in the DNA, and transactivation of gene

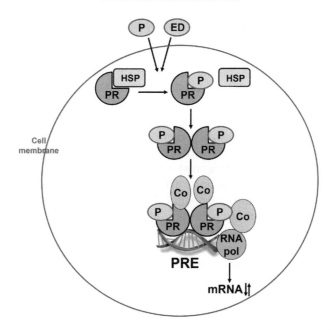

FIGURE 6.1 Genomic action of PR. Progesterone (P) binds to intracellular PR, resulting in the release of receptor-associated HSPs, dimerization, and binding to PREs in DNA. Transactivation of gene expression involves the binding of coregulators (Co) and RNA polymerase (RNApol), resulting in alteration to mRNAs. EDs may interfere in this pathway by binding to intracellular PR and setting off a similar sequence of events, but with altered consequences to mRNA levels.

expression [1] (Figure 6.1). PR exists in two isoforms that differ in their N-terminal regions, with PR-B being the full-length form and the shorter PR-A isoform lacking the B-upstream region. The two isoforms are produced from the same gene by different upstream promoters and are most often co-expressed within cells. Both act as ligand-activated transcription factors [1]. Since the PR gene requires estrogen for its expression [2], it acts mainly as a downstream effector of estrogen signaling. In addition to genomic actions, PR can act through nongenomic pathways, and ligand-independent activation can also occur in a cell-type and promoter-specific manner [1].

6.2.2 Assay Systems

Assays for disrupters of progesterone action are analogous to those described for estrogen disruption. Competitive binding assays can be used to measure the displacement of radiolabeled progesterone from PR. Reporter gene assays can be used to measure the transactivation of progesterone-responsive reporter genes in cells containing PR either endogenously or following transfection of the PR gene into the cells. This author has reported progestin regulation of a reporter gene stably transfected into T47D human breast cancer cells that contain endogenous PR [3]. The reporter gene was based on the progesterone-responsive mouse mammary tumor virus long terminal repeat response element and regulation was demonstrated using the synthetic progestin R5020 [3]. However, the complication is that these cells also contain GRs and androgen receptors (ARs), which act through the same response element [3]. In order to distinguish actions on PR from GR or AR, therefore, it is either necessary to use specific inhibitors or to develop assay systems that possess only one type of receptor. The PR-CALUX reporter assay has been developed to contain PR and a progestin-responsive luciferase reporter gene in human osteoblast cells, and this model has been used to identify antiprogestagenic activity of some brominated flame-retardant chemicals [4]. Using yeast-based reporter assays that contain only PR and a progestin-responsive reporter, some organochlorine pesticides [5] together with nonylphenol [6] have been reported to give PR antagonist activity. A reporter assay using human embryonic kidney cells has confirmed antagonist activity to human PR not only from a range of organochlorine pesticides, but also bisphenol A [7]. Such assays have been extended to measuring antiprogestagenic activity in indoor domestic dust [8].

Progesterone acts with estrogens as a key regulator of proliferation and differentiation in reproductive tissues, but with progesterone often opposing estrogen action. Any disruption to the balance between levels of progesterone and estrogen, therefore, can disrupt endocrine homeostasis. Measurement of effects of environmental chemicals on synthesis of progesterone is a sensitive assay to detecting potential endocrine disruption due to hormonal imbalance. Alligators from the contaminated environment in Lake Apopka, near Orlando, Florida, following a chemical spill have shown reproductive and developmental abnormalities, and this has been linked to altered steroid hormone levels, including progesterone [9]. In animal models, disruption of progesterone synthesis has been reported using co-cultured porcine granulosa and thecal cells in the presence of some organochlorine compounds [10], and dose–response measurements of caffeine in male rats has been shown to reduce plasma progesterone levels [11].

6.3 GLUCOCORTICOID RECEPTOR

6.3.1 Mechanisms of Action

Unlike the defined reproductive effects of progesterone, glucocorticoids have very wide regulatory actions in all cells, including modulating immune response, mediating stress responses, controlling glucose metabolism, and maintaining body fluid homeostasis [12,13]. The main human hormone cortisol (hydrocortisone) is produced from the adrenal cortex and acts at target cells through intracellular GRs. The domain structure of GR includes an N-terminal transactivation domain, a central DBD, and a C-terminal LBD in line with other steroid hormone receptors. During evolution, however, the ancestral corticosteroid receptor has diverged into the GR (NR3C1) and mineralocorticoid receptor (MR, NR3C2), which share 94% amino acid homology in the DBD and 56% in the LBD. Evidence suggests a proinflammatory role for MR that contrasts with the anti-inflammatory role of GR [12]. Furthermore, alternative translation sites can also give rise to different GR proteins that may regulate cellular sensitivity to glucocorticoids [12]. Through genomic pathways, cortisol binds to GRs and the ligand-receptor complexes dimerize and then bind to specific glucocorticoid response elements in the DNA to upregulate expression of anti-inflammatory proteins. Through indirect genomic pathways, cortisol can bind to other transcription factors in the cytosol, preventing their nuclear translocation and so downregulating expression of pro-inflammatory proteins [12,13]. Because of their anti-inflammatory roles, a range of synthetic glucocorticoids are now used to treat diseases caused by an overactive immune response in order to suppress allergic, inflammatory, asthmatic, and autoimmune disorders.

6.3.2 Assay Systems

Assays for disruption of glucocorticoid action are analogous to those for estrogen action (Chapter 3). Competitive binding assays can be used to measure the displacement of radiola-beled cortisol (or the synthetic glucocorticoid dexamethasone) from GRs. Reporter gene assays can be used to measure the transactivation of glucocorticoid-responsive reporter genes transfected into cells, and such assays have shown GR antagonist responses in human HeLa cells with a metabolite of the fungicide vinclozolin [14] and in Chinese hamster ovary cells with several organophosphate flame retardants [15]. Other studies have suggested that cellular levels of GRs can be reduced by exposure to the fungicide hexachlorobenzene [16] and that the ability of GRs to bind to DNA can be compromised following the binding of some monomethylated metabolites of arsenic [17]. Adrenocortical cell lines can be used to investigate the effects of environmental chemicals on glucocorticoid synthesis. The physiological consequences of disruption of glucocorticoid action can vary; therefore, in vivo assays can use a variety of end points ranging from levels of cortisol, levels of GR, and effects on the expression of genes characteristic of the hypothalamus–pituitary–gonad (HPG) axis. Disruption of the hypothalamus–pituitary–interrenal axis by polychlorinated biphenyls (PCBs) through modulation to GRs has been reported in Arctic char, which are coldwater fish native to Arctic waters [18].

6.4 PEROXISOME PROLIFERATOR-ACTIVATED RECEPTORS

6.4.1 Mechanisms of Action

PPARs are another group of nuclear hormone receptors that act as ligand-activated transcription factors. Originally identified as orphan receptors, they are now known to bind to a wide range of polyunsaturated fatty acids and therefore act as lipid sensors which play a major role in maintaining lipid homeostasis and regulating glucose metabolism (energy balance). PPARs all possess a similar domain structure, with an N-terminal DBD and a C-terminal LBD. Interaction with ligands at the LBD results in translocation of the PPAR to the nucleus, where it heterodimerizes with another nuclear receptor, the retinoid X receptor (RXR), and binds through two zinc fingers in the DBD of the PPAR to specific peroxisome proliferator response elements (PPREs) found in the vicinity of promoters of PPAR-responsive genes [19,20] (Figure 6.2).

There are three receptors (PPARα, PPARβ/δ, and PPARγ), which differ in their ligand specificity, tissue distribution, and cellular functions [19]. A notable feature of the LBDs of PPARs is their size, which is three to four times larger than that of other nuclear receptors and therefore allows the binding of a wide variety of unsaturated fatty acids [19,20]. Essential fatty acids and eicosanoids (e.g., leukotrienes and prostaglandins) can also bind to PPARs, although these are required at high concentrations (around 100 μM) for PPAR activation [20].

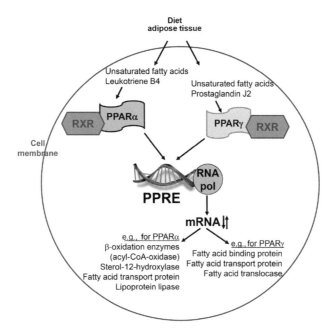

FIGURE 6.2   Genomic action of PPAR. Fatty acids bind to intracellular PPARα or PPARγ, which then heterodimerize with RXR and bind to PPREs in the DNA. Transactivation of gene expression involves binding of coregulators and RNA polymerase (RNApol) resulting in alteration to mRNAs. Some main target genes for PPARα and PPARγ are indicated. EDs may interfere in this pathway by binding to intracellular PPARs and setting off a similar sequence of events, but with altered consequences to gene expression.

PPARα and PPARβ/δ act mainly to facilitate the breakdown of lipids and energy combustion, while PPARγ functions in adipogenesis, and therefore energy storage. PPARα is most highly expressed in tissues that are active in fatty acid metabolism, such as liver and skeletal muscle, but also in intestinal mucosa and brown adipose tissue, where its activation acts to lower lipid levels. The main site of PPARγ expression is in white and brown adipose tissues, especially in adipocytes, where it functions in regulating lipid biosynthesis. PPARβ/δ is expressed more ubiquitously, but with relatively higher levels in the gastrointestinal tract, kidney, and skeletal muscle [20]. In view of the major role of PPARs in regulating lipid and glucose metabolism, disruption of their actions can be expected to have wide-ranging implications for human health, including in the development of diabetes and atherosclerosis.

6.4.2 Assay Systems

Assays used to predict the disruption of PPAR-mediated mechanisms of action are analogous to those used for other members of the nuclear receptor superfamily. Radiolabeled thiazolidinediones have been used in competitive PPAR ligand-binding assays [21,22]. Reporter gene assays can be used to measure transactivation of *PPRE*-driven reporter genes transfected into cells [21]. Such assays have demonstrated the ability of monophthalate esters and perfluorooctane-based chemicals to transactivate PPAR-regulated gene expression [23–25].

Tributyltin (TBT) was the first EDC shown by a range of assay systems, both in vitro and in vivo, to disrupt lipid metabolism and adipogenesis, and to do so through a PPAR/RXR-mediated mechanism [26]. It was after these studies that the "obesogen hypothesis" was formulated, postulating that environmental pollutants could promote the development of obesity [27,28]. Cell-based assays to test the disruption of PPAR regulation of lipid home-ostasis have been developed using the 3T3-L1 cell line. 3T3-L1 cells are mouse fibroblasts (pre-adipocytes) that can differentiate into adipocytes, and several EDCs have now been shown to enable this differentiation, including TBT [26], bisphenol A [29], nonylphenol [30], and several components of personal care products, including parabens and some musks [31]. Assays for obesogenic activity of EDCs in vivo have used measures of fat uptake in mice (including body weight and fat tissue deposits) and the amphibian *Xenopus*. Injection of TBT into pregnant mice between day 12 and 18 have shown effects from exposure in utero on the progeny after birth, including increased lipid accumulation in adipose deposits, liver, and testis of the neonates and increased epididymal adipose mass in the adults [26]. More recently a "humanized" *Xenopus* model has been developed by somatic gene transfer into muscle or brain of genes for human PPARγ and a *PPRE*-driven green fluorescent protein (GFP) reporter [32]. This offers several advantages, in that *Xenopus* tadpoles are easy to breed, exposure of embryos to EDCs is straightforward because embryos develop externally, and metabolizing enzymes needed for activation of compounds are similar to humans. Activation can then be visualized directly under the microscope from the GFP signal [32].

6.5 PREGNANE X RECEPTOR

6.5.1 Mechanisms of Action

PXR is another member of the nuclear receptor superfamily of ligand-activated transcription factors, also known as the *steroid and xenobiotic receptor* or *pregnane-activated receptor*. It is widely expressed in human cells, especially in the liver, small intestine, and colon, where it acts as a xenobiotic sensor regulating the expression of enzymes used for metabolism and elimination of foreign compounds. The PXR domain structure incorporates a DBD at the N-terminus, which facilitates binding to DNA response elements; and an LBD at the C-terminus, which is characterized by a notably large spherical cavity enabling interaction with a range of hydrophobic compounds containing polar groupings. The mechanism of action is similar to the PPARs in that the PXR also requires heterodimerization with RXR for transactivation of gene expression. Ligand binding to PXR results, then, in heterodimerization of the ligand–PXR complex with RXR and binding through the DBD of the PXR to PXR response elements in DNA to transactivate gene expression. Two main target genes are those of the multidrug resistance protein 1 and cytochrome P450 3A4, which both contain PXR response elements in their promoter regions. Cytochrome P450 3A4 is an important oxidative enzyme known to influence the clearance of not only many commonly used drugs, but also steroid hormones, the antiestrogen tamoxifen, and the component of the contraceptive pill ethinyl estradiol. Expression is also regulated by PXR of genes encoding other enzymes in oxidative metabolism (phase I), conjugation (phase II) and transport (phase III) of foreign compounds. Among these genes are those for glucuronyl transferases and sulfotransferases, which act to determine the bioavailability of steroid hormones as well as the elimination of xenobiotics [33,34].

6.5.2 Assay Systems

The ability of polybrominated diphenyl ethers (PBDEs) to act through PXR-mediated mechanisms has served to identify assays for these receptors. PXR-driven luciferase reporter gene assays in HepG2 liver cells demonstrated the induction of luciferase by PBDEs 47, 99, and 209 [35]. The compromised induction of CYP3a11 and 2b10 in PXR-knockout mice, as shown by Northern blotting analysis of the mRNAs and Western immunoblotting of the proteins [35], provided further evidence that the induction of these genes by PBDEs [36] was PXR-mediated in vivo as well.

6.6 ARYL HYDROCARBON RECEPTOR

6.6.1 Mechanisms of Action

The AhR is another cytosolic ligand-activated transcription factor that functions as a key regulator of cellular exposure to foreign compounds, but it is not a member of the nuclear receptor superfamily because it has some differences in its mechanism of action. It belongs to the family of basic helix-loop-helix/period AhR nuclear translocator single-minded (bHLH/PAS) family of transcriptional regulators and is both well conserved in evolution and ubiquitously expressed [37]. Although no known physiological ligand is known, it is strongly activated by binding of organic pollutant chemicals such as polychlorinated dibenzodioxins (dioxins), polychlorinated dibenzofurans, and PCBs as well as polycyclic aromatic hydrocarbons such as benzo(a)pyrene [37]. In the unliganded state, AhR resides in a complex with chaperone and repressor proteins. Ligand binding triggers conformational change, leading to dissociation of the repressive complex and heterodimerization with its obligatory partner, the AhR nuclear translocator (ARNT), which is facilitated by the PAS domain structure of the AhR. The dimer translocates to the nucleus and binds to DNA through a basic helix–loop–helix structure in the DBD of the AhR to specific response elements in the DNA termed *AhR response elements.* These short consensus sequences in the DNA (5′-T/GCGTG-3′) are also referred to as *dioxin response elements (DREs)* or *xenobiotic response elements* and are located in the region of the promoter of target genes. The recruitment of coactivating transcription factors leads to transactivation of gene expression [37] (Figure 6.3). The main target genes of the AhR are Phase I or Phase II drug-metabolizing cytochrome P450 enzymes, which suggests that the AhR functions as a sensor of foreign compounds, which leads to the upregulation of enzymes needed for metabolic reactions necessary for their clearance from the body. However, one main side effect is that some of these enzymes are also responsible for the breakdown (hydroxylation) [AhR hydroxylase (CYP1A1), CYP1B1, CYP1A2] or the synthesis [aromatase (CYP19A1)] of 17β-estradiol. Therefore, some xenobiotics can act as EDCs by influencing levels of endogenous steroid hormones through an AhR-mediated mechanism.

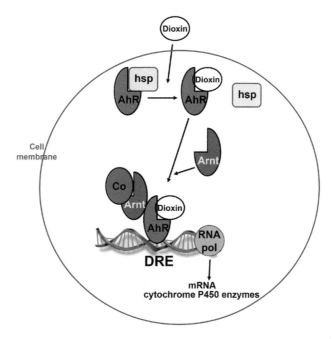

FIGURE 6.3 Genomic action of the AhR. Dioxin (or other organochlorine compounds) bind to intracellular AhR, which results in the release of associated repressor HSPs. The ligand–receptor complex heterodimerizes with ARNT and binds to DREs in the DNA. Transactivation of gene expression involves binding of coregulators (Co) and RNA polymerase (RNApol), resulting in alteration to mRNAs. Main target genes are those encoding cytochrome P450 enzymes. In this way, the AhR acts as a sensor for foreign compounds, enabling the expression of genes for their metabolism and clearance from the body.

6.6.2 Assay Systems

Assays for AhR-mediated mechanisms of action are analogous to those used for the nuclear receptor superfamily. Competitive binding assays can be used to measure displacement of radiolabeled dioxin from the AhR. Reporter gene assays can be used to measure transactivation of AhR-responsive reporter genes transfected into cells. Since CYP1A1, CYP1B1, and aromatase (CYP19A1) are well-defined target genes of the AhR, the effects of EDCs can be studied directly on the expression of these genes using real-time RTPCR.

6.7 PROSTAGLANDINS

Prostaglandins are short-lived lipid-signaling molecules that are produced and act locally. Their actions are, therefore, paracrine and autocrine rather than endocrine. Although originally isolated from the prostate, they are made in most tissues of the human body and mediate many essential physiological effects, such as early male sexual development, sexual behavior, induction of uterine contraction in labor, inflammatory responses, pain, calcium

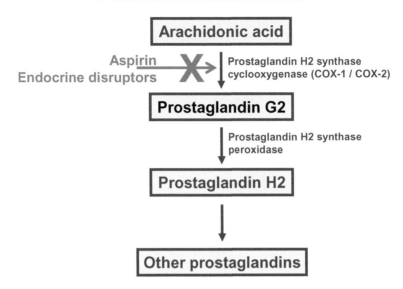

FIGURE 6.4   Prostaglandins are synthesized from arachidonic acid by cyclooxygenases (COX-1 and COX-2) and terminal prostaglandin synthases. COX-1 is responsible for the baseline synthesis of prostaglandins, while COX-2 produces increased levels of prostaglandins in inflammatory responses. EDs have been reported to interfere in both the expression and function of COX enzymes, which is similar to the mechanism of action of aspirin.

movement, and vasodilation. The deregulation of prostaglandin action has been implicated in the development of cancer, cardiovascular disease, and inflammatory conditions [38].

Prostaglandins are synthesized in cells from arachidonic acid by cyclooxygenases (COX-1 and COX-2) and terminal prostaglandin synthases. COX-1 is responsible for baseline synthesis of prostaglandins, while COX-2 produces increased levels of prostaglandins in inflammatory responses. Endocrine disruptors (EDs) have been reported to interfere in both the expression and function of COX enzymes (Figure 6.4). Exposure to dioxin has been reported to reduce the expression of COX-2 in the granulosa cells of the ovary, and this has been suggested as a potential mechanism by which dioxin blocks ovulation [39]. Acetyl salicylate (aspirin) is a commonly used analgesic that acts to relieve pain by inhibiting the COX-mediated conversion of arachidonic acid to prostaglandin, and it has now been shown that several EDs, including phthalates, parabens, benzophenones, and bisphenol A, can also interfere in this pathway by binding directly to the active site of cyclooxygenases and thus inhibiting prostaglandin synthesis [40]. Assays include the measurement by immunoassay of prostaglandins secreted from cultured SC5 mouse juvenile Sertoli cells, primary human mast cells, or ex vivo rat testis [40].

6.8 HOW MANY OTHER RECEPTORS MAY BE DISRUPTED?

This section of the book has described the ability of environmental compounds to act as EDCs through binding to a range of intracellular ligand-activated transcription factors. This disruptive action through receptor-mediated mechanisms is unprecedented in toxicology because not only can the compounds act at low (nanomolar or at most micromolar) concentrations when binding to receptors, but also the effects are directly targeted to gene expression in the nucleus because the receptors are themselves transcription factors. Since there are 48 members of the human nuclear receptor superfamily [41] that can bind not only EDCs but also a range of drugs used for therapeutic purposes [42], it would seem unlikely that the extent of disruption described at the current time in this book could represent anything other than just the tip of an iceberg. It would seem inevitable that each of these 48 members of the nuclear receptor superfamily, together with other ligand-activated transcription factors (as exampled from the AhR), could be disrupted. Furthermore, the disruption of the G-protein coupled estrogen receptor (GPER) (see Chapter 3) opens up a question of how many other G-protein coupled receptors might also be disrupted, and the extent of interaction between so many receptors will undoubtedly continue to unfold with time.

References

[1] Hagan CR, Lange CA. Molecular determinants of context-dependent progesterone receptor action in breast cancer. BMC Med 2014;12(32):1–9.

[2] Kastner P, Krust A, Turcotte B, Stropp U, Tora L, Gronemeyer H, et al. Two distinct estrogen-regulated promoters generate transcripts encoding the two functionally different human progesterone receptor forms A and B. EMBO J 1990;9:1603–14.

[3] Glover JF, Darbre PD. Multihormone regulation of MMTV-LTR in transfected T-47-D human breast cancer cells. J Steroid Biochem 1989;32:357–63.

[4] Hamers T, Kamstra JH, Sonnenveld E, Murk AJ, Kester MHA, Andersson PL, et al. *In vitro* profiling of the endocrine-disrupting potency of brominated flame retardants. Toxicol Sci 2006;92:157–73.

[5] Li J, Li N, Ma M, Giesy JP, Wang Z. *In vitro* profiling of the endocrine disrupting potency of organochlorine pesticides. Toxicol Lett 2008;183:65–71.

[6] Chatterjee S, Kumar V, Majumder CB, Roy P. Screening of some anti-progestin endocrine disrupters using a recombinant yeast based *in vitro* bioassay. Toxicol In Vitro 2008;22:788–98.

[7] Viswanath G, Halder S, Divya G, Majumder CB, Roy P. Detection of potential (anti)progestagenic endocrine disruptors using a recombinant human progesterone receptor binding and transactivation assay. Mol Cell Endocrinol 2008;295:1–9.

[8] Suzuki G, Tue NM, Malarvannan G, Sudaryanto A, Takahashi S, Tanabe S, et al. Similarities in the endocrine-disrupting potencies of indoor dust and flame retardants by using human osteosarcoma (U2OS) cell-based reporter gene assays. Environ Sci Technol 2013;47:2898–908.

[9] Hamlin HJ, Lowers RH, Albergotti LC, McCoy MW, Mutz J, Guillette LJ. Environmental influence on yolk steroids in American alligators (*Alligator mississippiensis*). Biol Reprod 2010;83:736–41.

[10] Wojtowicz AK, Kajta M, Gregorasczuk EL. DDT- and DDE-induced disruption of ovarian steroidogenesis in prepubertal porcine ovarian follicles: a possible interaction with the main steroidogenic enzymes and estrogen receptor β. J Physiol Pharmacol 2007;58:873–85.

[11] Tinwell H, Colombel S, Blanck O, Bars R. The screening of everyday life chemicals in validated assays targeting the pituitary–gonadal axis. Reg Toxicol Pharmacol 2013;66:184–96.

[12] Yang N, Ray DW, Matthews LC. Current concepts in glucocorticoid resistance. Steroids 2012;77:1041–9.

[13] Rose AJ, Herzig S. Metabolic control through glucocorticoid hormones: an update. Mol Cell Endocrinol 2013;380:65–78.

[14] Molina JMM, Hillenweck A, Jouanin I, Zalko D, Cravedi JP, Fernandez MF, et al. Steroid receptor profiling of vinclozolin and its primary metabolites. Toxicol Appl Pharmacol 2006;216:44–54.

[15] Kojima H, Takeuchi S, Itoh T, Iida M, Kobayashi S, Yoshida T. *In vitro* endocrine disruption potential of organophosphate flame retardants via human nuclear receptors. Toxicology 2013;314:76–83.

[16] Lelli SM, Ceballos NR, Mazzetti MB, Aldonatti CM, deViale LCSM. Hexachlorobenzene as hormonal disruptor—studies about glucocorticoids: their hepatic receptors, adrenal synthesis and plasma levels in relation to impaired gluconeogenesis. Biochem Pharmacol 2007;73:873–9.

[17] Gosse JA, Taylore VF, Jackson BP, Hamilton JW, Bodwell JE. Monomethylated trivalent arsenic species disrupt steroid receptor interactions with their DNA response elements at non-cytotoxic cellular concentrations. J Appl Toxicol 2014;34:498–505.

[18] Aluru N, Jorgensen EH, Maule AG, Vijayan MM. PCB disruption of the hypothalamus–pituitary–interrenal axis involves brain glucocorticoid receptor downregulation in anadromous Arctic charr. Am J Physiol Regul Integr Comp Physiol 2004;287:R787–93.

[19] Berger J, Moller DE. The mechanisms of action of PPARs. Annu Rev Med 2002;53:409–35.

[20] Grygiel-Gorniak B. Peroxisome proliferator-activated receptors and their ligands: nutritional and clinical implications—a review. Nutrition J 2014;13:17–27.

[21] Lehmann JM, Moore LB, Smith-Oliver TA, Wilkison WO, Willson TM, Kliewer SA. An antidiabetic thiazolidine-dione is a high affinity ligand for peroxisome proliferator-activated receptor γ. J Biol Chem 1995;270:12953–12956.

[22] Berger J, Bailey P, Biswas C, Cullinan CA, Doebber TW, Haves NS, et al. Thiazolidinediones produce a conformational change in peroxisomal proliferator-activated receptor-gamma: binding and activation correlate with antidiabetic actions in db/db mice. Endocrinology 1996;137:4189–95. 1996.

[23] Maloney EK, Waxman DJ. Transactivation of PPAR alpha and PPAR gamma by structurally diverse environmental chemicals. Toxicol Appl Pharmacol 1999;161:209–18.

[24] Hurst CH, Waxman DJ. Activation of PPAR alpha and PPAR gamma by environmental phthalate monoesters. Toxicol Sci 2003;74:297–308.

[25] Shipley JM, Hurst CH, Tanaka SS, DeRoos FL, Butenhof JL, Seacat AM, et al. Transactivation of PPARalpha and induction of PPARalpha target genes by perfluorooctane-based chemicals. Toxicol Sci 2004;80:151–60.

[26] Grun F, Watanabe H, Zamanian Z, Maedia L, Arima K, Cubacha R, et al. Endocrine-disrupting organotin compounds are potent inducers of adipogenesis in vertebrates. Mol Endocrinol 2006;20:2141–55.

[27] Grun F. The obesogen tributyltin. Vitam Horm 2014;94:277–325.

[28] Grun F, Blumberg B. Minireview: the case for obesogens. Mol Endocrinol 2009;23:1127–34.

[29] Masuno H, Kidani T, Sekiya K, Sakayama K, Shiosaka T, Yamamoto H, et al. Bisphenol A in combination with insulin can accelerate the conversion of 3T3-L1 fibroblasts to adipocytes. J Lipid Res 2002;43:676–84.

[30] Masuno H, Okamoto S, Iwanami J, Honda K, Shiosaka T, Kidani T, et al. Effect of 4-nonylphenol on cell proliferation and adipocyte formation in cultures of fully differentiated 3T3-L1 cells. Toxicol Sci 2003;75:314–20.

[31] Pereira-Fernandes A, Demaegdt H, Vandermeiren K, Hectors TLM, Jorens PG, Blust R, et al. Evaluation of a screening system for obesogenic compounds: screening of endocrine disrupting compounds and evaluation of the PPAR dependency of the effect. PLoS One 2013;8(e77481):1–17.

[32] Punzon I, Latapie V, LeMevel S, Hagneau A, Jolivet P, Palmier K, et al. Towards a humanized PPARγ reporter system for in vivo screening of obesogens. Mol Cell Endocrinol 2013;374:1–9.

[33] Qiao E, Ji M, Wu J, Ma R, Zhang X, He Y, et al. Expression of the PXR gene in various types of cancer and drug resistance (Review). Oncol Lett. 2013;5:1093–100.

[34] Smutny T, Mani S, Pavek P. Post-translational and post-transcriptional modifications of pregnane X receptor (PXR) in regulation of cytochrome P450 superfamily. Curr Drug Metab 2013;14:1059–69.

[35] Pacyniak EK, Cheng X, Cunningham ML, Crofton K, Klaassen CD, Guo GL. The flame retardants, polybrominated diphenyl ethers, are pregnane X receptor activators. Toxicol Sci 2007;97:94–102.

[36] Sanders JM, Burka LT, Smith CS, Black W, James R, Cunningham ML. Differential expression of CYP1A1, 2B and 3A genes in the F344 rat following exposure to a polybrominated diphenyl ether mixture or individual components. Toxicol Sci 2005;88:127–33.

[37] Feng S, Cao Z, Wang X. Role of aryl hydrocarbon receptor in cancer. Biochim Biophys Acta 2013;1836:197–210.

[38] Fitzgerald GA. COX-2 and beyond: approaches to prostaglandin inhibition in human disease. Nat Rev Drug Discov 2003;2:879–90.

[39] Mizuyachi K, Son DS, Rozman KK, Terranova PF. Alteration in ovarian gene expression in response to 2,3,7,8-tetrachlorodibenzo-p-dioxin: reduction of cyclooxygenase-2 in the blockage of ovulation. Reprod Toxicol 2002;16:299–307.

[40] Kristensen DM, Skalkam ML, Audouze K, Lesne L, Lethimonier CD, Frederiksen H, et al. Many putative endocrine disruptors inhibit prostaglandin synthesis. Environ Health Perspect 2011;119:534–41.

[41] Zhang Z, Burch PE, Cooney AJ, Lanz RB, Pereira FA, Wu J, et al. Genomic analysis of the nuclear receptor family: new insights into structure, regulation and evolution from the rat genome. Genome Res 2004;14:580–90.

[42] Simons SS, Edwards DP, Kumar R. Minireview: dynamic structures of nuclear hormone receptors: new promises and challenges. Mol Endocrinol 2014;28:173–82.

Nonmonotonic Responses in Endocrine Disruption

Laura N. Vandenberg

Abstract

There are a number of features of endocrine-disrupting chemicals (EDCs) that distinguish them from traditional toxicants. One such attribute is the ability of EDCs to induce nonmonotonic dose response curves (NMDRCs), where low and high doses can produce opposite effects. NMDRCs are often described as U- or inverted U-shaped, and they are a common feature in a number of scientific fields, including endocrinology, nutrition, and pharmacology. This chapter describes the mechanisms by which NMDRCs can manifest and some specific examples from the EDC literature. It also describes the recent debate over whether NMDRCs are "real," and whether they are common enough to influence chemical safety assessments for EDCs. Finally, this chapter concludes with a discussion about a related but distinct phenomenon known as *low-dose effects*. Together, these two features of EDCs suggest that the methods used to determine safe doses for human exposures are flawed.

Endocrine Disruption and Human Health.
DOI: http://dx.doi.org/10.1016/B978-0-12-801139-3.00007-7

7.1 INTRODUCTION

In the study of endocrine-disrupting chemicals (EDCs), two topics that are frequently raised and strongly debated are the related issues of nonmonotonicity and low-dose effects. This chapter will explain these concepts and why they are relevant not only for the study of EDCs, but also for the regulation of this class of chemicals. Importantly, although these topics are considered controversial by some scientists in some fields [1], scientists in a number of disciplines (including the fields of endocrinology, environmental health, and pharmacology) considered these to be mainstream, and even expected, characteristics of chemicals that interfere with hormone action [2–4]. Understanding the nuances of this debate, as well as both the scientific issues and policy implications of nonmonotonicity and low-dose effects, will be significant as this field moves forward.

7.2 WHAT IS NONMONOTONICITY?

One factor that plays an important role in the study of toxicants (including traditional toxic chemicals, hormones, and EDCs) and is also an essential step in the risk assessment process is determining whether there is a dose response for the end point being studied. The term *dose response* simply refers to the relationship between the applied dose (the amount of a substance administered to cultured cells, an animal, or a person) and the observed effect. The expectation for toxic substances is a monotonic dose–response relationship, where more of the toxin (a higher dose) will have more of an effect. This is a fundamental principle of toxicology dating back to Paracelsus, the founder of the field of toxicology. Paracelsus is often quoted as saying, "Dosis facit venenum," translated as "the dose makes the poison." However, more current translations of his texts instead quote him as stating, "solely the dose determines that a thing *is not a poison*" (emphasis added) [5], which offers a somewhat more nuanced approach to dose-response relationships.

Within the category of monotonic dose responses, there are different dose–response shapes, including linear relationships and sigmoid curves (Figure 7.1A); these are all classified as monotonic because the sign of the slope of the curve (positive or negative) does not change with an increasing or decreasing dose. In contrast, a nonmonotonic dose–response curve (NMDRC) is one where the sign of the slope (positive or negative) changes at some point across the dose range (Figure 7.1A) [6]. Nonmonotonic curves are often referred to as *U-shaped, inverted U-shaped, J-shaped, V-shaped*, or *biphasic*, but some nonmonotonic curves have slopes that change sign multiple times, giving an appearance like an *M* or *W* (Figure 7.1B).

NMDRCs, therefore, are characterized mathematically. Determining the slope of a line requires three data points, and thus the mathematical identification of an NMDRC requires at least five doses (Figure 7.1C). Yet, many experiments do not include five distinct dose groups, and even fewer studies calculate the slopes of the dose responses (and therefore can determine if the sign changes from positive to negative or vice versa). Thus, other criteria have been used to determine if a dose–response curve should be considered nonmonotonic.

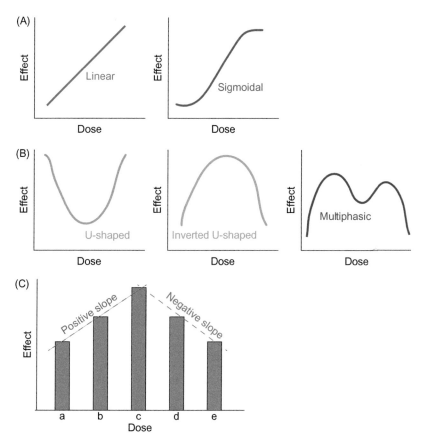

FIGURE 7.1   Monotonic and NMDRCs. (A) Hypothetical examples of monotonic dose–response curves, including linear and sigmoidal curves. (B) Hypothetical examples of NMDRCs, including U-shaped, inverted U-shaped, and multiphasic (M-shaped) curves. (C) Three data points are needed to calculate the slope of a line, and five data points are needed to determine whether an NMDRC is present. In this example, the slope is calculated from the responses at doses a, b, and c; it has a positive sign. The slope is also calculated from the responses at doses c, d, and e; in this case, it has a negative sign.

These include (1) a significant difference observed at a lower dose relative to untreated controls, but no significant difference observed at a higher dose relative to untreated controls; (2) a significant difference observed at a low dose relative to untreated controls, and a significant difference in the opposite direction observed at a higher dose relative to untreated controls; (3) a significant difference observed at a low dose relative to untreated controls, as well as a significant difference between the low-dose group and a high-dose group, regardless of whether there is a significant difference between the high-dose group and the untreated control (Figure 7.2). There are also statistical analyses that can be used to determine whether experimental results are linear/monotonic or nonmonotonic (see Ref. [7] and its associated supplemental materials for details).

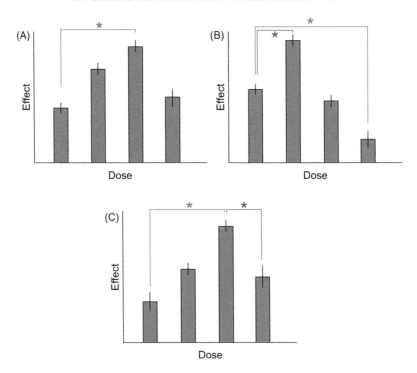

FIGURE 7.2 Methods for determining nonmonotonicity when five treatment groups are not present. Nonmonotonicity is defined as a curve where the sign of the slope (positive or negative) changes at some point across the dose range. Calculating a slope requires three data points, and thus determining whether an NMDRC is present requires a minimum of five treatment groups (see Figure 7.1C). Yet, many studies do not include five treatment groups, and the slope of the curve is rarely calculated in any experiment. Nonmonotonicity can also be inferred if (A) a significant difference is observed at a low dose relative to untreated controls, but no significant difference is observed at a higher dose relative to untreated controls; (B) a significant difference is observed at a low dose relative to untreated controls, and a significant difference in the opposite direction is observed at a higher dose relative to untreated controls; and/or (C) a significant difference is observed at a low dose relative to untreated controls, and a significant difference is also observed between the low-dose group and the high-dose group.

Nonmonotonic responses defy the dogma that "the dose makes the poison" because they provide examples where more of a compound actually elicits less of a response than lower doses (see Figure 7.1B). Perhaps it is because of this dogma (or perhaps because they seem unintuitive), NMDRCs are often dismissed as "implausible," "unproven," "controversial," and "improbable" [1,8,9]. Yet, as discussed later in this chapter, nonmonotonicity is both accepted and well understood in a number of mainstream scientific disciplines, including pharmacology, endocrinology, and nutrition [4,10,11]. Equally important, from the perspective of toxicology, NMDRCs do not defy Paracelsus's actual theory that "solely the dose determines that a thing is not a poison" because this statement does not imply that more of a dose must always induce more of an effect.

7.3 NONMONOTONICITY IN PHARMACOLOGY, ENDOCRINOLOGY, AND NUTRITION

There are a number of scientific fields where compounds that defy the "dose makes the poison" concept are common. One example, from the fields of pharmacology and endocrinology, is often referred to as "flare" [12]. In this situation, drugs like tamoxifen, a common treatment for breast cancer that acts as an estrogen receptor antagonist, stimulates growth of the tumor at low concentrations but inhibits growth of the tumor—and can actually help to shrink it—at high doses [13,14]. Flare provides a well-characterized example of an NMDRC where low doses induce the opposite effect of high doses [15,16]. Another example of nonmonotonicity observed in the field of pharmacology comes from the drug Lupron, which is used as a fertility drug in women [17]. At low doses, Lupron stimulates follicle-stimulating hormone (FSH) and thus induces ovulation, but at high doses, the drug suppresses ovulation [18].

NMDRCs are common in the field of endocrinology; in fact, nonmonotonicity is considered a principle of endocrinology and is expected for many end points [3,4,19]. For example, numerous studies have shown that the rodent mammary gland has biphasic responses to estrogens, where lower doses induce growth parameters but higher doses do not [20–22]. Isolated breast cells in culture also display NMDRCs in response to estrogens, where the total cell number is highest at moderate doses [23,24]. In a recent example from epidemiological endocrinology, studies show that both low and high endogenous testosterone levels increase the risk of disease and death in men, leading medical professionals to propose that there is an "optimal window" of hormone concentration [25].

The concept of an "optimal window" is quite common in the field of nutrition as well (Figure 7.3). It is widely understood that moderate levels of many nutrients are ideal for the maintenance of health [26]. Many vitamin deficiencies and vitamin overdoses (very low and high doses) have overlapping symptoms. For example, both very low and very high consumption of vitamin B3 can induce skin conditions, mental confusion, and even death [27].

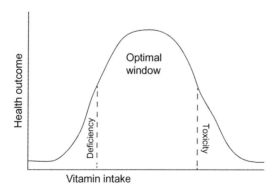

FIGURE 7.3   The concept of an "optimal window" of vitamin concentration. Low concentrations are associated with vitamin deficiencies, whereas high concentrations are associated with vitamin toxicity. These examples of nonmonotonic associations between vitamin consumption and health outcomes are common in the field of nutrition.

7.4 MECHANISMS FOR NONMONOTONICITY

Scientists working in the field of endocrinology have been instrumental in understanding the mechanisms that contribute to these nonintuitive responses, specifically for hormones. Much of this work has been conducted in cultured cells, simplified systems that allow these mechanisms to be dissected at the subcellular level.

One of the most common mechanisms for NMDRCs is the presence of two competing and overlapping monotonic curves that act on a common end point. For example, increasing doses of estrogen are associated with proliferation of breast cells (although it is often said that estrogens induce proliferation in breast cells, it is more accurate to say that estrogens relieve an inhibition of cell proliferation—see Refs. [28,29] for a full discussion). Increasing doses of estrogen also increase cell death; high doses of this hormone are overtly toxic, and this toxicity is independent of actions via the estrogen receptor [23,30]. When looking at total cell number, these individual monotonic curves are not observed—instead, total cell number manifests as an NMDRC (Figure 7.4). Although cytotoxicity has been implicated in many of these overlapping monotonic curves, in fact other similar responses, like the competing effects of cell proliferation and inhibition of cell proliferation, also have been observed and are distinct from cell death [31–33]. These dual actions of hormones are not limited to cell culture conditions. In the developing mammary gland, for example, estrogens induce proliferation, manifested as ductal growth [34], while simultaneously inducing apoptosis, manifested as lumen formation (allowing solid epithelial structures to become ducts) [35].

Another mechanism by which NMDRCs can manifest is the presence of multiple receptors for a hormone (like the progesterone receptor isoforms PR-A and PR-B, which are expressed in different tissues and have different roles in diseases [36,37]). In some circumstances, actions at these different receptors can have competing effects on a common end point. For example, in the uterus, estrogens induce proliferation via estrogen receptor α but

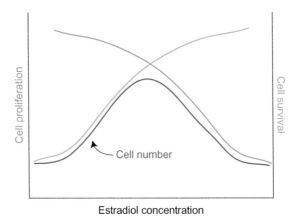

FIGURE 7.4   Nonmonotonic curves can manifest due to two overlapping monotonic responses that act on a common end point. In this hypothetical example, increasing doses of estrogen are associated with increases in cell proliferation (green line) and decreases in cell survival (orange line). When the end point being observed is total cell number (blue line), an NMDRC is apparent.

induce apoptosis via estrogen receptor β [38]. Thus, increasing doses of this single hormone induces two competing actions, which can manifest as an inverted U-shaped relationship between dose and organ size.

Another mechanism that has been implicated in nonmonotonicity is receptor selectivity, where lower doses of a hormone bind with high affinity to one receptor, but at higher doses, the same hormone can bind to multiple receptors, including receptors for which it has relatively low affinity. For example, estrogens bind to a variety of estrogen receptors, including membrane-bound estrogen receptors, and can induce effects via these receptors at exceptionally low doses [39–41]. But, perhaps surprisingly, high doses of estrogens can bind to other nuclear receptors, including thyroid hormone receptors (TRs) and androgen receptors (ARs) [42]. Thus, the effects of estrogens observed at these high doses are expected to be quite different from the effects at low doses due to the different downstream signaling pathways associated with these different receptors.

Other mechanisms that have been dissected for specific hormone receptors include receptor desensitization and receptor downregulation. With receptor desensitization, repeated or prolonged exposure to hormones causes biochemical inactivation of the receptor [43,44]; thus increased doses cannot induce greater effects. Although receptor desensitization has been observed for many hormones, including glucagon, FSH, prostaglandins, and chorionic gonadotropin, this process is typically associated with G-protein coupled receptors (GPERs) [45]. Receptor downregulation may be a more common process [46] and occurs due to the kinetics of ligand–receptor binding and movement of the receptor within the cell. When a nuclear receptor is bound by ligand, it translocates to the nucleus and binds to specific response elements on DNA. But this is not a permanent effect, and thus the receptors must be inactivated and degraded [47]. As the hormone concentration increases, receptor degradation also increases; at high doses, degradation outpaces the ability of the cell to produce new receptors, and thus the effects of increasing doses are diminished compared to lower doses [47]. This process is even more complicated in vivo, where signaling from one hormone receptor can influence the stability of other receptors [48]. Still other mechanisms that produce NMDRCs have been studied, including the actions of cell- and tissue-specific cofactors [49,50], the interactions of different cell types within a single organ [51,52], and endocrine negative feedback loops [53,54], among others.

Identifying which mechanism is responsible for each individual nonmonotonic response is a complex undertaking, and in many cases, it has not been done. There are two important takeaway messages from this. The first is that extensive work has identified a number of different mechanisms that can produce NMDRCs, and thus these types of responses should be considered biologically plausible, at least for molecules that interact with receptors [10]. The second is that comprehending the mechanism of action is always a separate issue from observing a phenomenon [3], and thus our lack of *understanding* of all mechanisms should not influence our *acceptance* of NMDRCs.

7.5 NONMONOTONICITY FOR EDCs

Nonmonotonicity is not uncommon for many end points after exposures to hormones. This is considered one of the principles of endocrinology. Similarly, it has been proposed that NMDRCs should be expected for EDCs because these compounds follow many of the same biological "rules" as natural signaling molecules like hormones [3,4,10,19]. In 2012, a group of 12 scientists with a range of interests from cancer biology to epidemiology to conservation science performed an in-depth review of the EDC literature [10]. A portion of this review was dedicated to examining the case of nonmonotonicity, ultimately identifying hundreds of examples of NMDRCs. Importantly, these examples of nonmonotonicity, many of which were U- or inverted U-shaped, were observed in in vitro and laboratory animal experiments and in human populations. Ultimately, the authors concluded that NMDRCs "are remarkably common in studies of natural hormones and EDCs." In an editorial highlighting this large review, the director of the U.S. National Institute of Environmental Health Sciences, a part of the National Institutes of Health (NIH), wrote "The question is no longer whether nonmonotonic dose responses are 'real' and occur frequently enough to be a concern; clearly these are common phenomena with well-understood mechanisms. Instead the question is which dose-response shapes should be expected for specific environmental chemicals and under what specific circumstances" [55].

A number of examples can illustrate the breadth and depth of the end points and chemicals that have NMDRCs. In cultured cells, similar to what has been observed for breast cells treated with natural estrogens, a biphasic relationship is common for the effects of estrogen-mimicking compounds on total cell number [24,56–59]. This response has been observed for pharmaceutical hormones [like diethylstilbestrol (DES) and ethinyl estradiol] and chemicals used in plastics [bisphenol A (BPA)], detergents and surfactants (octylphenol and nonylphenol), phytoestrogens and natural antioxidants (daidezin and carpelastofuran), and insecticides [dichlorodiphenyltrichloroethane (DDT)]. In laboratory animals, NMDRCs were observed for the effects of synthetic estrogens on uterine weight [60,61] and prostate weight [62,63]; the effects of herbicides on the growth, survival, and metamorphosis parameters in several species of frogs and toads [64–66]; and the effects of phytocompounds on behavioral end points [67,68], among many others.

Perhaps most surprising was the number of examples of nonmonotonicity in the environmental epidemiology literature. Considering the known mechanisms for inducing NMDRCs, it is expected that in large human populations, many factors would make it difficult to observe nonmonotonic relationships between EDC exposures and health outcomes. In fact, comparisons of the methods that are used by environmental epidemiologists suggest that the ways exposures are compared (continuous versus quartiles versus sextiles) can significantly influence the detection of NMDRCs [69]. Although NMDRCs have been reported for a large range of end points, including bone mineral density [70], telomere length in leukocytes [71], risk of endometriosis [72], and mental development score in infants [73], the strongest evidence for nonmonotonicity in human populations are numerous studies examining the relationship between persistent organic pollutants [like polychlorinated biphenyls (PCBs), organochlorine pesticides, and dioxins] and aspects of metabolic syndrome [including risk of diabetes, body mass index (BMI), and triglyceride levels] [74–77].

Although the 2012 review of the EDC literature concluded that NMDRCs were "common" [10], there was no attempt to determine what percentage of all dose–response curves are nonmonotonic. The conclusion that these responses are "common" was based instead on the large number of chemicals that were shown to induce NMDRCs—the authors identified examples for more than 70 different EDCs [10]. Assessing the frequency of NMDRCs in the literature as a whole is a tremendous (and perhaps impossible) undertaking. A few smaller studies, however, have attempted to quantify the frequency of nonmonotonicity. In one study, a sample of the toxicology literature was analyzed and U- and inverted U-shaped curves were observed in 12–24% of all dose–response studies [78]. Although this study examined toxicology studies rather than EDC studies in particular, it provides further evidence that nonmonotonicity is common. In a second review, NMDRCs were analyzed for more than 100 in vitro studies for BPA, a well-studied EDC [79]. Nonmonotonic responses were observed in greater than 20% of all dose response experiments, again suggesting that these curves are common. It has also been noted that these assessments may underestimate the true frequency of NMDRCs because there are likely to be biases against publishing "unexpected" dose responses, especially in fields where "the dose makes the poison" is the dogma [78].

7.6 ONGOING DEBATE ON EDCs AND NONMONOTONICITY

After the publication of the 2012 review of the EDC literature, a short commentary was published by a group of industry-funded consultants, which raised a number of challenges to the conclusions that were reached [80]. A summary of these challenges—and the responses provided to refute these challenges [3]—are provided in Table 7.1. A number of additional venues for debate were also opened up by the publication of these papers, including an international meeting of scientific experts from academia, industry, and government. Although consensus was not the goal of this meeting (and was not achieved), the vast majority of attendees at this meeting agreed that NMDRCs "exist at some dose range" [81].

Following that meeting, the U.S. Environmental Protection Agency (EPA) published a draft "State of Science" report that aimed to assess nonmonotonicity for EDCs that affect estrogen, androgen, and thyroid hormone signaling pathways [82]. In that report, the EPA panel concluded that NMDRCs occur in estrogen, androgen, and thyroid hormone systems and are "not unexpected" in vitro. Yet, they also stated that NMDRCs were "not commonly identified" in vivo. Like with the 2012 EDC review by academic experts [10], the use of the word *common* raised significant problems because without a systematic approach to quantifying the totality of the dose–response literature, it is not possible to say what the frequency of NMDRCs is for EDCs, and therefore whether or not they are truly common. The response to the EPA's draft report from the scientific community was not positive; a large number of issues were raised in public comments (summarized in Table 7.2). The EPA requested a review of its draft report by the National Academy of Sciences (NAS), and this expert panel concluded that the report "failed to establish (or enforce) a clear set of methods for collecting and analyzing the evidence on NMDR curves to ensure that the groups conducted their assessments in a clear, consistent, and therefore replicable manner" [83]. Reiterating many of the points raised in public comments (Table 7.2), the NAS panel wrote that "EPA's approach to evaluating whether NMDR curves exist for endocrine disruptors was not systematic, consistent, or transparent" and concluded that "[a]lthough it is clear that the [EPA] authors spent enormous time and energy in developing [their] evaluation, it is fundamentally compromised."

TABLE 7.1   Challenges to the Hypothesis that NMDRCs Occur for EDCs

Challenge	Response
NMDRCs are not reproducible.	There are a number of examples of very reproducible NMDRCs, including the effects of estrogen and synthetic estrogens on breast cell number. For the EDC BPA, nonmonotonic responses have been observed in at least five independent laboratories.
The frequency of NMDRCs is not known.	Although the frequency of NMDRCs is not known for the entirety of the EDC literature, smaller assessments have quantified NMDRCs in the toxicology literature and find them in 10–24% of all dose–response experiments.
NMDRCs do not occur in "guideline studies"; i.e., the kinds of studies used by risk assessors in chemical safety assessments.	First, guideline studies typically examine three to four doses and thus are not optimally designed to detect NMDRCs. Yet, there are numerous examples where findings suggestive of nonmonotonicity are dismissed or ignored in guideline studies, for end points that include mortality, incidence of carcinomas, and organ weight.
NMDRCs are observed in some tissues, but not others.	It is not clear how this challenges findings of NMDRCs, just as the selective appearance of tumors in some tissues but not others would not prevent the classification of a compound as a carcinogen. It is well known that tissue-based factors influence how different organs respond to hormones.
NMDRCs do not occur in the range of human exposures to EDCs.	Epidemiology studies revealing NMDRCs immediately dispute this claim. In animals, it is unclear why NMDRCs must occur in the range of human exposures to be important, since high- to low-dose extrapolation also occurs at doses that can fall outside the range of human exposures.
A mechanism has not been demonstrated for each NMDRC observed.	Many mechanisms have been detailed that explain how NMDRCs can manifest. Although a specific mechanism is often not attributed to each observation of an NMDRC, this does not negate the observation itself.
The examples of NMDRCs do not include end points that are considered adverse.	The definitions of what constitutes an "adverse effect" vary considerably between different groups and typically require expert judgment (and thus often lack transparency in how end points are determined to be adverse or not). Certainly, the end points examined in most epidemiology studies would be considered adverse, and many other end points examined in animal studies would be as well.

What is clear from this ongoing debate is that there are many issues that complicate the question of whether NMDRCs are common, and even what that means. Interestingly, one question that has not received much attention is: How frequently must NMDRCs occur for them to be considered important in chemical safety assessments? The next section of this chapter will explore why challenging the dogma of "the dose makes the poison" has significant implications for how the risk assessment process is conducted for EDCs.

7.7 HOW DOES NONMONOTONICITY INFLUENCE CHEMICAL SAFETY ASSESSMENTS?

When chemicals are tested for toxicity, they are typically examined at very high doses—and in fact, hazard assessments require that doses be used that produce overt, obvious signs of toxicity. These signs of toxicity can include death, significant loss of body weight, and

TABLE 7.2   Criticisms of the EPA's Assessment of NMDRCs in Studies of EDCs

Issue	Brief explanation
Errors in data analysis and misrepresentation of study findings	• Studies that clearly ruled out cytotoxicity were noted as showing evidence of cytotoxicity. • Studies that included negative and positive controls were considered inconclusive because of a lack of appropriate controls. • Studies that specifically ruled out contamination were dismissed due to concerns about contamination.
Misrepresentation of the conclusions of other expert panels	• The report misinterprets the conclusions of the UNEP/WHO state-of-science 2012 document. • The report incorrectly characterizes the findings of a 2002 EPA/NTP expert panel on low doses.
Reliance on outdated literature	• The report suggests that specific findings could not be replicated. In fact, they have been replicated—the inability to replicate is limited to attempts made by industry groups, a data set that has been considered flawed by numerous expert groups.
Examination of extremely limited data, and a lack of justification for which studies were included or excluded	• The report did not use consistent methods to identify or assess the literature. • The methods used in the literature review process were not adequately described. • The methods used in the different sections of the report varied significantly without any explanation or justification.
Makes repeated assessments of the frequency of NMDRCs without corroborating data	• Statements that NMDRCs were "more common" for one type of study compared to another type of study are not justified, nor supported by literature. • The conclusion that NMDRCs are not common is never explained nor quantified.
EPA failed to obtain expertise from outside the risk assessment community	• All of the contributors to this draft report were associated with the EPA or Food and Drug Administration (FDA), and there are concerns about the conflict of interest inherent in an agency assessing whether their dogma and status quo methods for chemical safety assessments are adequate.
Sections of the report lack citations	• Entire pages of the report lack references, so it is not possible for the reader to determine which evidence was used to form specific conclusions.
EPA fails to acknowledge the disconnect between the presence of an NMDRC and the identification of a chemical as an EDC	• One conclusion from the report is that the EPA's testing methods are perfectly capable of identifying EDCs, so the presence of NMDRCs are not important because they do not interfere with this process. This illustrates a lack of understanding of how the identification of EDCs is distinct from the identification of safe doses of EDCs.

other clinical signs. High doses that are tested include an LD_{50}, the lethal dose at which 50% of the animals die; the maximum tolerated dose (MTD), the dose at which toxicity but not death is observed; the lowest observed adverse effect level (LOAEL), the lowest concentration that still causes an adverse effect; and the no observed adverse effect level (NOAEL), the highest dose at which no adverse effects are induced (Figure 7.5A). During a chemical safety assessment, the NOAEL is usually divided by 10, 100, or 1000 depending on the level of uncertainty attributed to the data. Uncertainty factors typically take into account whether humans could be more sensitive than the animals used in toxicology studies, whether children will be more sensitive to chemical exposure than adults, and whether genetic

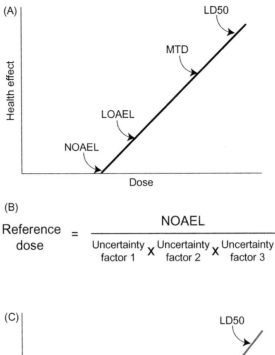

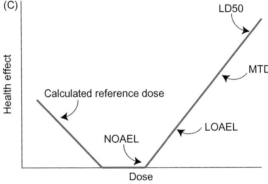

FIGURE 7.5   High-dose testing and low-dose extrapolation is not appropriate if NMDRC occur. (A) High doses—typically in the mg/kg range—are usually tested in traditional toxicology assessments. These high doses include the LD50, MTD, LOAEL, and NOAEL. (B) The reference dose, often considered the safe dose for humans or wildlife, is calculated by dividing the NOAEL by a number of uncertainty factors that are selected based on characteristics of the chemical and its uses. (C) In some circumstances, the reference dose could be hazardous if nonmonotonic relationships exist between dose and effect.

variability within the human population will lead some people to be more sensitive than others. After these uncertainty factors are applied and the NOAEL is divided, the resulting value is referred to as a "reference dose" (Figure 7.5B), which is generally considered safe for humans (or another target species). In this way, high-dose testing is extrapolated, using simple calculations, to obtain a lower, "safe" dose. This lower dose is rarely if ever tested.

What if there is a nonmonotonic relationship between dose and effect? In some circumstances, the dose that is deemed "safe" using extrapolations from high-dose testing, or lower doses, could be hazardous (Figure 7.5C). At the very least, NMDRCs challenge the dogma from chemical safety assessments that suggests that high-dose testing is sufficient to identify safe lower doses. How frequent must NMDRCs occur to challenge current risk assessment practices? This is a question that will need to be considered and answered by scientists and risk assessors alike.

7.8 LOW DOSE, A RELATED ISSUE

Discussions of nonmonotonicity almost always include the concept of *low dose*. Although related and important to the understanding of EDCs, the concepts of *nonmonotonicity* and *low dose* are actually distinct. The term *low dose* actually has a number of meanings [84]: (1) a dose below those used in traditional toxicology studies (i.e., doses below the NOAEL); (2) a dose in the range of typical human exposure; (3) a dose that produces circulating blood levels in experimental compounds that mimic the levels measured in humans. In this way, the term *low dose* sets a cutoff, and any effects observed below that cutoff would be considered "low-dose effects," regardless of what shape the dose response curve follows. NMDRCs could occur in the low-dose range, but they are not defined by the concentrations being tested; nonmonotonicity is strictly determined by whether the slope of the curve changes sign.

How is it that effects could be observed at doses below the NOAEL? The first explanation is that the type of study that is used to identify the NOAEL (and thus establish the cutoff for a low dose) does not examine every possible end point. Thus, it is possible that the effects observed at the low doses would also be observed at higher doses, if one were to look for them. The second explanation is that there is a nonmonotonic relationship between dose and the end point being examined.

Like nonmonotonicity, low-dose effects are expected for hormones, which operate in the body in extremely low concentrations—often in the part-per-billion or part-per-trillion concentration range [10]. At these low doses, hormones can maintain homeostasis and normal physiology in adults, and in developing individuals, they can induce the differentiation of tissues, reorganize specific regions of the brain, and change physiology and behavior [85]. In fact, studies from both litter-bearing rodents and human twins have revealed that exceptionally low differences in hormone exposures during fetal development (Figure 7.6) can shape a large number of end points, including organ size, reproductive success, and risk of adult diseases like breast cancer [86–88].

The presence of low-dose effects, regardless of how the low-dose cutoff is established, is strongly debated for EDCs [1,2,4,8–10,80]. The question of whether they exist is a relatively easy one to address: to state that they do not exist requires that the entire field of environmental epidemiology, which examines associations between chemical exposures (in human populations—and therefore at low doses) and health effects, be ignored or dismissed. In laboratory animals, there are now hundreds of studies that meet at least one of the definitions of a low-dose study [4,10,89–91]. Although some of these findings could be debated as to whether they have examined adverse, relevant end points, this does not negate that these phenomena are real.

Like NMDRCs, the presence of low-dose effects challenges current chemical safety assessment dogma. Many of the environmental epidemiology studies examine human populations where exposures are below the reference (safe) dose, yet they find associations

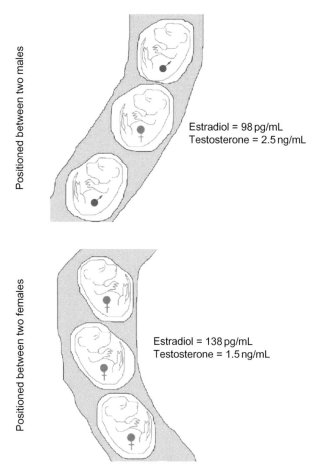

FIGURE 7.6   Small differences in hormone concentration are observed in rodents depending on their intrauterine position between male and female siblings. For example, female rodents positioned between two male fetuses will have slightly higher circulating testosterone levels, whereas females positioned between two female fetuses will have slightly higher circulating estradiol levels.

between exposures to these low doses and diseases or conditions of concern. If the safe dose is truly safe, how could this happen? It is exceedingly unlikely that all of these epidemiology studies are confounded by other environmental factors (like diet, stress, exercise, use of pharmaceuticals, etc.) What is much more likely is that the methods used to determine chemical safety are flawed [19,92–94].

7.9 CONCLUSIONS

NMDRCs and low-dose effects are considered principles of endocrinology and are expected in the study of hormones. These concepts are also widely accepted in other scientific disciplines, but they continue to be debated in the fields of toxicology and risk assessment. The mechanisms by which NMDRCs and low-dose effects occur are well understood for hormones. Because EDCs follow many of the same biological rules as hormones, it is not surprising that there are many examples of nonmonotonic responses, and effects observed at low doses, for these compounds. There are some unanswered questions in the study of these phenomena, but the question of whether they exist should be considered settled. Instead, exploration is needed as to whether these phenomena are significant enough to challenge current chemical safety assessment practices and how future safety assessments should be conducted instead.

References

[1] Lamb IV JC, Boffetta P, Foster WG, Goodman JE, Hentz KL, Rhomberg LR, et al. Critical comments on the WHO-UNEP State of the Science of Endocrine Disrupting Chemicals—2012. Regul Toxicol Pharmacol 2014;69:22–40.
[2] Bergman A, Heindel JJ, Kasten T, Kidd KA, Jobling S, Neira M, et al. The impact of endocrine disruption: a consensus statement on the state of the science. Environ Health Perspect 2013;121:A104–6.
[3] Vandenberg LN, Colborn T, Hayes TB, Heindel JJ, Jacobs DR, Lee DH, et al. Regulatory decisions on endocrine disrupting chemicals should be based on the principles of endocrinology. Reprod Toxicol 2013;38C:1–15.
[4] Zoeller RT, Brown TR, Doan LL, Gore AC, Skakkebaek NE, Soto AM, et al. Endocrine-disrupting chemicals and public health protection: a statement of principles from the Endocrine Society. Endocrinology 2012;153:4097–110.
[5] Borzelleca JF. Paracelsus: herald of modern toxicology. Toxicol Sci 2000;53:2–4.
[6] Kohn MC, Melnick RL. Biochemical origins of the non-monotonic receptor-mediated dose-response. J Mol Endocrinol 2002;29:113–23.
[7] Do RP, Stahlhut RW, Ponzi D, Vom Saal FS, Taylor JA. Non-monotonic dose effects of in utero exposure to di(2-ethylhexyl) phthalate (DEHP) on testicular and serum testosterone and anogenital distance in male mouse fetuses. Reprod Toxicol 2012;34:614–21.
[8] Dietrich DR, Aulock SV, Marquardt H, Blaauboer B, Dekant W, Kehrer J, et al. Scientifically unfounded precaution drives European Commission's recommendations on EDC regulation, while defying common sense, well-established science and risk assessment principles. Chem Biol Interact 2013;205:A1–5.
[9] Nohynek GJ, Borgert CJ, Dietrich D, Rozman KK. Endocrine disruption: fact or urban legend? Toxicol lett 2013;223:295–305.
[10] Vandenberg LN, Colborn T, Hayes TB, Heindel JJ, Jacobs Jr. DR, Lee DH, et al. Hormones and endocrine-disrupting chemicals: low-dose effects and nonmonotonic dose responses. Endocr Rev 2012;33:378–455.
[11] Gore AC, Heindel JJ, Zoeller RT. Endocrine disruption for endocrinologists (and others). Endocrinology 2006;147:S1–S3.
[12] McLeod DG. Hormonal therapy: historical perspective to future directions. Urology 2003;61:3–7.
[13] Arnold DJ, Markham MJ, Hacker S. Tamoxifen flare. JAMA 1979;241:2506.
[14] Plotkin D, Lechner JJ, Jung WE, Rosen PJ. Tamoxifen flare in advanced breast cancer. JAMA 1978;240:2644–6.
[15] Veldhuis JD, Santen RJ. Tamoxifen flare. JAMA 1979;241:2506–7.
[16] Wallach HW. Tamoxifen flare. JAMA 1979;242:27.
[17] Berin I, Stein DE, Keltz MD. A comparison of gonadotropin-releasing hormone (GnRH) antagonist and GnRH agonist flare protocols for poor responders undergoing in vitro fertilization. Fertil Steril 2010;93:360–3.
[18] Feldberg D, Farhi J, Ashkenazi J, Dicker D, Shalev J, Ben-Rafael Z. Minidose gonadotropin-releasing hormone agonist is the treatment of choice in poor responders with high follicle-stimulating hormone levels. Fertil Steril 1994;62:343–6.
[19] Myers JP, Zoeller RT, vom Saal FS. A clash of old and new scientific concepts in toxicity, with important implications for public health. Environ Health Perspect 2009;117:1652–5.
[20] Vandenberg LN, Wadia PR, Schaeberle CM, Rubin BS, Sonnenschein C, Soto AM. The mammary gland response to estradiol: monotonic at the cellular level, non-monotonic at the tissue-level of organization? J Steroid Biochem Mol Biol 2006;101:263–74.

[21] Wadia PR, Vandenberg LN, Schaeberle CM, Rubin BS, Sonnenschein C, Soto AM. Perinatal bisphenol A exposure increases estrogen sensitivity of the mammary gland in diverse mouse strains. Environ Health Perspect 2007;115:592–8.

[22] Skarda J, Kohlerova E. Mouse bioassay for *in vivo* screening of oestrogen and progesterone antagonists. J Vet Med A Physiol Pathol Clin Med 2006;53:145–53.

[23] Welshons WV, Thayer KA, Judy BM, Taylor JA, Curran EM, vom Saal FS. Large effects from small exposures: I. Mechanisms for endocrine-disrupting chemicals with estrogenic activity. Environ Health Perspect 2003;111:994–1006.

[24] Shioda T, Chesnes J, Coser KR, Zou L, Hur J, Dean KL, et al. Importance of dosage standardization for interpreting transcriptomal signature profiles: evidence from studies of xenoestrogens. Proc Natl Acad Sci USA 2006;103:12033–8.

[25] Ruige JB, Ouwens DM, Kauman JM. Beneficial and adverse effects of testosterone on the cardiovascular system in men. J Clin Endocrinol Metab 2013;98:4300–10.

[26] Querfeld U, Mak RH. Vitamin D deficiency and toxicity in chronic kidney disease: in search of the therapeutic window. Pediatr Nephrol 2010;25:2413–30.

[27] Chawla J, Kvarnberg D. Hydrosoluble vitamins. Handb Clin Neurol 2014;120:891–914.

[28] Soto AM, Sonnenschein C. The role of estrogens on the proliferation of human breast tumor cells (MCF-7). J Steroid Biochem 1985;23:87–94.

[29] Soto AM, Sonnenschein C. The two faces of Janus: sex steroids as mediators of both cell proliferation and cell death. J Natl Cancer Inst 2001;93:1673–5.

[30] Soto AM, Maffini MV, Schaeberle CM, Sonnenschein C. Strengths and weaknesses of *in vitro* assays for estrogenic and androgenic activity. Best Pract Res Clin Endocrinol Metab 2006;20:15–33.

[31] Soto AM, Lin T-M, Sakabe K, Olea N, Damassa DA, Sonnenschein C. Variants of the human prostate LNCaP cell line as a tool to study discrete components of the androgen-mediated proliferative response. Oncol Res 1995;7:545–58.

[32] Geck P, Maffini MV, Szelei J, Sonnenschein C, Soto AM. Androgen-induced proliferative quiescence in prostate cancer: the role of AS3 as its mediator. Proc Natl Acad Sci USA 2000;97:10185–90.

[33] Amara JF, Dannies PS. 17 beta-estradiol has a biphasic effect on gh cell growth. Endocrinology 1983;112:1141–3.

[34] Nandi S. Endocrine control of mammary gland development and function in the C3H/ He Crgl mouse. J Natl Cancer Inst 1958;21:1039–63.

[35] Humphreys RC, Krajewska M, Krnacik S, Jaeger R, Weiher H, Krajewski S, et al. Apoptosis in the terminal end bud of the murine mammary gland: a mechanism of ductal morphogenesis. Development 1996;122:4013–22.

[36] Attia GR, Zeitoun K, Edwards D, Johns A, Carr BR, Bulun SE. Progesterone receptor isoform A but not B is expressed in endometriosis. J Clin Endocrinol Metab 2000;85:2897–902.

[37] Kariagina A, Aupperlee MD, Haslam SZ. Progesterone receptor isoform functions in normal breast development and breast cancer. Crit Rev Eukaryot Gene Expr 2008;18:11–33.

[38] Morani A, Warner M, Gustafsson JA. Biological functions and clinical implications of oestrogen receptors alfa and beta in epithelial tissues. J Intern Med 2008;264:128–42.

[39] Watson CS, Bulayeva NN, Wozniak AL, Finnerty CC. Signaling from the membrane via membrane estrogen receptor-alpha: estrogens, xenoestrogens, and phytoestrogens. Steroids 2005;70:364–71.

[40] Watson CS, Gametchu B. Membrane-initiated steroid actions and the proteins that mediate them. Proc Soc Exp Biol Med 1999;220:9–19.

[41] Powell CE, Soto AM, Sonnenschein C. Identification and characterization of membrane estrogen receptor from MCF7 estrogen-target cells. J Steroid Biochem Mol Biol 2001;77:97–108.

[42] Sohoni P, Sumpter JP. Several environmental oestrogens are also anti-androgens. J Endocrinol 1998;158:327–39.

[43] Freedman NJ, Lefkowitz RJ. Desensitization of G protein-coupled receptors. Recent Prog Horm Res 1996;51:319–51.

[44] Bohm SK, Grady EF, Bunnett NW. Regulatory mechanisms that modulate signalling by G-protein-coupled receptors. Biochem J 1997;322:1–18.

[45] Lohse MJ. Molecular mechanisms of membrane receptor desensitization. Biochim Biophys Acta 1993;1179:171–88.

[46] Shankaran H, Wiley HS, Resat H. Receptor downregulation and desensitization enhance the information processing ability of signalling receptors. BMC Syst Biol 2007;1:48.

[47] Ismail A, Nawaz Z. Nuclear hormone receptor degradation and gene transcription: an update. IUBMB Life 2005;57:483–90.

[48] Kinyamu HK, Archer TK. Estrogen receptor-dependent proteasomal degradation of the glucocorticoid receptor is coupled to an increase in mdm2 protein expression. Mol Cell Biol 2003;23:5867–81.

[49] Carroll JS, Meyer CA, Song J, Li W, Geistlinger TR, Eeckhoute J, et al. Genome-wide analysis of estrogen receptor binding sites. Nat Genet 2006;38:1289–97.

[50] Maffini M, Denes V, Sonnenschein C, Soto A, Geck P. APRIN is a unique Pds5 paralog with features of a chromatin regulator in hormonal differentiation. J Steroid Biochem Mol Biol 2008;108:32–43.

[51] Haslam SZ. Mammary fibroblast influence on normal mouse mammary epithelial cell responses to estrogen *in vitro*. Cancer Res 1986;46:310–6.

[52] McGrath CM. Augmentation of the response of normal mammary epithelial cells to estradiol by mammary stroma. Cancer Res 1983;43:1355–60.

[53] Lesser B, Bruchovsky N. Effect of duration of the period after castration on the response of the rat ventral prostate to androgens. Biochem J 1974;142:429–31.

[54] Bruchovsky N, Lesser B, Van Doorn E, Craven S. Hormonal effects on cell proliferation in rat prostate. Vitam Horm 1975;33:61–102.

[55] Birnbaum LS. Environmental chemicals: evaluating low-dose effects. Environ Health Perspect 2012;120:A143–4.

[56] Habauzit D, Boudot A, Kerdivel G, Flouriot G, Pakdel F. Development and validation of a test for environmental estrogens: checking xeno-estrogen activity by CXCL12 secretion in BREAST CANCER CELL LINES (CXCL-test). Environ Toxicol 2010;25:495–503.

[57] Welshons WV, Nagel SC, Thayer KA, Judy BM, vom Saal FS. Low-dose bioactivity of xenoestrogens in animals: fetal exposure to low doses of methoxychlor and other xenoestrogens increases adult prostate size in mice. Toxicol Ind Health 1999;15:12–25.

[58] Pedro M, Lourenco CF, Cidade H, Kijoa A, Pinto M, Nascimento MS. Effects of natural prenylated flavones in the phenotypical ER (+) MCF-7 and ER (−) MDA-MB-231 human breast cancer cells. Toxicol Lett 2006;164:24–36.

[59] Soto AM, Fernandez MF, Luizzi MF, Oles Karasko AS, Sonnenschein C. Developing a marker of exposure to xenoestrogen mixtures in human serum. Environ Health Perspect 1997;105:647–54.

[60] Shelby MD, Newbold RR, Tully DB, Chae K, Davis VL. Assessing environmental chemicals for estrogenicity using a combination of *in vitro* and *in vivo* assays. Environ Health Perspect 1996;104:1296–300.

[61] Newbold RR, Jefferson WN, Padilla-Banks E, Haseman J. Developmental exposure to diethylstilbestrol (DES) alters uterine response to estrogens in prepubescent mice: low versus high dose effects. Reprod Toxicol 2004;18:399–406.

[62] Putz O, Schwartz CB, Kim S, LeBlanc GA, Cooper RL, Prins GS. Neonatal low- and high-dose exposure to estradiol benzoate in the male rat: I. Effects on the prostate gland. Biol Reprod 2001;65:1496–505.

[63] vom Saal FS, Timms BG, Montano MM, Palanza P, Thayer KA, Nagel SC, et al. Prostate enlargement in mice due to fetal exposure to low doses of estradiol or diethylstilbestrol and opposite effects at high doses. Proc Natl Acad Sci USA 1997;94:2056–61.

[64] Storrs SI, Kiesecker JM. Survivorship patterns of larval amphibians exposed to low concentrations of atrazine. Environ Health Perspect 2004;112:1054–7.

[65] Brodeur JC, Svartz G, Perez-Coll CS, Marino DJ, Herkovits J. Comparative susceptibility to atrazine of three developmental stages of *Rhinella arenarum* and influence on metamorphosis: non-monotonous acceleration of the time to climax and delayed tail resorption. Aquat Toxicol 2009;91:161–70.

[66] Freeman JL, Beccue N, Rayburn AL. Differential metamorphosis alters the endocrine response in anuran larvae exposed to T3 and atrazine. Aquat Toxicol 2005;75:263–76.

[67] Boccia MM, Kopf SR, Baratti CM. Phlorizin, a competitive inhibitor of glucose transport, facilitates memory storage in mice. Neurobiol Learn Mem 1999;71:104–12.

[68] Wisniewski AB, Cernetich A, Gearhart JP, Klein SL. Perinatal exposure to genistein alters reproductive development and aggressive behavior in male mice. Physiol Behav 2005;84:327–34.

[69] Lee DH, Porta M, Jacobs Jr. DR, Vandenberg LN. Chlorinated persistent organic pollutants, obesity, and type 2 diabetes. Endocr Rev 2014;35:557–601.

[70] Cho M-R, Shin J-Y, Hwang J-H, Jacobs DR, Kim S-Y, Lee D-H. Associations of fat mass and lean mass with bone mineral density differ by levels of persistent organic pollutants: National Health and Nutrition Examination Survey 1999–2004. Chemosphere 2011;82:1268–76.

[71] Shin J-Y, Choi YY, Jeon H-S, Hwang J-H, Kim S-A, Kang JH, et al. Low-dose persistent organic pollutants increased telomere length in peripheral leukocytes of healthy Koreans. Mutagenesis 2010;25:511–6.

[72] Trabert B, De Roos AJ, Schwartz SM, Peters U, Scholes D, Barr DB, et al. Non-dioxin-like polychlorinated biphenyls and risk of endometriosis. Environ Health Perspect 2010;118:1280–5.

[73] Claus Henn B, Ettinger AS, Schwartz J, Tellez-Rojo MM, Lamadrid-Figueroa H, Hernandez-Avila M, et al. Early postnatal blood manganese levels and children's neurodevelopment. Epidemiology 2010;21:433–9.

[74] Lee D-H, Lee IK, Porta M, Steffes M, Jacobs DR. Relationship between serum concentrations of persistent organic pollutants and the prevalence of metabolic syndrome among non-diabetic adults: results from the National Health and Nutrition Examination Survey 1999–2002. Diabetologia 2007;50:1841–51.

[75] Lee D-H, Steffes MW, Sjodin A, Jones RS, Needham LL, Jacobs DR. Low dose of some persistent organic pollutants predicts type 2 diabetes: a nested case-control study. Environ Health Perspect 2010;118:1235–42.

[76] Lee DH, Steffes MW, Sjodin A, Jones RS, Needham LL, Jacobs Jr. DR. Low dose organochlorine pesticides and polychlorinated biphenyls predict obesity, dyslipidemia, and insulin resistance among people free of diabetes. PLoS One 2011;6:e15977.

[77] Lim JS, Lee D-H, Jacobs DR. Association of brominated flame retardants with diabetes and metabolic syndrome in the U.S. population, 2003–2004. Diabetes Care 2008;31:1802–7.

[78] Davis JM, Svendsgaard DJ. Nonmonotonic dose-response relationships in toxicological studies Calabrese EJ, editor. Biological effects of low level exposures: dose–response relationships. Boca Raton, FL: Lewis Publishers; 1994. pp. 67–85.

[79] Vandenberg LN. Non-monotonic dose responses in studies of endocrine disrupting chemicals: bisphenol A as a case study. Dose Response 2013;12:259–76.

[80] Rhomberg LR, Goodman JE. Low-dose effects and nonmonotonic dose-responses of endocrine disrupting chemicals: has the case been made? Regul Toxicol Pharmacol 2012;64:130–3.

[81] Beausoleil C, Ormsby JN, Gies A, Hass U, Heindel JJ, Holmer ML, et al. Low dose effects and non-monotonic dose responses for endocrine active chemicals: science to practice workshop: workshop summary. Chemosphere 2013;93:847–56.

[82] EPA. State of the science evaluation: nonmonotonic dose responses as they apply to estrogen, androgen, and thyroid pathways and EPA testing and assessment procedures. Available at: <http://epa.gov/ncct/download_files/edr/NMDR.pdf>; 2013.

[83] NRC Research Council National Review of the environmental protection agency's state-of-the-science evaluation of nonmonotonic dose–response relationships as they apply to endocrine disruptors. Washington, DC: The National Academies Press; 2014.

[84] Melnick R, Lucier G, Wolfe M, Hall R, Stancel G, Prins G, et al. Summary of the National Toxicology Program's report of the endocrine disruptors low-dose peer review. Environ Health Perspect 2002;110:427–31.

[85] Diamanti-Kandarakis E, Bourguignon JP, Guidice LC, Hauser R, Prins GS, Soto AM, et al. Endocrine-disrupting chemical: an Endocrine Society scientific statement. Endocr Rev 2009;30:293–342.

[86] Lummaa V, Pettay JE, Russell AF. Male twins reduce fitness of female co-twins in humans. Proc Natl Acad Sci USA 2007;104:10915–20.

[87] Swerdlow AJ, De Stavola BL, Swanwick MA, Maconochie NES. Risks of breast and testicular cancers in young adult twins in England and Wales: evidence on prenatal and genetic aetiology. Lancet 1997;350:1723–8.

[88] Ryan BC, Vandenbergh JG. Intrauterine position effects. Neurosci Biobehav Rev 2002;26:665–78.

[89] Vandenberg LN, Ehrlich S, Belcher SM, Ben-Jonathan N, Dolinoy DC, Hugo ER, et al. Low dose effects of bisphenol A: an integrated review of in vitro, laboratory animal and epidemiology studies. Endocrine Disruptors 2013;1:e25078.

[90] Richter C, Birnbaum LS, Farabollini F, Newbold RR, Rubin BS, Talsness CE, et al. In vivo effects of bisphenol A in laboratory rodent studies. Reprod Toxicol 2007;24:199–224.

[91] WHO. State of the science of endocrine disrupting chemicals—2012. An assessment of the state of the science of endocrine disruptors prepared by a group of experts for the United Nations Environment Programme (UNEP) and WHO (WHO/UNEP, ed.). Available at: <http://unep.org/pdf/9789241505031_eng.pdf>; 2013.

[92] Myers JP, vom Saal FS, Akingbemi BT, Arizono K, Belcher S, Colborn T, et al. Why public health agencies cannot depend upon 'Good Laboratory Practices' as a criterion for selecting data: the case of bisphenol-A. Environ Health Perspect 2009;117:309–15.

[93] vom Saal FS, Akingbemi BT, Belcher SM, Crain DA, Crews D, Guidice LC, et al. Flawed experimental design reveals the need for guidelines requiring appropriate positive controls in endocrine disruption research. Toxicol Sci 2010;115:612–3.

[94] vom Saal FS, Myers JP. Good laboratory practices are not synonymous with good scientific practices, accurate reporting, or valid data. Environ Health Perspect 2010;118:A60.

CONCERNS FOR HUMAN HEALTH

8

Endocrine Disruption and Female Reproductive Health

Philippa D. Darbre

OUTLINE

8.1 Introduction   144

8.2 Major Targets of Endocrine
    Disruption for Female
    Reproductive Health   145

8.3 Sources of Endocrine Disruption
    for Female Reproductive Health   147

8.4 Exposure to DES and Consequences
    for Female Reproductive Health   148

8.5 Pubertal Development   149
    8.5.1 Physiological Changes in Puberty   149
    8.5.2 Estrogens in Hair Products That
          Advance Pubertal Changes   150
    8.5.3 Epidemiological Evidence for
          Alterations to Pubertal Timing   150

8.6 Disorders of the Ovary   151
    8.6.1 Premature Ovarian Failure   151
    8.6.2 Irregularity of Menstrual
          Cycles and Fecundity   151
    8.6.3 Menopause   152
    8.6.4 Polycystic Ovary Syndrome   152

8.7 Uterine Disorders   153
    8.7.1 Uterine Fibroids   153
    8.7.2 Endometriosis   153

8.8 Benign Breast Disease   154

8.9 Final Comments   155

References   156

Abstract

This chapter provides an overview of evidence suggesting a role for endocrine-disrupting chemicals (EDCs) in altered timing of female puberty, disorders of ovarian function, and benign abnormalities of the uterus and breast. Evidence that prenatal exposure to exogenous estrogen can affect female reproductive health after birth is demonstrated by the development of rare vaginal cancers and other adverse reproductive outcomes in daughters born to women who had taken diethylstilbestrol (DES) during pregnancy. The reversibility of a case of abnormal menstrual bleeding in a 3-year old girl by ceasing the use of

Endocrine Disruption and Human Health.
DOI: http://dx.doi.org/10.1016/B978-0-12-801139-3.00008-9

an estrogen-containing hair lotion demonstrates the potent effects of exogenous estrogens used in personal care products on the pubertal process. However, evidence that EDCs contribute to other conditions rests on animal models, experimental cell cultures, and correlative epidemiology. It is likely that most reproductive abnormalities arise from long-term, low-dose exposure to complex mixtures of EDCs, which makes identification of sources of causative agents a challenge.

8.1 INTRODUCTION

The reproductive health of women depends on maintaining coordinated responses of a network of endocrine signals that function primarily to ensure successful procreation but also have other wide-ranging influences on the female body, including not only secondary reproductive tissues such as the breast, but also nonreproductive tissues such as the bone, brain, and cardiovascular system. Consequences of any disrupting influences can be expected, therefore, not only to influence fertility, but to have wide repercussions for female health more generally. Furthermore, since women have the responsibility of carrying the baby through the very delicate formative stages of embryonic and fetal life until birth, consequences of the choices made by the mother can have repercussions for the future reproductive health of the child. In this context, it is essential to remember that the placenta is itself an endocrine organ and that the placenta allows the transfer of materials from mother to child. This chapter will address the consequences of endocrine disruption for puberty and menopause, for ovarian function, and for benign abnormalities of female reproductive tissues, including ovary [premature ovarian failure (POF), polycystic ovary], uterus (fibroids, endometriosis), and breast (cysts, fibroadenoma) (Figure 8.1). Issues surrounding

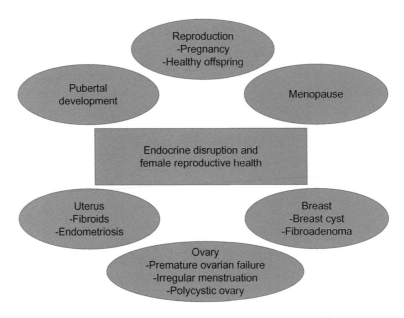

FIGURE 8.1   Consequences of endocrine disruption for female reproductive health.

the development of cancers of reproductive tissues will be discussed in a later chapter of this book (Chapter 10). The consequences of fetal exposure to endocrine-disrupting chemicals (EDCs) for adult disease and transgenerational influences of EDCs will be themes throughout this entire section of this book (Chapters 8–15).

8.2 MAJOR TARGETS OF ENDOCRINE DISRUPTION FOR FEMALE REPRODUCTIVE HEALTH

Estrogens and progesterone are essential hormones in the reproductive health of women. The rise in estrogen synthesis from the ovary heralds the start of reproductive life at puberty, and the reduction in estrogen synthesis at menopause closes the reproductive life of a woman. During the reproductive years, estradiol and progesterone are produced from the ovary in a cyclical manner during the various phases of the menstrual cycle (Figure 8.2), and this is under neuroendocrine control (Figure 8.3). Secretion of gonadotropin-releasing hormone (GnRH) from the hypothalamus and luteinizing hormone (LH)/follicle-stimulating hormone (FSH) from the pituitary regulate the secretion of estradiol from the granulosa cells of the ovary and progesterone from the corpus luteum (Figure 8.3). For each 28-day cycle, ovulation occurs at the midpoint and levels of estradiol rise once during the first half of the cycle and once again during the second half of the cycle. Progesterone levels rise only in the second half of the cycle following formation of the corpus luteum (Figure 8.2). If after ovulation, the oocyte is fertilized, then implantation interrupts these cyclical changes in order

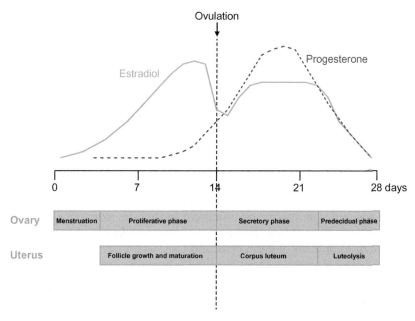

FIGURE 8.2   A schematic diagram showing changes in relative levels of secretion of estradiol and progesterone during the 28 days of the menstrual cycle. Ovulation occurs on day 14.

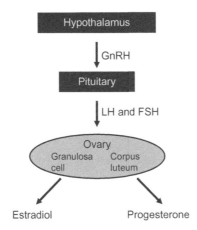

FIGURE 8.3   Neuroendocrine control of secretion of estradiol and progesterone from the ovary. GnRH from the hypothalamus and LH/FSH from the pituitary regulate production of estradiol from the granulosa cells of the ovary and progesterone from the corpus luteum.

to establish a pregnancy, and the increase in levels of progesterone relative to estrogens is essential not only for maintenance of the pregnancy, but also for many of the physiological changes in the female body during pregnancy, including differentiation of the mammary glands in preparation for lactation. The rise in levels of human chorionic gonadotropin in early pregnancy are essential to the establishment and maintenance of the embryo, and during later pregnancy, the altered hormonal milieu of the breast causes lobuloalveolar structures to form and the increase in levels of prolactin become essential for the establishment of lactation. All these elegant endocrine controls are essential for female reproductive health, and any disruption to hormonal homeostasis, especially to the balance between levels of estrogen and progesterone or their cycling, will have consequences both for the processes of fertility/pregnancy/childbirth and for female health more generally.

One of the most important considerations for endocrine disruption and female reproductive health is the timing of exposure. While exposure to EDCs may be expected to affect adult life, there is increasing evidence that some adult female reproductive health problems may be programmed by exposures in the early embryo or fetus in utero [1]. The in utero exposure may be all that is needed for the development of adverse consequences in adult life without any need for subsequent exposure, and furthermore, the consequences may pass to future generations again without any requirement for further exposure. This places considerable responsibility on the mother to ensure a safe uterine environment for her developing child during the very delicate formative stages of embryonic and fetal development. In this context, it is important to remember that the development of germ cells into follicles for egg production occurs in early embryonic/fetal life and that a woman is born with her full complement of follicles. Unlike sperm, follicles are not produced during adult life; rather, they only undergo further development of what is already there, and therefore any damage sustained in utero already would be present in adult life. Much of the support for the fetal origin of adult disease comes from the use of the synthetic estrogen diethylstilbestrol (DES) in pregnancy, which is now known to have consequences not only for the mother, but also for her children (see Section 8.4).

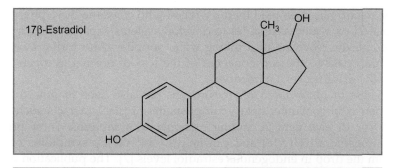

FIGURE 8.4   The chemical structures of diethylstilbestrol and ethinyl estradiol compared with 17β-estradiol.

8.3 SOURCES OF ENDOCRINE DISRUPTION FOR FEMALE REPRODUCTIVE HEALTH

There has been an unprecedented rise over recent decades in the global use of synthetic hormones both as oral contraceptives to enable freedom of sexual activity without consequent pregnancy and as hormone replacement therapy (HRT) to counter menopausal symptoms. Use of these pharmaceuticals has become engrained as an integral part of the social fabric of society and are taken by many women without any regard to the wider implications of the long-term use of such drugs not only for their own long-term endocrine health, but also for the distribution of the drugs into the environment. Ethinyl estradiol (Figure 8.4), the main synthetic estrogen in oral contraceptives, is now detectable in waterways in the United States [2] and Europe [3] and is known to have adverse effects on reproduction in fish [4,5]. Little regard has been paid by the women who consume these pharmaceuticals to the burdens placed on water companies to develop systems capable of adequately removing these drugs for the recycling of drinking water supplies. And furthermore, inadequate attention has been paid to the consequences of the loss of normal estrogen/progesterone homeostasis in the drive for sexual freedom.

The effectiveness of plant-based phytoestrogens has also been embraced by the populations of women who consume dietary supplements of plant extracts such as soy, black cohosh, red clover, or aloe vera to counter menopausal symptoms. These phytoestrogens have potent estrogenic activity [6] and can help to relieve the symptoms of menopause, which arise from the drop in endogenous estradiol levels [7]. The publication of a study of a million women that linked HRT to increased risk of breast cancer [8] served to drive many women to seek more "natural" alternatives to the synthetic hormones of HRT [7].

In addition to the pharmaceuticals and plant products, the many environmental contaminants with endocrine-disrupting properties found in diet, the domestic environment, and personal care products have potential to further add to the threat to female reproductive health. A large body of literature testifies to the reproductive effects of environmental EDCs on female reproduction in wildlife [5], but many hundreds of these same chemicals now have been measured in human body tissues. Since the effects of exposure to chemicals cannot be tested directly in humans, it is a sad fact that consequences are often first assessed following accidents or inadvertent exposure. The long-term consequences of exposure of women to high doses of estrogen has become visible following the exposure of many women to the synthetic estrogen DES, which was administered from the 1940s to the 1970s to prevent miscarriage, and the consequences extend from not only the women exposed, but also to their offspring who were exposed in utero (see Section 8.4) [9].

8.4 EXPOSURE TO DES AND CONSEQUENCES FOR FEMALE REPRODUCTIVE HEALTH

DES is a synthetic nonsteroidal estrogen that was first synthesized in 1938 [10] and then prescribed to several million women between 1940 and 1971 to prevent the threat of miscarriage in the first trimester [11]. The structure of DES can be seen to share many similarities to that of 17β-estradiol (Figure 8.4), which explains its potent estrogenic activity. In 1971, it was reported to have caused a rare vaginal tumor in daughters born to women who had taken DES during pregnancy and therefore who had been exposed in utero [12], and as a result, further prescription ceased. However, it is estimated that 5–10 million people in the United States, 300,000 in the United Kingdom, and 200,000 in France were exposed either through taking the drug during pregnancy or through exposure in utero [9]. Over the following years, in vivo studies have shown that DES causes tumors in estrogen-sensitive tissues in several animal species and can cause tumors in adult animals following prenatal exposure [9]. Neonatal exposure can irreversibly damage the reproductive system in other ways that also result in early puberty and reduced fertility [9]. Long-term follow-up studies of the daughters born to DES-treated mothers have demonstrated that in utero exposure of women to DES is associated with an increased lifetime risk of a wide range of adverse reproductive health outcomes, listed in Table 8.1 [13]. Animal studies demonstrate that effects of DES exposure in utero can pass down to the F2 and F3 generations through

TABLE 8.1   Adverse Health Outcomes in Women Exposed to DES In Utero

Health outcome	Cumulative risk		Hazard ratio	95% Confidence interval
	Unexposed women (%)	Women exposed in utero (%)		
Infertility	15.5	33.3	2.37	2.05–2.75
Spontaneous abortion	38.6	50.3	1.64	1.42–1.88
Preterm delivery	17.8	53.3	4.68	3.74–5.86
Loss of second-trimester pregnancy	1.7	16.4	3.77	2.56–5.54
Ectopic pregnancy	2.9	14.6	3.72	2.58–5.38
Preeclampsia	13.7	26.4	1.42	1.07–1.89
Stillbirth	2.6	8.9	2.45	1.33–4.54
Early menopause	1.7	5.1	2.35	1.67–3.31
Grade 2 or greater cervical intraepithelial neoplasia	3.4	6.9	2.28	1.59–3.27
Breast cancer at 40 years of age or older	2.2	3.9	1.82	1.04–3.18

As Published by Hoover et al. in 2011 [13].
$n = 4653$ for exposed women; $n = 1927$ for unexposed controls.

heritable changes in gene expression (from histone modification, DNA methylation, or microRNA expression) [9]. Although it is too early to yet ascertain any F2 or F3 transgenerational effects in the DES-exposed daughters, the consequences documented in the F1 generation demonstrate that exposure to a synthetic estrogen in the fetal life of a woman can have consequences for her health in later adult life, even without any further exposure after birth. However, the fact that not every DES-exposed daughter had adverse symptoms emphasizes the diversity in response between individuals and demonstrates the difficulty in identifying causative agents where varied susceptibility influences outcomes.

8.5 PUBERTAL DEVELOPMENT

8.5.1 Physiological Changes in Puberty

Puberty is an endocrine-regulated developmental process of late childhood in which alterations lead to maturation of secondary sexual characteristics and to the attainment of reproductive capacity [14]. Changes occur in reproductive hormones, most notably in an increase in estrogen in the female, but there are also increases in progesterone and adrenal hormones. Profound changes occur in amount and regional distribution of body fat, which is significant because fat can both produce and store steroid hormones. Many EDCs are also fat soluble, and body fat therefore can act as a depot for complex mixtures of environmental chemicals from a range of external sources. The onset of puberty is also associated with physiological insulin resistance, making it a sensitive time for disruption of insulin homeostasis, and it is also a time of complex psychological and behavioral changes.

8.5.2 Estrogens in Hair Products That Advance Pubertal Changes

A pertinent report was published in 2008 of the case of a 36-month old girl who presented with vaginal bleeding, uterus enlargement, and thelarche (breast development) following exposure to ethinyl estradiol contained in her mother's hair lotion [15]. The child was in the habit of playing with her mother's hair, her mother's combs, and the empty lotion bottles. Analysis of long scalp hairs revealed ethinyl estradiol concentrations of $10.6\,\mu g/g$ in the girl's hair and $46.6\,\mu g/g$ in the mother's hair, although nothing was detectable in their blood or urine. Six months after discontinuation of the estrogen-containing hair lotion, the girl's hyperestrogenic symptoms resolved, which serves as a reminder of the potent effects of exogenous synthetic estrogens used in personal care products on the pubertal process [15]. However, what is also important about such a case is that the clinical symptoms could be reversed, therefore enabling the causative factor to be unequivocally identified.

This was not an isolated case. Another report of premature thelarche, pubic hair, or both has been published in four African-American girls that also experienced relief after their mothers ceased using estrogen- or placenta-containing hair products on the girls [16].

8.5.3 Epidemiological Evidence for Alterations to Pubertal Timing

Much research has focused on the timing of puberty because both thelarche (breast development) and menarche (occurrence of first menstruation) occur at an earlier age in girls today (13 years) compared to a century ago (17 years), and studies over recent decades suggest a further linear decline in age of puberty in many Western countries [17–19]. Heritable patterns in the age of menarche demonstrate genetic determinants [20], but there are also environmental factors because many studies now attest to children adopted into Western lifestyles from undeveloped countries having a reduced age of puberty. An early study reported the median menarcheal age of 107 girls adopted from India by families in Sweden to be 11.6 years, significantly lower than in Swedish and most Indian studies. Five girls had menarche before the age of 9 years, the earliest at 7.3 years [21]. Studies of adoption into a range of other Western countries report similar findings [17–18]. Improved nutrition and better living conditions may have contributed to the decline of age at menarche, but the speed of the transition indicates an influence of endocrine-disrupting elements from the environment.

On the basis of average age of onset of puberty in current decades, abnormally precocious puberty has been defined as occurring at less than 8 years of age [17]. Outbreaks of precocious puberty have been reported in Italy [22] and in Puerto Rico [23]. In a school in Milan, Italy, girls aged 3–5 (21.6%) and aged 6–7 (67.1%) had significantly enlarged breast growth compared to age-matched controls in other schools; and although the cause was never established, the outbreak was suspected to relate to an uncontrolled supply of poultry and beef [22]. Since age-matched Puerto Rican girls living in the United States do not have precocious puberty and other nationalities living in Puerto Rico do [24], studies have tried to identify causative exposure to specific EDCs in Puerto Rico; but so far, only phthalates have been shown to be associated as raised in the serum of those with precocious puberty [25]. Significantly raised levels of phthalates [dimethyl, diethyl, dibutyl, and di-(2-ethylhexyl)] and its major metabolite mono-(2-ethylhexyl)phthalate were identified in 28 (68%) samples from thelarche patients ($n = 41$). Of the control samples ($n = 35$) analyzed, only one showed significant levels of diisooctyl phthalate [25]. Following on from this study, many other measurements have been made of urinary or serum levels of chlorinated pesticides [dichlorodiphenyltrichloroethane (DDT), dichlorodiphenyldichloroethylene (DDE)], polychlorinated biphenyls (PCBs), dioxins, polybrominated biphenyls, bisphenol A (BPA), lead, and cadmium in girls with precocious puberty compared to age-matched controls, but no simple picture has emerged [18].

8.6 DISORDERS OF THE OVARY

The function of the ovary is to produce eggs for fertilization. The differentiation of germ cells in the ovaries begins in the first trimester of pregnancy, and during later stages of pregnancy, immature follicles (primordial) are formed such that a woman is born with a full complement of follicles. Each egg (oocyte) is contained within an ovarian follicle, and in a cycling adult ovary, there are follicles at different stages of development. Primordial follicles can develop into preovulatory follicles and then antral follicles by a process termed *folliculogenesis.* It is the antral follicles that contain the oocyte surrounded by granulosa and thecal cells, which are the major source of ovarian steroids and which are capable of ovulation. After ovulation or expulsion of the oocyte from the follicle, the remaining granulosa and thecal cells become luteal cells and the remaining follicular structure becomes the corpus luteum. It is the corpus luteum that then produces progesterone, which is necessary for successful implantation of a fertilized oocyte and for maintenance of pregnancy. Disruption of ovarian function by EDCs can lead to a range of adverse outcomes, such as anovulation, infertility, estrogen deficiency, POF, and ovarian cyst development [26].

8.6.1 Premature Ovarian Failure

POF occurs in about 1% of women under the age of 40 and leads to reproductive disorders and early menopause [27]. The mechanisms may involve improper prenatal development of the fetal gonad or disruption of the postnatal processes of folliculogenesis, causing blockage of follicle maturation, premature activation of the follicle, or increased apoptosis. However, a potential precursor is the development of multioocyte follicles (MOFs), and exposure to some EDCs has been shown to cause MOFs in animal models. Neonatal exposure to DES has been shown to cause MOFs in mice, which seems to be an ERβ-mediated mechanism because it was not different in ERalpha knockout mice but was reduced in ERbeta knockout mice [28]. Early postnatal exposure to parabens has been shown to inhibit the early phase of folliculogenesis in rats, which could be mediated through their ability to also stimulate messenger RNA (mRNA) for the anti-Müllerian hormone (AMH) [29]. In addition, 4-vinylcyclohexene diepoxide can destroy selectively primordial follicles in rats and mice [30]. Exposure of adult mice and rats to methoxychlor can cause ovarian atrophy, again due to the inhibition of folliculogenesis [31].

8.6.2 Irregularity of Menstrual Cycles and Fecundity

Interference in hormonal regulation of the menstrual cycle may result in irregular or altered cycle length that could reduce fecundity (ability to conceive in a menstrual cycle). Studies in humans have shown that exposure to organochlorine compounds or pesticides can interfere with length and regularity of the menstrual cycle. A study of Taiwanese mothers showed that those with longer (>33 days) or irregular menstrual cycles had higher total levels of polychlorinated dibenzo-*p*-dioxins, dibenzofurans, and biphenyls in placental tissue [32]. In Sweden, the major route of exposure to persistent organochlorine compounds is through consumption of fatty fish from the Baltic Sea, and women who consumed higher levels of this fish were found to have shorter menstrual cycles [33]. A study of women applying pesticides on farms in Iowa and North Carolina were found to have longer cycles and increased odds of missed periods than women who had never worked with pesticides, and this increased further for women working with hormonally active pesticides [34]. Animal studies support these findings and show that even exposure in utero to phytoestrogens, BPA, or DES can increase the length of the menstrual cycle in adult female mice [35].

8.6.3 Menopause

Menopause occurs during the late 40s or early 50s of a woman's life and is characterized by a cessation of ovarian function that leads to the absence of menstruation. Age at menopause has implications for both fertility and risk of hormone-related chronic diseases. A study of exposure to pesticides has reported a significant delay in menopause for women who had worked mixing and applying pesticides compared to those who had never used pesticides [36].

For some women, the hormonal changes that occur during menopause resulting in lack of energy, hot flushes, and mood changes can severely disrupt normal life, and they seek use of hormone replacement therapies. The risks associated with synthetic hormones [8] has driven women to seek alternative, more "natural" approaches [7]. The effectiveness of self-dosing on a range of plant extracts that contain potent phytoestrogens such as soy, red clover, or black cohosh testify to the ability of these products to alleviate menopausal symptoms. However, the long-term consequences need evaluation [7]. For example, one 5-year study of 376 healthy postmenopausal women showed that those who received 150 mg/day of isoflavones had a significant increase of endometrial hyperplasia [37].

8.6.4 Polycystic Ovary Syndrome

Polycystic ovary syndrome (PCOS) is one of the most common female endocrine disorders; the World Health Organization (WHO) in 2010 estimated that it affects 116 million women worldwide, which amounts to 3.4% of the global female population [38]. In general, it occurs in 5–10% of women of reproductive age and is thought to be a leading cause of female subfertility. It is characterized by multiple ovarian cysts, which are immature follicles where development has been arrested and are visible using ultrasound imaging. Symptoms include irregular menstruation, reduced numbers of menstrual periods, and insulin resistance, and it is associated with excess production of ovarian androgens, especially testosterone. PCOS shows familial clustering and greater coincidence in monozygotic than dizygotic twins, which indicates inherited susceptibility; and this susceptibility seems to operate in an autosomal-dominant manner. However, there is also an environmental component, and there are serious concerns as to whether endocrine disrupters (particularly BPA) might play a role in the etiology of this condition.

Animal models have shown that exposure to BPA during the prenatal period in mice [39] and sheep [40] and the neonatal period in rats [41] can disrupt ovarian function as the animals reach adulthood, and the studies in mice and rats specifically noted the development of a large number of ovarian cysts. In human populations, serum levels of BPA have been reported to be increased in women with PCOS [42], and increased levels of BPA in PCOS women have been shown to correlate positively with higher levels of testosterone and androstenedione [43]. It is, therefore, possible that BPA plays a role in the pathogenesis of PCOS [44].

8.7 UTERINE DISORDERS

The uterus is an endocrine-sensitive organ that functions as the site where the fetus develops during gestation. Effects of endocrine disruption could be anticipated, therefore, to result in uterine abnormalities. Uterine fibroids and endometriosis are the most common benign uterine disorders and the potential for EDCs to affect these conditions is discussed next.

8.7.1 Uterine Fibroids

Uterine fibroids are common benign tumors that affect up to 25% of white women and 70% of black women and can cause infertility and abnormal bleeding [1]. They arise in the myometrium as benign tumors of uterine smooth muscle tissue termed *leiomyomas*, mainly between puberty and menopause. Fibroid growth is strongly dependent on estrogen and progesterone, and therefore the potential exists for EDCs to play a role in their development [1]. A recent study has reported raised levels of some PCB congeners in the omental (lower abdominal) fat in women with fibroids [45]. Another study has reported raised levels of BPA in the urine of women with fibroids compared to those without [46]. In vitro studies have demonstrated that BPA can increase not only the growth of uterine leiomyoma cells [47], but also enable their migration and invasion [48]. In vivo studies have reported that neonatal exposure (days 1–5) to BPA in mice results in leiomyomas in adulthood (18 months) [49].

8.7.2 Endometriosis

Endometriosis is a condition in which cells from the lining of the uterus (endometrium) grow outside the uterine cavity, most commonly in the peritoneum or pelvic region. The main symptoms of this disease include pelvic pain and abnormalities to menstruation, and it can be associated with infertility. This condition occurs in around 6–10% of women, but the causes remain to be established. It has been associated with genetic predisposition and the use of Caesarian section at childbirth, but endometrial tissue is strongly influenced by estrogen, and this condition is associated with low progesterone levels and involves immune modulation. Therefore, it is thought that there is a likely environmental EDC component and that environmental organochlorinated pollutants (in particular dioxins and PCBs) may be involved because they are known to modulate both endocrine and immune function [50]. Studies in monkeys have shown that exposure to 2,3,7,8-tetrachlorodibenzo-*p*-dioxin increases the incidence and severity of endometriosis in a dose-dependent manner and that the dioxin-exposed monkeys have immune abnormalities similar to those in women with endometriosis [51]. Studies in rats support these results [52], and mouse models show that other polyhalogenated aromatic hydrocarbons that can bind to the aryl hydrocarbon receptor (AhR) can also cause endometriosis [53] and that mice are particularly susceptible when exposed during the perinatal period [54]. Many studies have been conducted to measure levels of organochlorine compounds in urine or serum in patients with or without endometriosis, but any differences remain inconsistent.

Animal models also attest to the ability of other EDCs to cause endometriosis. Perinatal exposure of female mice to BPA has been shown in one study to cause endometrial hyperplasia [49], and in other studies to lead to the development of endometriosis [55,56]. However, translation to human exposure studies has been less conclusive in that measurement of urinary BPA levels were higher in women with endometriosis in one study [57] but not another [58]. One study reported raised levels of BPA in the serum of infertile women, and there also were raised levels of PPARγ in those women with endometriosis in the infertile group [59]. One study showed an association of endometriosis with raised levels of some phthalate metabolites [60]. Further follow-up of DES-exposed daughters has suggested that they also have a higher incidence of endometriosis [61].

8.8 BENIGN BREAST DISEASE

Among breast diseases, breast cancer has the highest profile and attracts the greatest attention because of its associated mortality, but in terms of incidence, it represents only about 5% of clinical abnormalities of the breast. Other major breast abnormalities include fibroadenomas and breast cysts [62]. Gross cystic breast disease is the most common benign breast disorder estimated to affect up to 7% of Western women [62]. In this condition, palpable cysts over 3 mm in diameter arise from dilation and/or obstruction of terminal duct lobular units and are associated with retention of fluid and secretory material of the lining epithelial cells [63]. Fibroadenomas are benign tumors composed of fibrous and glandular tissue, which also arise in terminal duct lobular units. Both these conditions occur most frequently prior to menopause, indicating their hormonal dependence. The reasons for such high levels of benign breast diseases remain unknown, but it has been suggested that EDCs may be contributory environmental factors [64,65], and animal models have demonstrated that many EDCs can disrupt normal mammary gland development in rodents [66].

It is interesting to note that many benign breast conditions, such as fibroadenomas, cysts [67], and phyllodes tumors [68], occur at a disproportionately high rate in the upper outer quadrant of the breast, and it has been pointed out previously that this is also the site of application of EDCs in underarm cosmetics [64,65]. Cultural practices over recent decades have made underarm sweating socially unacceptable, and in response, many people in the population apply antiperspirant and deodorant products many times a day to the underarm. This leaves the associated chemical constituents (including any EDCs) on the skin, which allows continuous exposure and consequent absorption at low levels into underlying tissues [64,65].

On the basis that aluminum-based antiperspirant salts act to stop underarm perspiration by blocking sweat ducts under the arm [69], and breast cysts arise from blocked breast ducts [62,63] in the adjacent region of the body, it has been suggested that breast cysts might arise from antiperspirant use if sufficient aluminum were absorbed into underlying breast tissues over long-term usage [64,65]. Levels of aluminum have been found to be substantially raised in breast cyst fluid compared to blood serum [70], which demonstrates the presence of high levels of aluminum in the vicinity of the cysts, even although the source of the aluminum cannot be identified from this study.

Immunohistochemical studies of breast fibroadenomas have reported raised levels of AhRs, which may be indicative of a sensitivity of these cells to environmental chemicals [71]. Studies are now needed to investigate whether specific environmental chemicals may be related to the development of these benign tumors.

8.9 FINAL COMMENTS

This chapter has provided an overview of the emerging evidence that EDCs may affect female reproductive health. The challenge remains to identify the causative factors for such a range of adverse health outcomes in different tissues. The reversibility of the effects of components in hair lotions on initiating early menstruation is very important since it enables the environmental causative factor to be identified unequivocally, but very few cases are so easy to solve or are even reversible at all. The adverse consequences associated with the use of DES in pregnancy have served to demonstrate that exposure to a potent estrogen can have adverse effects not only for the mother, but for the daughters exposed in utero, and therefore have highlighted the potential of a fetal origin for adult disease. However, the fact that not all daughters had symptoms (or even the same symptoms) emphasizes the variability in responses that can be expected even from known causative agents.

At the current time, most research has focused on studying associations of single chemicals with a particular disease outcome. However, future research will need to take much more account of the ability of mixtures of EDCs at low doses over the long term to give rise to adverse consequences. Many EDCs have overlapping properties, and therefore small concentrations of hundreds of chemicals may work together to achieve a significant effect that would not be visible for each component alone. This has been demonstrated in cell culture experiments for estrogenic activity of mixtures of parabens [72] and other xenoestrogens [73] and in fish in vivo for mixtures of xenoestrogens [74]. Furthermore, since varied lifestyles will result in different exposures to EDCs, it can be expected that specific outcomes may be generated by different EDC mixtures. Measurements of EDCs in the urine or blood of women with specific clinical symptoms is a useful first approach, but it has several pitfalls, in that many different EDCs may be able to generate the same outcome (and as a result, there will not be raised levels of any one EDC in all cases of a specific outcome). Furthermore, levels in urine or blood may not always reflect levels in the target tissues of the ovary, uterus, or breast.

A report in 1946 from West Australian farmers that sheep grazing on certain clovers become infertile [75] should have served as an early warning of endocrine disruption, but perhaps it has been too often dismissed as something that happens only to sheep in the countryside in a distant land. Many female reproductive health problems are increasing in conjunction with the increasing release into the environment of industrial chemicals with analogous properties, and many of these chemicals have been established as entering the human body by being present in urine or blood. At the moment, the research seems to progress on "bandwagons," but the real need is to find more ways of reversing conditions by precautionary intervention so that causative agents and mixtures can be identified and then avoided. There is also an urgent need to educate women about the importance of understanding the need to alter their lifestyles to avoid potentially damaging chemical exposure during pregnancy.

References

[1] McLachlan JA, Simpson E, Martin M. Endocrine disrupters and female reproductive health. Best Pract Res Clin Endocrinol Metab 2006;20:63–75.

[2] Kolpin DW, Furlong ET, Meyer MT, Thurman EM, Zaugg SD, Barber LB, et al. Pharmaceuticals, hormones, and other organic wastewater contaminants in US streams, 1999–2000: a national reconnaissance. Environ Sci Technol 2002;36:1202–11.

[3] Johnson AC, Dumont E, Williams RJ, Oldenkamp R, Cisowska I, Sumpter JP. Do concentrations of ethinyl-estradiol, estradiol, and diclofenac in European rivers exceed proposed EU environmental quality standards? Environ Sci Technol 2013;47:12297–304.

[4] Caldwell DJ, Mastrocco F, Hutchinson TH, Lange R, Heijerick D, Janssen C, et al. Derivation of an aquatic predicted no-effect concentration for the synthetic hormone, 17 alpha-ethinyl estradiol. Environ Sci Technol 2008;42:7046–54.

[5] Berkman A, Heindel JJ, Jobling S, Kidd KA, Zoeller RT, editors. State of the science of endocrine disrupting chemicals—2012. United Nations Environment Programme and the World Health Organization; 2013.

[6] Woods HF (chairman). Phytoestrogens and health. London: Food Standards Agency Publication. Crown Copyright, <http://cot.food.gov.uk/pdfs/phytoreport0503>; 2003.

[7] Moreira AC, Silva AM, Santos MS, Sardao VA. Phytoestrogens as alternative replacement therapy in menopause: what is real, what is unknown? J Steroid Biochem Mol Biol 2014;143C:61–71.

[8] Beral V, Million Women Study Collaborators Breast cancer and hormone replacement in the Million Women Study. Lancet 2003;362:419–27.

[9] Harris RM, Waring RH. Diethylstilboestrol—a long-term legacy. Maturitas 2012;72:108–12.

[10] Dodds EC, Goldberg L, Lawson W, Robinson R. Estrogenic activity of certain synthetic compounds. Nature 1938;141:247–8.

[11] Smith OW. Diethylstilboestrol in the prevention and treatment of complications of pregnancy. Am J Obstet Gynecol 1948;56:821–34.

[12] Herbst AL, Ulfelder H, Poskanzer DC. Adenocarcinoma of the vagina: association of maternal stilboestrol therapy with tumor appearance in young women. N Engl J Med 1971;284:878–81.

[13] Hoover RN, Hyer M, Pfeiffer RM, Adam E, Bond B, Cheville AL, et al. Adverse health outcomes in women exposed *in utero* to diethylstilboestrol. N Engl J Med 2011;365:1304–14.

[14] Bourguignon JP, Parent AS. The impact of endocrine disruptors on female pubertal timing Diamanti-Kandarakis E, Gore AC, editors. Endocrine disruptors and puberty. New York, NY: Humana Press, Springer; 2012. pp. 325–37.

[15] Guaneri MP, Brambilla G, Loizzo A, Colombo I, Chiumello G. Estrogen exposure in a child from hair lotion used by her mother: clinical and hair analysis data. Clin Toxicol 2008;46:762–4.

[16] Twary CM. Premature sexual development in children following the use of estrogen- or placenta-containing hair products. Clin Pediatr (Phila) 1998;37:733–9.

[17] Parent AS, Teilman G, Juul A, Skakkebaek NE, Toppari J, Bourguignon JP. The timing of normal puberty and the age limits of sexual precocity: variations around the world, secular trends, and changes after migration. Endocr Rev 2003;24:668–93.

[18] World Health Organization Endocrine disrupters and child health: possible developmental early effects of endocrine disrupters on child health. Geneva, Switzerland: WHO; 2012. <www.who.int>.

[19] Diamanti-Kandarakis E, Gore AC, editors. Endocrine disruptors and puberty. New York, NY: Humana Press, Springer; 2012. pp. 1–378.

[20] Kaprio J, Rimpela A, Winter T, Viken RJ, Rimpela M, Rose RJ. Common genetic influences on BMI and age at menarche. Hum Biol 1995;67:739–53.

[21] Proos LA, Hofvander Y, Tuvemo T. Menarcheal age and growth pattern of Indian girls adopted in Sweden. I. Menarcheal age. Acta Paediatr Scand 1991;80:852–8.

[22] Fara GM, DelCorvo G, Bernuzzi S, Bigatello A, DiPietro C, Scaglioni S, et al. Epidemic of breast enlargement in an Italian school. Lancet 1979;2:295–7.

[23] Comas AP. Precocious sexual development in Puerto Rico. Lancet 1982;1:1299–300.

[24] Freni-Titulaer LW, Cordero JF, Haddock L, Lebron G, Martinez R, Mills JL. Premature thelarche in Puerto Rico: a search for environmental factors. Am J Dis Child 1986;140:1263–7.

[25] Colon I, Caro D, Bourdony CJ, Rosario O. Identification of phthalate esters in the serum of young Puerto Rican girls with premature breast development. Environ Health Perspect 2000;108:895–900.

[26] Craig ZR, Wang W, Flaws JA. Endocrine-disrupting chemicals in ovarian function: effects on steroidogenesis, metabolism and nuclear signalling. Reproduction 2011;142:633–46.

[27] Nelson LM. Clinical practice. Primary ovarian insufficiency. N Engl J Med 2009;360:606–14.

[28] Kirigaya A, Kim H, Hayashi S, Chambon P, Watanabe H, Lquchi T, et al. Involvement of estrogen receptor beta in the induction of polyovular follicles in mouse ovaries exposed neonatally to diethylstilbestrol. Zoolog Sci 2009;26:704–12.

[29] Ahn HJ, An BS, Jung EM, Yang H, Choi KC, Jeung EB. Parabens inhibit the early phase of folliculogenesis and steroidogenesis in the ovaries of neonatal rats. Mol Reprod Dev 2012;79:626–36.

[30] Kappeler CJ, Hoyer PB. 4-Vinylcyclohexene diepoxide: a model chemical for ovotoxicity. Syst Biol Reprod Med 2012;58:57–62.

[31] Martinez EM, Swartz WJ. Effects of methoxychlor on the reproductive system of the adult female mouse. Gross and histologic observations. Reprod Toxicol 1991;5:139–47.

[32] Chao HR, Wang SL, Lin LY, Lee WJ, Papke O. Placental transfer of polychlorinated dibenzo-p-dioxins, dibenzo-furans, and biphenyls in Taiwanese mothers in relation to menstrual cycle characteristics. Food Chem Toxicol 2007;45:259–65.

[33] Axmon A, Rylander L, Stromberg U, Hagmar L. Altered menstrual cycles in women with a high dietary intake of persistent organochlorine compounds. Chemosphere 2004;56:813–9.

[34] Farr SL, Cooper GS, Cai J, Savitz DA, Sandler DP. Pesticide use and menstrual cycle characteristics among premenopausal women in the Agricultural Health Study. Am J Epidemiol 2004;160:1194–204.

[35] Nikaido Y, Yoshizawa K, Danbara N, Tsujita-Kyutoku M, Yuri T, Uehara N, et al. Effects of maternal xenoestrogen exposure on development of the reproductive tract and mammary gland in female CD-1 mouse offspring. Reprod Toxicol 2004;18:803–11.

[36] Farr SL, Cai J, Savitz DA, Sandler DP, Hoppin JA, Cooper GS. Pesticide exposure and timing of menopause: the Agricultural Health Study. Am J Epidemiol 2006;163:731–42.

[37] Unfer V, Casini ML, Costabile L, Mignosa M, Gerli S, DiRenzo GC. Endometrial effects of long-term treatment with phytoestrogens: a randomized double-blind, placebo-controlled study. Fertil Steril 2004;82:145–8.

[38] Vos T, Flaxman AD, Naghavi M, Lozano R, Michaud C, Ezzati M, et al. Years lived with disability (YLDs) for 1160 sequelae of 289 diseases and injuries 1990–2010: a systematic analysis for the Global Burden of Disease Study 2010. Lancet 2012;380(9859):2163–96.

[39] Newbold RR, Jefferson WN, Padilla-Banks E. Prenatal exposure to bisphenol A at environmentally relevant doses adversely affects the murine female reproductive tract later in life. Environ Health Perspect 2009;117:879–85.

[40] Padmanabhan V, Sarma HN, Savabieasfahani M, Steckler TL, Veiga-Lopez A. Developmental reprogramming of reproductive and metabolic dysfunction in sheep: native steroids vs. environmental steroid receptor modulators. Int J Androl 2010;33:394–404.

[41] Fernández M, Bourguignon N, Lux-Lantos V, Libertun C. Neonatal exposure to bisphenol a and reproductive and endocrine alterations resembling the polycystic ovarian syndrome in adult rats. Environ Health Perspect 2010;118:1217–22.

[42] Tsutsumi O. Assessment of human contamination of estrogenic endocrine-disrupting chemicals and their risk for human reproduction. J Steroid Biochem Mol Biol 2005;93:325–30.

[43] Kandari E, Chatzigeorgiou A, Livadas S, Palioura E, Economou F, Koutsilieris M, et al. Endocrine disruptors and polycystic ovary syndrome (PCOS): elevated serum levels of bisphenol A in women with PCOS. J Clin Endocrinol Metab 2011;96:E480–4.

[44] Rutkowska A, Rachon D. Bisphenol A (BPA) and its potential role in the pathogenesis of the polycystic ovary syndrome (PCOS). Gynecol Endocrinol 2014;30:260–5.

[45] Trabert B, Chen Z, Kannan K, Peterson CM, Pollack AZ, Sun L, et al. Persistent organic pollutants (POPs) and fibroids: results from the ENDO study. J Expo Sci Environ Epidemiol 2014 [EPub ahead of print].

[46] Shen Y, Xu Q, Ren M, Feng X, Cai Y, Gao Y. Measurement of phenolic environmental estrogens in women with uterine leiomyoma. PLoS One 2013;8:e796838. 1–5.

[47] Shen Y, Shen Y, Ren ML, Feng X, Cai YL, Gao YX, et al. An evidence *in vitro* for the influence of bisphenol A on uterine leiomyoma. Eur J Obstet Gynecol Reprod Biol 2014;178:80–3. [EPub ahead of print].

[48] Wang KH, Kao AP, Chang CC, Lin TC, Kuo TC. Bisphenol A at environmentally relevant doses induces cyclooxygenase-2 expression and promotes invasion of human mesenchymal stem cells derived from uterine myoma tissue. Taiwan J Obstet Gynecol 2013;52:246–52.

3. CONCERNS FOR HUMAN HEALTH

[49] Newbold RR, Jefferson WN, Padlila-Banks E. Long-term adverse effects of neonatal exposure to bisphenol A on the murine female reproductive tract. Reprod Toxicol 2007;24:253–8.

[50] Porpora MG, Resta S, Fuggetta E, Storelli P, Megiorni F, Manganaro L, et al. Role of environmental organochlorinated pollutants in the development of endometriosis. Clin Exp Obstet Gynecol 2013;40:565–7.

[51] Rier SE, Martin DC, Bowman RE, Dmowski WP, Becker JL. Endometriosis in rhesus monkeys (*Macaca mulatta*) following chronic exposure to 2,3,7,8-tetrachlorodibenzo-*p*-dioxin. Fundam Appl Toxicol 1993;21:433–41.

[52] Cummings AM, Metcalf JL. Induction of endometriosis in mice: a new model sensitive to estrogen. Reprod Toxicol 1995;9:233–8.

[53] Johnson KL, Cummings AM, Birnbaum LS. Promotion of endometriosis in mice by polychlorinated dibenzo-*p*-dioxins, dibenzofurans, and biphenyls. Environ Health Perspect 1997;105:750–5.

[54] Cummings AM, Hedge JM, Birnbaum LS. Effect of perinatal exposure to TCDD on the promotion of endometriotic lesion growth by TCDD in adult female rats and mice. Toxicol Sci 1999;52:45–9.

[55] Signorile PG, Spugnini EP, Mita L, Mellone P, D'Avino A, Bianco M, et al. Pre-natal exposure of mice to bisphenol A elicits an endometriosis-like phenotype in female offspring. Gen Comp Endocrinol 2010;168:318–25.

[56] Signorile PG, Spugnini EP, Citro G, Viceconte R, Vincenzi B, Baldi F, et al. Endocrine disruptors *in utero* cause ovarian damages linked to endometriosis. Front Biosci (Elite Ed) 2012;4:1724–30.

[57] Cobellis L, Colacurci N, Trabucco E, Carpentiero C, Grumetto L. Measurement of bisphenol A and bisphenol B levels in human blood sera from healthy and endometriotic women. Biomed Chromatogr 2009;23:1186–90.

[58] Itoh H, Iwasaki M, Hanaoka T, Sasaki H, Tanaka T, Tsugane S. Urinary bisphenol-A concentration in infertile Japanese women and its association with endometriosis: a cross-sectional study. Environ Health Prev Med 2007;12:258–64.

[59] Caserta D, Bordi G, Ciardo F, Marci R, La Rocca C, Tait S, et al. The influence of endocrine disruptors in a selected population of infertile women. Gynecol Endocrinol 2013;29:444–7.

[60] Buck Louis GM, Peterson CM, Chen Z, Croughan M, Sundaram R, Stanford J, et al. Bisphenol A and phthalates and endometriosis: the Endometriosis: Natural History, Diagnosis and Outcomes Study. Fertil Steril 2013;100:162–9.

[61] Missmer SA, Hankinson SE, Spiegelman D, Barberi RL, Michels KB, Hunter DJ. *In utero* exposures and the incidence of endometriosis. Fertil Steril 2004;82:1501–8.

[62] Haagensen CD. Diseases of the breast, 2nd ed. Philadelphia, PA: WB Saunders; 1971.

[63] Mannello F, Tonti GAM, Papa S. Human gross cyst breast disease and cystic fluid: bio-molecular, morphological, and clinical studies. Breast Cancer Res Treat 2006;97:115–29.

[64] Darbre PD. Hypothesis: underarm cosmetics are a cause of breast cancer. Eur J Cancer Prev 2001;10:389–93.

[65] Darbre PD. Underarm cosmetics and breast cancer. J Appl Toxicol 2003;23:89–95.

[66] Fenton SE, Beck LM, Borde AR, Rayner JL. Developmental exposure to environmental endocrine disruptors and adverse effects on mammary gland development Diamanti-Kandarakis E, Gore AC, editors. Endocrine disruptors and puberty. New York, NY: Humana Press, Springer; 2012. pp. 201–24.

[67] Rimsten A. Symptoms and signs in benign and malignant tumours of the breast. Ups J Med Sci 1976;81:54–60.

[68] Stebbing JF, Nash AG. Diagnosis and management of phyllodes tumour of the breast: experience of 33 cases at a specialist centre. Ann R Coll Surg Engl 1996;77:181–4.

[69] Laden K, Felger CB. Antiperspirants and deodorants: cosmetic science and technology series, vol. 7. New York, NY: Marcel Dekker; 1988.

[70] Mannello F, Tonti GA, Darbre PD. Concentration of aluminium in breast cyst fluids collected from women affected by gross cystic breast disease. J Appl Toxicol 2008.

[71] Bidgoli SA, Ahmadi R, Zavarhei MD. Role of hormonal and environmental factors on early incidence of breast cancer in Iran. Sci Total Environ 2010;408:4056–61.

[72] Charles AK, Darbre PD. Combinations of parabens at concentrations measured in human breast tissue can increase proliferation of MCF-7 human breast cancer cells. J Appl Toxicol 2013;33:390–8.

[73] Rajapakse N, Silva E, Kortenkamp A. Combining xenoestrogens at levels below individual no-observed-effect concentrations dramatically enhances steroid hormone action. Environ Health Perspect 2002;110:917–21.

[74] Brian JV, Harris CA, Scholze M, Backhaus T, Booy P, Lamoree M, et al. Accurate prediction of the response of freshwater fish to a mixture of estrogenic chemicals. Environ Health Perspect 2005;113:721–8.

[75] Bennetts HW, Underwood ET, Shier FL. A specific breeding problem of sheep on subterranean clover pastures in Western Australia. Aust Vet J 1946;22:2–12.

Endocrine Disruption and Male Reproductive Health

Philippa D. Darbre

Abstract

This chapter provides an overview of the dependence of development and maintenance of the male phenotype (masculinization) on testicular hormones and emphasizes its vulnerability to endocrine disruption, particularly in perturbations to the balance of androgen to estrogen. Evidence for consequences to male reproductive health following fetal exposure to excess estrogen is demonstrated from the outcome

Endocrine Disruption and Human Health.
DOI: http://dx.doi.org/10.1016/B978-0-12-801139-3.00009-0

for sons whose mothers were treated with diethylstilbestrol (DES) during pregnancy. Evidence that exposure to exogenous estrogens can affect adult life is provided by the reported cases of gynecomastia (inappropriate breast growth) following exposure to estrogenic chemicals in dermally applied creams. Several male reproductive health problems, including hypospadias and cryptorchidism (urogenital tract malformations), abnormalities of spermatogenesis (declining sperm counts and sperm quality), alterations to puberty, and development of prostatic hyperplasia, are increasing in Westernized countries. These are suspected to arise from exposure to endocrine disruptors, and epidemiological studies aim to identify culprit chemicals. However, such an array of reproductive abnormalities are most likely to arise from exposure to complex mixtures of chemicals rather than single chemicals and probably to different mixtures in different locations, which makes proving the sources of causative chemicals a daunting task.

9.1 INTRODUCTION

Male sexuality is determined genetically at the time of fertilization by the presence of a Y chromosome in the spermatozoan as it fuses with the X-chromosome-containing ovum, and the sex-determining region of the Y chromosome (SRY) then drives the bipotential gonad of the embryo to become a testis through hormone-independent mechanisms [1,2]. However, once the early testis is formed, development of the full male phenotype, including further testicular development (masculinization), becomes completely dependent on a complex network of endocrine signals, particularly hormones secreted from the testes [2]. Individuals who lack any gonads are phenotypically female [1] and endocrine intervention is required to modify the default female phenotype to become male [2]. This makes both development and maintenance of masculinization vulnerable to endocrine-disrupting influences at all developmental stages from early embryo to adulthood; in particular, disruption of early embryonic developmental processes may have consequences for male reproductive health in adult life [2]. This chapter will address the consequences of endocrine disruption for development of the urogenital tract and for sperm production. It will discuss the ability of endocrine-disrupting chemicals (EDCs) to bring about inappropriate breast growth (gynecomastia), alterations to puberty, and hyperplasia in prostatic tissue (Figure 9.1). Issues surrounding the development of cancers in reproductive tissues (prostate cancer, testicular cancer, breast cancer) will be discussed in Chapter 10.

9.2 WHAT ARE THE ENDOCRINE TARGETS FOR DISRUPTION OF MALE REPRODUCTIVE HEALTH?

Testicular hormones are essential for the development and maintenance of the male phenotype. Genetic studies have shown that the Y chromosome is the initial determinant of maleness because even with many additional X chromosomes, the karyotype XXXXXY is phenotypically male, whereas without the Y chromosome, even the karyotype X remains phenotypically female. However, an ability to respond to endocrine signals is essential for masculinization [2]. During early embryonic life, the bipotential gonad develops into testes which secrete anti-Müllerian hormone (AMH), testosterone and insulin-like factor-3 (Insl3) (Figure 9.2). AMH is made by the fetal Sertoli cells and causes the degeneration of the Müllerian duct (which would otherwise develop into the female fallopian tubes, uterus, and vagina). Testosterone is secreted from the fetal Leydig cells and causes the Wolffian duct to

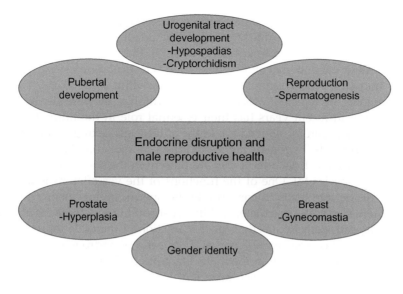

FIGURE 9.1   Diagram outlining the consequences of endocrine disruption for male reproductive health.

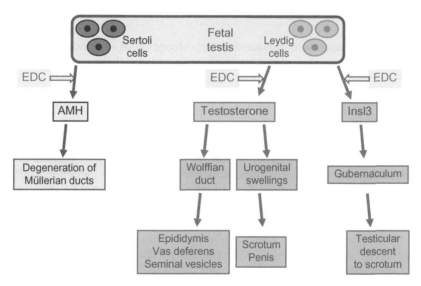

FIGURE 9.2   Endocrine regulation of masculinization showing the sites of production of the three key hormones and their effects on target tissues. EDCs could disrupt the production or action of any of these hormones.

differentiate into the epididymis, vas deferens, and seminal vesicles and the urogenital swellings to develop into the scrotum and penis, and it also inhibits the development of the breast primordia [2]. In androgen insensitivity syndrome, where there are mutations in the androgen receptor (AR) gene, despite a normal XY karyotype and the presence of testes synthesizing testosterone, the individuals develop female secondary sex characteristics because they cannot respond to the testosterone [1]. The third testicular hormone Insl3 is also produced by the fetal Leydig cells, and following studies in knockout mice [3], this is now recognized as responsible for development of the gubernaculum, which guides testicular descent into the scrotum, a prerequisite for normal spermatogenesis and fertility in adulthood [2].

Although estrogens are referred to as the female hormones, they are also synthesized and present in men; only in recent years has their essential role in the normal function of the male reproductive tract been recognized [4]. In the adult testis, estrogens are synthesized by Leydig cells and germ cells. Estrogens are also formed by the aromatization of testosterone in fat and muscle tissues. Estrogen receptors are present in the testis, efferent ductules, and epididymis of most species [4]. One of the functions of the vas efferens is to absorb water from the lumen of the rete testis to concentrate the sperm, giving them a longer lifespan and providing more sperm per ejaculate, and this absorption of water is regulated by estrogens [4]. Therefore, estrogens are needed for the function of the male reproductive system, but too much estrogen becomes feminizing, and the ratio of androgen to estrogen is a key determinant of reproductive health in the male. Disruption of this delicate balance between androgens and estrogens can alter masculinization.

9.3 SOURCES AND TIMING OF ENDOCRINE DISRUPTION FOR MALE REPRODUCTIVE HEALTH

Environmental exposures to compounds with estrogenic or antiandrogenic activity have the potential to disrupt the androgen:estrogen ratio in men if they enter the body in sufficient quantities. Many such compounds have been identified, which may enter through oral exposure in diet; inhalation from domestic, urban, or rural environments; or transdermal through increasing use of body care products by men (see Chapters 1 and 2). Pharmaceuticals provide another source of exposure, including the increasing use of mild analgesics with antiandrogenic activity [5].

Apart from the source of exposure, timing is another equally important consideration. Although early embryonic stages of sex determination are hormone independent, after the testes have formed, the embryonic endocrine-dependent processes of masculinization are inherently susceptible to disruption of the action of any of the three testicular hormones (i.e., AMH, Insl3, testosterone) [2] and may be disrupted through transplacental transfer from the mother. Animal models have shown that exposure to certain phthalate esters in utero can suppress testosterone and Insl3 secretion by fetal Leydig cells, giving rise to reproductive abnormalities in the adult [2]. In the human, exposure to the synthetic estrogen diethylstilbestrol (DES), prescribed to mothers during pregnancy between 1940 and 1971, has revealed increased incidence of reproductive abnormalities in the sons who were exposed *in utero* (see the next section of this chapter).

Another sensitive time frame for male reproductive development is in the early postnatal period, and modern life provides many external endocrine-disrupting influences for newborn boys. Estrogenic and antiandrogenic chemicals contained in personal care products (such as baby wipes and diaper creams) are applied continuously to the genital area during early life, and absorption may be enhanced in cases of diaper rash, which damages the skin. Dietary exposure to certain parabens in the early postnatal period have been shown to impair reproductive health in rodents (see Section 9.7). Cultural practices of feeding soy-based milk products to baby boys remains an unresolved concern. Soy contains plant phytoestrogens, which have the estrogenic potency to affect the postnatal development of the male reproductive system [6].

9.4 EXPOSURE TO DES IN UTERO AND FETAL ORIGIN OF ENDOCRINE DYSFUNCTION IN MEN

As described in Chapter 8, DES is a synthetic estrogen that was widely prescribed to women between 1940 and 1971 to prevent threatened miscarriage in the first trimester [7]. Long-term follow-up studies of sons born to DES-treated mothers have demonstrated that in utero exposure is associated with increased lifetime risk of adverse reproductive health outcomes for the sons as well as the daughters [8]. Prenatal DES exposure was associated with increased risk of cryptorchidism, epididymal cyst formation, and testicular inflammation, and the risk was greater for sons exposed prior to the 11th week of pregnancy (Table 9.1) [8]. No significant associations have been observed with varicocele; structural abnormalities of the penis (including hypospadias); urethral stenosis; inflammation of the urethra, prostate, or epididymis; or benign prostatic hypertrophy [8]. Since it is inherently difficult to relate specific chemical exposures of women in early pregnancy to outcomes in their sons, especially

TABLE 9.1   Adverse Health Outcomes in Men Exposed to DES In Utero

Health outcome	Timing of exposure in utero	Risk ratio
Epididymal cyst	Any	2.5
	Before week 11	3.5
	After week 11	2.0
Cryptorchidism	Any	1.9
	Before week 11	2.9
	After week 11	1.1
Urethral stenosis		1.3
Abnormality of penis, including hypospadias		1.1
Varicocele		0.9
Inflammation of testes	Any	2.5
	Before week 11	3.0
	After week 11	2.1
Inflammation of urethra		1.5
Inflammation of prostate		1.1
Inflammation of epididymis		1.0
Benign prostatic hypertrophy		1.2

Source: As Published by Palmer et al. in 2009 [8].

3. CONCERNS FOR HUMAN HEALTH

if they are not manifest until adulthood, the inadvertent exposure of so many boys to DES in utero provides a unique view of the effects in the human population of early embryonic exposure to a potent estrogen on subsequent male reproductive health. Although an increased risk of some reproductive abnormalities was observed, the fact that not all sons were obviously affected underlines the variation between individual responses. Whether the variation relates to individual susceptibility of the sons or to doses delivered from the mother through the placenta to the sons remains unknown, but it serves to demonstrate the difficulty in identifying endocrine-disrupting influences that may not manifest uniformly across the population.

9.5 EXPOSURE TO EDCs IN ADULT LIFE AND GYNECOMASTIA

The ability of external environmental estrogenic compounds to affect male reproductive health in adult life is demonstrated from the reported case of the "mortician's mystery," published in the *New England Journal of Medicine* in 1988 [9]. This paper describes the case of an embalmer who presented as a mysterious case of gynecomastia (inappropriate breast growth in the adult man) and hypogonadotropic hypogonadism (diminished function of gonads), with signs of estrogen excess but with undetectable levels of endogenous estrogens. His pubertal development had been uneventful and he fathered seven children, but over the previous 10 years, he had suffered progressive loss of libido, decrease in testicular size, and marked breast development. Over these 10 years, he had been working as an embalmer, applying creams to corpses without wearing gloves. The paper describes evidence that the creams contained estrogenic components and that by 1 year after cessation of exposure to the embalming creams through simply wearing gloves, the symptoms had reversed, including an increase in size of his testes. This demonstrates a clear case where long-term topical exposure to estrogenic components of embalming creams (sometimes termed "the embalmer's curse") can result in endocrine disruption to the adult male, but which are reversible after ceasing the exposure.

Another equally poignant report describes gynecomastia in three prepubertal boys who had normal serum levels of endogenous steroids. All the boys had been using topical personal care products containing lavender or tea-tree oils, and the symptoms resolved some months after ceasing exposure to these products. Interestingly, both lavender oil and tea-tree oil were shown by in vitro studies to possess estrogenic activity [10].

The development of breast tissue is inhibited by testosterone, but it is stimulated by estrogens; therefore, the condition of gynecomastia is usually assumed to be caused by excess estrogen levels. Such studies aid the understanding of endocrine-disrupting influences because the reversibility of the condition in adult life enables identification of the specific causative environmental factors.

9.6 UROGENITAL TRACT MALFORMATIONS

9.6.1 Hypospadias and Cryptorchidism

Hypospadias and cryptorchidism are common birth defects in the male urogenital tract (Figure 9.3). Hypospadias result from abnormal development of the urethra (which carries urine from the body) such that it opens on the underside, the shaft, or the perineum rather than the tip of the penis (Figure 9.3). Cryptorchidism is a common birth defect characterized

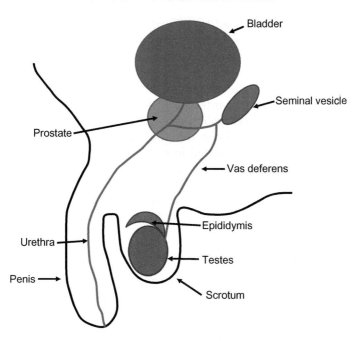

FIGURE 9.3   Diagram of the male reproductive system. The urogenital tract is composed of the testes (where sperm are made), located in the scrotum; epididymis/vas deferens (along which sperm pass); and the penis, which has a single duct (urethra) that releases not only sperm but also urine from the bladder. Male accessory sex glands include the prostate and seminal vesicles, which produce the fluids (semen) added to the sperm as they travel down the ducts.

by maldescent of the testes, resulting in the absence of one or both testes from the scrotum (Figure 9.3). The incidence of both conditions has been reported to be increasing over recent decades in the Western world, although with some differences between countries in magnitude and temporal trends [11–17], and there is an association between the two conditions because a record of cryptorchidism is associated with an increased risk of hypospadias and vice versa [18]. The rapid pace of the increase in these conditions suggests environmental rather than genetic determinants [19] and the consistently lower rates noted in Finland compared to Denmark has sparked debate as to whether specific environmental factors might explain the differences between these two Nordic countries [20].

The dependence of urogenital tract development on endocrine signaling (see Section 9.2) implicates a fetal origin of these birth defects. Endocrine disruption in the embryo could lead to the emergence of the urethral orifice in an inappropriate location on the ventral surface of the penis, scrotum, or perineum (hypospadias). The process of testicular descent could be disrupted in the fetus either during the transabdominal phase (second trimester), mediated by Insl3, or during the inguinoscrotal phase (third trimester), mediated by androgens. This has led to the hypothesis that these malformations might be caused by exposure to endocrine disruptors in utero, and in particular to compounds with estrogenic or antiandrogenic activity that might change the androgen/estrogen balance. Animal models have provided a proof of principle in that rats exposed in utero to dibutyl phthalate develop hypospadias and cryptorchidism [21]. However, apart from the higher risk of cryptorchidism in sons exposed to DES in utero (see Section 9.4), direct testing in humans cannot be done and studies have to rely on an epidemiological approach. A lifestyle approach has shown that living near hazardous-waste landfill sites can be correlated with risk of hypospadias in five European countries [22]. Cryptorchidism has been correlated in Spain with living close to intensive farming where pesticides are used [23], in Denmark with mothers working in gardening [24], and in the Netherlands with paternal pesticide exposure [25]. In Denmark, maternal use of mild analgesics, especially during the second trimester of pregnancy, has been dose-dependently correlated with cryptorchidism [26]. Further studies have been collated in a recent review, and there are some reports of an association between higher levels of mixtures of pesticides or mixtures of polybrominated diphenyl ether (PBDE) flame retardants in the mother's milk of cryptorchid boys [19]. Interestingly, single chemicals did not reach significance but some mixtures did, which implies that multiple chemicals may be acting together before an effect can be reached [19].

9.6.2 Anogenital Distance

Anogenital distance (AGD) is the distance from the anus to the base of the penis, and reduction in this length is an indicator of abnormal male reproductive tract masculinization. AGD, together with penile length, provide accessible end-point markers for male reproductive health. In the rodent model, perineal growth depends on dihydrotestosterone (DHT) and males with a shortened AGD have increased risk of hypospadias and cryptorchidism [27]. Prenatal exposure of male rodents to dioxins [28], phthalates [29], n-butylparaben [30], or bisphenol A (BPA) [31] has been reported to cause shortening of AGD. In humans, AGD and penile length have both been reported to be reduced in boys with hypospadias or cryptorchidism [32]. Women with raised levels of phthalates in their urine during pregnancy have been reported to be more likely to have sons with shorter AGD and penile length [33,34]. In similar studies, AGD has also been inversely associated with prenatal exposure to dichlorodiphenyldichloroethylene (DDE) [35], to BPA [36] and to plasma dioxinlike activity in maternal blood at delivery [37]. In real life, however, exposure is never to a single EDC, but rather to complex mixtures from a range of environmental sources, and assessment of the effects of mixtures poses the next and greater challenge. In rats, pioneering mixture studies have been carried out using four antiandrogenic chemicals [di(2-ethylhexyl)phthalate (DEHP), vincolzolin, prochlaraz, and finsateride] mixed at individual no observed adverse effect levels (NOAELs). Exposure of mothers to these chemicals in combination gave significant reductions in AGD in male offspring [38].

9.7 SPERM COUNTS AND SPERM QUALITY AS INDICATORS OF FERTILITY

From puberty until the end of life, spermatogenesis in the testes and epididymis produces mature spermatozoa, which are added to fluids from the seminal vesicle and prostate to form semen. Semen quality is a measure of the ability of semen to accomplish fertilization and includes both quantity of sperm (sperm count) and quality of sperm. Many papers have now reported a decline not only in sperm count, but also in sperm quality (motility and morphology) over the past 50 years in Western countries [39–43]. A striking difference was noted in particular between higher sperm counts in men in Finland compared with Denmark, where 18% of young men from the general population have been reported to have a sperm concentration below 20×10^6/mL, which is considered by the World Health Organisation (WHO) as abnormal [20].

Animal models have shown that maternal exposure to butylparaben during gestation and lactation can result in reproductive disorders in male offspring by postnatal day 49 [44]. Whether the effects resulted from butylparaben crossing the placenta during gestation, passing in breast milk during suckling, or a combination of both were not determined in this study, but the sensitivity of early postnatal male rodents to the development of reproductive disorders when exposed to butylparaben via the dietary route has been confirmed in subsequent studies [45]. Further rodent studies have reported that repeat oral dosage in the diet of butylparaben or propylparaben [45–47], but not methylparaben or ethylparaben [48], to juvenile rodents can result in alterations to spermatogenesis, testosterone secretion, and epididymal weight. Investigating the potential for effects in the human population, urinary levels of parabens were measured from those attending an infertility clinic and studied in relation to markers of sperm quality. Higher levels of butylparaben were not associated with usual markers of sperm count, motility, or morphology but were reported to be associated with sperm DNA damage as measured using a comet assay [49]. Similar studies reported also a correlation between sperm DNA damage and urinary levels of BPA [50,51]. These studies are highly relevant because baby boys have been exposed to oral BPA in early postnatal life through the use of plastic baby bottles; and many Western countries have now taken steps to remove BPA from these products. Since parabens are now known to penetrate skin [52], the wisdom of topical application of parabens in baby wipes and baby creams to the genital area of baby boys during this sensitive time frame has been questioned, and some countries have called for removal of parabens from these products [52].

Male infertility is a global health problem affecting around 1 in 20 of the male population [53], but whether falling sperm counts equate with reduced fertility remains to be established [54]. Poor semen quality may reflect a lack of selection pressure on male fertility in Western societies, and this is likely to be exacerbated by increasing use of assisted reproductive technology [54]. Male offspring of DES-treated mothers do not suffer infertility [55] despite DES influencing semen quality [56,57], and therefore, any influence from environmental factors remains an open question [54].

9.8 TESTICULAR DYSGENESIS SYNDROME

Traditionally, different male reproductive health problems would have been treated by different medical practitioners: hypospadias and cryptorchidism would have been treated by pediatric endocrinologists, urologists, and surgeons, while semen quality would have been assessed in fertility clinics. This would have impeded any link being made. However, recent observations of parallel trends has suggested a link not only between hypospadias, cryptorchidism, and declining semen quality, but also with the increasing incidence of testicular cancer [58–60] (see Chapter 10), which would have presented to yet another location, cancer clinics. This has led to the hypothesis that this collection of adverse trends in male

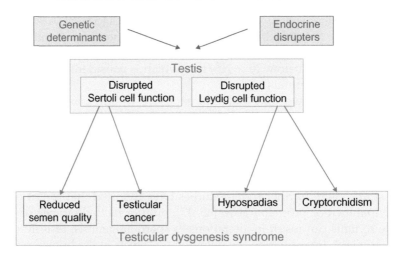

FIGURE 9.4   TDS [61]. Disturbance in early fetal life to Sertoli cell function may lead to reduced semen quality and testicular cancer in adult life. Disturbance in early fetal life to Leydig cell function may lead to hypospadias and cryptorchidism after birth.

reproductive health may be a single entity with a common origin in fetal life, which has been termed *testicular dysgenesis syndrome (TDS)* (Figure 9.4) [61]. While there are genetic determinants, it has been suggested that the increasing coincident trends may indicate common environmental factors, and especially those which lead to androgen insufficiency or disturbance to the androgen/estrogen balance in fetal life [61]. Exposure to compounds with estrogenic activity has been one plausible hypothesis, which has stemmed from the increased risk of these end points following exposure to DES in utero [62]. However, it is clear that not all DES-exposed sons had symptoms and that there are other sources of susceptibility/heterogeneity that need to be identified [62]. An alternative hypothesis has suggested that culprit chemicals might not be those with estrogenic activity, but rather those with antiandrogenic activity [63,64]. Although these hypotheses have underlying differences in mechanism, there is some overlap because many environmental chemicals with estrogenic activity also possess antiandrogenic activity and vice versa. Animal models have shown that rats exposed in utero to dibutyl phthalate developed cryptorchidism, hypospadias, infertility, and testicular abnormalities [21], and phthalates possess both estrogenic [65] and antiandrogenic [66] activities.

9.9 PUBERTAL DEVELOPMENT

9.9.1 Physiological Changes in Puberty

Puberty is an endocrine-regulated developmental process of late childhood that involves not only physical changes as secondary sexual characteristics mature and the reproductive organs become functional, but also psychological and behavioral changes [67]. In boys, this begins around 10–12 years of age and is complete by around 15–17 years of age. In 1970, Tanner and Marshall put forward a series of clinical measures to track the onset, progress, and duration of puberty in boys [68]. Tanner staging uses genital development (size and morphology of testes, scrotum, and penis) and growth of pubic hair (type of hair and location of hair growth), and this has provided a method to monitor early (precocious) or late-onset puberty. Timing of puberty does have a genetic component, and there are ethnic variations as well [69]. It can also be influenced by differences in nutrition (especially the resulting changes in body mass) [69,70]. However, since these developmental changes involve a complex interplay of pituitary, adrenal, thyroid, and sex hormones, endocrine disruption could have adverse consequences in this critical time period for boys.

9.9.2 Pubertal Timing and EDCs

In contrast to the many studies in girls, there are fewer studies reporting the effects of EDCs on trends in puberty in boys at the current time. Animal models have shown that exposure to several EDCs, including DES, PCBs, BPA, DDE, methoxychlor, phthalate, and tributyltin (TBT), can alter pubertal development in rodents. However, in contrast to the early onset in females, these compounds cause a delay in pubertal onset in males and are accompanied by dysfunction of testicular steroidogenic pathways and perturbation in secondary sexual maturation [71]. Furthermore, critical periods of vulnerability vary for different compounds, which, for example, was peripubertal for estrogenic compounds such as DES and ethynylestradiol, but gestational for PCBs [71]. In humans, some studies have suggested that exposure to PCBs and dioxins [72] and to endosulfan [73] can delay the onset of puberty and age of attaining pubertal milestones.

9.10 PROSTATIC HYPERPLASIA

Benign prostatic hyperplasia (BPH) is associated with an unregulated proliferation of connective tissue, smooth muscle tissue, and glandular epithelium that results in enlargement of the prostate gland such that it may compress the urethra and cause bladder outlet obstruction and lower urinary tract symptoms [74]. Autopsy has shown that BPH increases after the age of 40 and occurs in up to 90% of men over age 80 [75]. Androgens have been implicated in the development of BPH, and the use of the antiandrogen flutamide or 5α-reductase inhibitors, which block the conversion of testosterone to the more active DHT, can be effective in reducing prostate size [76]. However, not all men respond to this treatment, implying that there are also other factors. One possibility may be an altered balance between stimulatory and inhibitory growth factors [74]. However, testosterone is the primary circulating androgen in men, and testosterone can be converted by CYP19A1/aromatase into 17β-estradiol and the prostate is an estrogen target tissue [76–78]. It is known that as men age, they develop an increased ratio of estrogen to androgen [79], which mirrors the age-dependence of BPH, and reduction in estrogens through loss of aromatase can inhibit prostate proliferation [77,80].

Using rodent models, exposure to estrogens in early life has been shown to lead to abnormal prostate growth in later life [81]. Experiments published in 1997 reported an enlarged prostate in male mice whose mothers were fed low levels of estradiol or DES between days

11 and 17 of gestation [82]. A 50% increase in free serum estradiol in the male fetuses gave a 30% enlarged prostate, but further increase of two- to eightfold in serum-free estradiol did not, demonstrating that the effect was dependent on low levels rather than high dosage [82]. Further experiments showed that mothers fed BPA at a low dose of either 2 or $20\,\mu g/kg/$ day also gave birth to male offspring with enlarged prostates at 6 months of age [83]. These reports opened questions concerning a role for environmental estrogenic chemicals in BPH, and studies using human prostate stemlike cells have shown that exposure to BPA can alter their growth properties both in vitro and in vivo [84], suggesting that the experiments of 1997 in rodents may be relevant for humans.

9.11 GENDER IDENTITY

One unresolved issue concerns whether EDCs may be affecting gender identity; that is, how a man feels about himself regardless of physical characteristics [85]. Effects of EDC exposure in wildlife include documented development of extensive hermaphroditism with growth of ovarian tissue within testes and sexual abnormalities in male behavior. The question is whether this also can occur in humans. A study in 1995 reported that the central subdivision of the bed nucleus of the stria terminalis, a brain area that is essential for sexual development, is larger in men than women, and that the female brain structure was present in genetically male transsexuals [86]. This suggests that transgenderism is physiological in origin, and according to this study, it may be related to events during prenatal neurological development [86]. Therefore, it might be expected that hormone-dependent regulation of the brain would be subject to endocrine disruption and studies of sexually dimorphic nonreproductive behaviors can be influenced by environmental contaminants [87,88].

9.12 FINAL COMMENTS

Understanding of the dependence of the development and maintenance of the male phenotype on correct functioning of testicular hormones provides a sound basis for the concern that interference from environmental endocrine disruptors would affect these processes if sufficient appropriate compounds enter the human body. The challenge for the future is identifying the specific chemicals or mixtures of chemicals that may act together at low doses over the long term to affect specific tissues at specific times of life. Studies conducted under the National Health and Nutrition Examination Survey (NHANES) have provided evidence that many hundreds of EDCs are widely present in adults and children across the United States, demonstrating that the human body now contains complex mixtures of chemicals originating from environmental exposures that would not have occurred a century ago. However, demonstrating the presence of chemicals in the human body is only the starting point; what is now needed is to understand the specific concentrations of specific EDCs necessary for any adverse effects in different tissues at different stages of life.

Animal models have provided a proof of principle that exposure in utero to some environmental chemicals (most notably certain phthalates) can indeed disrupt male development, with reproductive consequences in the adult animal that are similar to those in the adult human. The only direct evidence in humans of adverse effects from exposure to exogenous estrogens during fetal development comes from the reproductive abnormalities reported in sons born to mothers who were given DES during the first trimester of pregnancy, and the fact that not all sons had symptoms (or even the same symptoms) illustrates the heterogeneity in response even from a relatively even source of exposure to a single compound. Whether higher doses or altered specific timing of doses would have caused effects in unaffected sons will never be known because DES is no longer prescribed.

The reversible nature of gynecomastia and other reproductive symptoms in adult men following cessation of exposure to specific sources of dermally applied estrogenic compounds are important not only in demonstrating that exposure to exogenous estrogens in adult life can have adverse effects on reproductive health, but also in identifying the specific chemical culprits. Since gynecomastia does not arise in every mortician who uses embalming creams without gloves or in every man who uses personal care products with lavender and tea-tree oils, there must again be individual susceptibilities involved; and understanding the nature of those susceptibilities in terms of dosage, absorption, metabolism, and clearance would be very important information that could enable more personalized reproductive medical advice.

The many studies carried out to date all point to the need for future research to make a paradigm shift away from assuming that a single chemical must be found at higher levels in all those suffering from a specific condition in order for there to be a functional association, partly because of the varied individual responses, but also because of the potential for multiple compounds to complement one another in their actions. Differing lifestyles will result in varied deposition of chemical mixtures in individuals, and different combinations of specific chemicals may cause similar adverse effects. There seems little doubt anymore that endocrine disruption is occurring, but the central question remains as to which chemical exposures might be causative for which conditions and how to begin to identify the specific sources of the culprit complex mixtures so that prevention can become a viable option. The reversibility of cases of gynecomastia provides a real hope that if the source can be eliminated for that individual, then symptoms can be reversed. However, the nonreversible nature of conditions such as hypospadias or cryptorchidism will require a more generalized precautionary approach to avoiding gestational exposure. More specific information will be needed before educational material can give advice to those with the ultimate responsibility (namely, the mother on behalf of her sons) about what substances to avoid—and this reminds us that in environmental matters, we are not always in control of our own destinies.

References

[1] Gilbert SF. Chromosomal sex determination in mammals Developmental biology, 6th ed. Sunderland, MA: Sinauer Associates; 2000. [Chapter 17].

[2] Sharpe RM. Pathways of endocrine disruption during male sexual differentiation and masculinisation. Best Pract Res Clin Endocrinol Metab 2006;20:91–110.

[3] Adham IM, Agoulnik AI. Insulin-like 3 signalling in testicular descent. Int J Androl 2004;27:257–65.

[4] Hess RA. Estrogen in the adult male reproductive tract: a review. Reprod Biol Endocrinol 2003;1(52):1–14.

[5] Kristensen DM, Hass U, Lesne L, Lottrup G, Jacobsen PR, Lethimonier CD, et al. Intrauterine exposure to mild analgesics is a risk factor for development of male reproductive disorders in human and rat. Hum Reprod 2013;26:235–44.

[6]   Woods HF. (chairman). Phytoestrogens and health. London: Food Standards Agency Publication. Crown Copyright, <http://cot.food.gov.uk/pdfs/phytoreport0503>; 2003.

[7]   Harris RM, Waring RH. Diethylstilboestrol—a long-term legacy. Maturitas 2012;72:108–12.

[8]   Palmer JR, Herbst AL, Noller KL, Boggs DA, Troisi R, Titus-Ernstoff L, et al. Urogenital abnormalities in men exposed to diethylstilboestrol *in utero*: a cohort study. Environ Health 2009;8(37):1–6.

[9]   Finkelstein JS, McCully WF, MacLaughlin DT, Godine JE, Crowley WF. The Mortician's mystery. N Engl J Med 1988;318:961–5.

[10] Henley DV, Lipson N, Korach KS, Bloch CA. Prepubertal gynecomastia linked to lavender and tea tree oils. N Engl J Med 2007;356:479–85.

[11] Chilvers C, Pike MC, Forman D, Fogelman K, Wadsworth ME. Apparent doubling of frequency of unde-scended testis in England and Wales in 1962–81. Lancet 1984;2:330–2.

[12] Matlai P, Beral V. Trends in congenital malformations of external genitalia. Lancet 1985;1:108.

[13] Paulozzi LJ, Erickson JD, Jackson RJ. Hypospadias trends in two US surveillance systems. Pediatrics 1997;100:831–4.

[14] Paulozzi LJ. International trends in rates of hypospadias and cryptorchidism. Environ Health Perspect 1999;107:297–302.

[15] Toppari J, Kaleva M, Virtanen HE. Trends in the incidence of cryptorchidism and hypospadias, and method-ological limitations of registry-based data. Hum Reprod Update 2001;7:282–6.

[16] Boisen KA, Kaleva M, Main KM, Virtanen HE, Haavisto AM, Schmidt IM, et al. Difference in prevalence of congenital cryptorchidism in infants between two Nordic countries. Lancet 2004;363:1264–9.

[17] Boisen K, Chellakooty M, Schmidt IM, Kai CM, Damgaard IN, Suomi AM, et al. Hypospadias in a cohort of 1072 Danish newborn boys: prevalence and relationship to placental weight, anthropometrical measurements at birth, and reproductive hormone levels at three months of age. J Clin Endocrinol Metab 2005;90:4041–6.

[18] Weidner IS, Moller H, Jensen TK, Skakkebaek NE. Risk factors for cryptorchidism and hypospadias. J Urol 1999;161:1606–9.

[19] Virtanen HE, Adamsson A. Cryptorchidism and endocrine disrupting chemicals. Mol Cell Endocrinol 2012;355:208–20.

[20] Bay K, Asklund C, Skakkebaek NE, Andersson AM. Testicular dysgenesis syndrome: possible role of endocrine disrupters. Best Pract Res Clin Endocrinol Metab 2006;20:77–90.

[21] Fisher JS, Macpherson S, Marchetti N, Sharpe RM. Human "testicular dysgenesis syndrome": a possible model using *in-utero* exposure of the rat to dibutylphthalate. Hum Reprod 2003;18:1383–94.

[22] Dolk H, Vrijheid M, Armstrong B, Abramsky L, Bianchi F, Garne E, et al. Risk of congenital anomalies near hazardous-waste landfill sites in Europe: the EUROHAZCON study. Lancet 1998;352:423–7.

[23] García-Rodríguez J, García-Martín M, Nogueras-Ocaña M, de Dios Luna-del-Castillo J, Espigares García M, Olea N, et al. Exposure to pesticides and cryptorchidism: geographical evidence of a possible association. Environ Health Perspect 1996;104:1090–5.

[24] Weidner IS, Moller H, Jensen TK, Skakkebaek NE. Cryptorchidism and hypospadias in sons of gardeners and farmers. Environ Health Perspect 1998;106:793–6.

[25] Pierik FH, Burdorf A, Deddens JA, Juttman RE, Weber RF. Maternal and paternal risk factors for cryptorchi-dism and hypospadias: a case-control study in newborn boys. Environ Health Perspect 2004;112:1570–6.

[26] Kristensen DM, Hass U, Lesné L, Lottrup G, Jacobsen PR, Desdoits-Lethimonier C, et al. Intrauterine exposure to mild analgesics is a risk factor for development of male reproductive disorders in human and rat. Hum Reprod 2011;26:235–44.

[27] Welsh M, Saunders PTK, Fisken M, Scott LB, Sharpe RM. Identification in rats of a programming window for reproductive tract masculinisation, disruption of which leads to hypospadias and cryptorchidism. J Clin Invest 2008;118:1479–90.

[28] FAO/WHO (Food and Agriculture Organization/World Health Organization). Evaluation of certain food addi-tives and contaminants. Fifty-Seventh Report of the Joint FAO/WHO Expert Committee on Food Additives, Rome, Italy; 2002.

[29] Mylchreest E, Wallace DG, Cattley RC, Foster PM. Dose-dependent alterations in androgen-regulated male reproductive development in rats exposed to di(*n*-butyl) phthalate during late gestation. Toxicol Sci 2000;55:143–51.

[30] Zhang L, Dong L, Ding S, Qiao P, Wang C, Zhang M, et al. Effects of *n*-butylparaben on steroidogenesis and spermatogenesis through changed E2 levels in male offspring. Environ Toxicol Pharmacol 2014;37:705–17.

[31] Christiansen S, Axelstad M, Boberg J, Vinggaard AM, Pedersen GA, Hass U. Low-dose effects of bisphenol A on early sexual development in male and female rats. Reproduction 2014;147:477–87.

[32] Thankamony A, Lek N, Carroll D, Williams M, Dunger DB, Acerini CL, et al. Anogenital distance and penile length in infants with hypospadias or cryptorchidism: comparison with normative data. Environ Health Perspect 2014;122:207–11.

[33] Swan SH, Main KM, Liu F, Stewart SL, Kruse RL, Calafat AM, et al. The Study for Future Families Research Team. Decrease in anogenital distance among male infants with prenatal phthalate exposure. Environ Health Perspect 2005;113:1056–61.

[34] Bustamante-Montes LP, Hernandez-Valero MA, Flores-Pimentel D, Garcia-Fabila M, Amaya-Chavez A, Barr DB, et al. Prenatal exposure to phthalates is associated with decreased anogenital distance and penile size in male newborns. J Dev Orig Health Dis 2013:4.

[35] Torres-Sanchez L, Zepeda M, Cebrian ME, Belkind-Gerson J, Garcia-Hernandez RM, Belkind-Valdovinos U, et al. Dichlorodiphenyldichloroethylene exposure during the first trimester of pregnancy alters the anal position in male infants. Ann NY Acad Sci 2008;1140:155–62.

[36] Miao M, Yuan W, He Y, Zhou Z, Wang J, Gao E, et al. *In utero* exposure to bisphenol-A and anogenital distance of male offspring. Birth Defects Res A Clin Mol Teratol 2011;91:867–72.

[37] Vafeiadi M, Agramunt S, Papadopoulou E, Besselink H, Mathianaki K, Karakosta P, et al. *In utero* exposure to dioxins and dioxin-like compounds and anogenital distance in newborns and infants. Environ Health Perspect 2013;121:125–30.

[38] Christiansen S, Scholze M, Dalgaard M, Vinggaard AM, Axelstad M, Kortenkamp A, et al. Synergistic disruption of external male sex organ development by a mixture of four antiandrogens. Environ Health Perspect 2009;117:1839–46.

[39] Carlsen E, Giwercman A, Keiding N, Skakkebaek NE. Evidence for decreasing quality of semen during past 50 years. BMJ 1992;305:609–13.

[40] Auger J, Kunstmann JM, Czyglik F, Jouannet P. Decline in semen quality among fertile men in Paris during the past 20 years. N Engl J Med 1995;332:281–5.

[41] Irvine S, Cawood E, Richardson D, MacDonald E, Aitken J. Evidence of deteriorating semen quality in the United Kingdom: birth cohort study in 577 men in Scotland over 11 years. BMJ 1996;312:467–71.

[42] Andersen AG, Jensen TK, Carlsen E, Jorgensen N, Andersson AM, Krarup T, et al. High frequency of suboptimal semen quality in an unselected population of young men. Hum Reprod 2000;15:366–72.

[43] Swan SH, Elkin EP, Fenster L. The question of declining sperm density revisited: an analysis of 101 studies published 1934–1996. Environ Health Perspect 2000;108:961–6.

[44] Kang KS, Che JH, Ryu DY, Kim TW, Li GX, Lee YS. Decreased sperm number and motile activity on the F1 offspring maternally exposed to butyl *p*-hydroxybenzoic acid (butyl paraben). J Vet Med Sci 2002; 64:227–35.

[45] Oishi S. Effects of butylparaben on the male reproductive system in rats. Toxicol Ind Health 2001;17:31–9.

[46] Oishi S. Effects of propylparaben on the male reproductive system. Food Chem Toxicol 2002;40:1807–13.

[47] Oishi S. Effects of butylparaben on the male reproductive system in mice. Arch Toxicol 2002;76:423–9.

[48] Oishi S. Lack of spermatotoxic effects of methyl and ethyl esters of *p*-hydroxybenzoic acid in rats. Food Chem Toxicol 2004;42:1845–9.

[49] Meeker JD, Yang T, Ye X, Calafat AM, Hauser R. Urinary concentrations of parabens and serum hormone levels, semen quality parameters, and sperm DNA damage. Environ Health Perspect 2010;119:252–7.

[50] Meeker JD, Calafat AM, Hauser R. Urinary bisphenol A concentrations in relation to serum thyroid and reproductive hormone levels in men from an infertility clinic. Environ Sci Technol 2010;44:1458–63.

[51] Meeker JD, Ehrlich S, Toth TL, Wright DL, Calafat AM, Trisini AT, et al. Semen quality and sperm DNA damage in relation to urinary bisphenol A in men from an infertility clinic. Reprod Toxicol 2010;30:532–9.

[52] Darbre PD, Harvey PH. Paraben esters: review of recent studies of endocrine toxicity, absorption, esterase and human exposure, and discussion of potential human health risks. J Appl Toxicol 2008;28:561–78.

[53] McLachlan RI, deKrester DM. Male infertility: the case for continued research. Med J Aust 2001;174:116–7.

[54] Aitken RJ. Falling sperm counts twenty years on: where are we now? Asian J Androl 2013;15:204–7.

[55] Wilcox AJ, Baird DD, Weinberg CR, Hornsby PP, Herbst AL. Fertility in men exposed prenatally to diethylstilbestrol. N Engl J Med 1995;332:1411–6.

[56] Stenchever MA, Williamson RA, Leonard J, Karp LE, Ley B, Shy K, et al. Possible relationship between *in utero* diethylstilbestrol exposure and male fertility. Am J Obstet Gynecol 1981;140:186–93.

[57] Whitehead ED, Letter E. Genital abnormalities and abnormal semen analyses in male patients exposed to diethylstilbestrol *in utero*. J Urol 1981;125:47–50.

[58] Adami HO, Bergstrom R, Mohner M, Aalonski W, Storm H, Ekbom A, et al. Testicular cancer in nine northern European countries. Int J Cancer 1994;59:33–8.

[59] Moller H. Trends in sex-ratio, testicular cancer and male reproductive hazards: are they connected? Acta Pathol Microbiol Immunol Scand 1998;106:232–8.

[60] Richiardi L, Bellocco R, Adami HO, Torrang A, Barlow L, Hakulinen T, et al. Testicular cancer incidence in eight northern European countries: secular and recent trends. Cancer Epidemiol Biomarkers Prev 2004;13:2157–66.

[61] Skakkebaek NE, Rajpert-De Meyts E, Main KM. Testicular dysgenesis syndrome: an increasingly common developmental disorder with environmental aspects. Hum Reprod 2001;16:972–8.

[62] Martin OV, Shialis T, Lester JN, Scrimshaw MD, Boobis AR, Voulvoulis N. Testicular dysgenesis syndrome and the estrogen hypothesis: a quantitative meta-analysis. Environ Health Perspect 2008;116:149–57.

[63] Luccio-Camelo DC, Prins GS. Disruption of androgen receptor signalling in males by environmental chemicals. J Steroid Biochem Mol Biol 2011;127:74–82.

[64] Kortenkamp A, Scholze M, Ermler S. Mind the gap: can we explain declining male reproductive health with known antiandrogens? Reproduction 2014;147:515–27.

[65] Jobling S, Reynolds T, White R, Parker MG, Sumpter JP. A variety of environmentally persistent chemicals, including some phthalate plasticizers, are weakly estrogenic. Environ Health Perspect 1995;103:582–7.

[66] Takeuchi S, Iida M, Kobayashi S, Jin K, Matsuda T, Kojima H. Differential effects of phthalate esters on transcriptional activities via human estrogen receptors alpha and beta, and androgen receptor. Toxicology 2005;210:223–33.

[67] Diamanti-Kandarakis E, Gore AC, editors. Endocrine disruptors and puberty. New York, NY: Humana Press, Springer; 2012.

[68] Marshall WA, Tanner JM. Variations in the pattern of pubertal changes in boys. Arch Dis Child 1970;45:13–23.

[69] Garry VF, Truran P. Secular trends in pubertal timing: a role for environmental chemical exposure? Diamanti-Kandarakis E, Gore AC, editors. Endocrine disruptors and puberty. New York, NY: Humana Press, Springer; 2012.

[70] Sorensen K, Aksglaede L, Petersen JH, Juul A. Recent changes in pubertal timing in healthy Danish boys: associations with body mass index. J Clin Endocrinol Metab 2010;95:263–70.

[71] Wu X, Zhang N, Lee MM. The influence of endocrine disruptors on male pubertal timing. Diamanti-Kandarakis E, Gore AC, editors. Endocrine disruptors and puberty. New York, NY: Humana Press, Springer; 2012.

[72] Den Hond E, Roels HA, Hoppenbrouwers K, Nawrot T, Thijs L, Vandermeulen C, et al. Sexual maturation in relation to polychlorinated aromatic hydrocarbons: Sharpe and Skakkebaek's hypothesis revisited. Environ Health Perspect 2002;110:771–6.

[73] Saiyed H, Dewan A, Bhatnagar V, Shenoy U, Shenoy R, Rajmohan H, et al. Effect of endosulfan on male reproductive development. Environ Health Perspect 2003;111:1958–62.

[74] Roehrborn CG. Pathology of benign prostatic hyperplasia. Int J Impotence Res 2008;20:S11–8.

[75] Berry SJ, Coffey DS, Walsh PC, Ewing LL. The development of human benign prostatic hyperplasia with age. J Urol 1984;132:474–9.

[76] Prins GS, Korach KS. The role of estrogens and estrogen receptors in normal prostate growth and disease. Steroids 2008;73:233–44.

[77] Nicholson TM, Ricke WA. Androgens and estrogens in benign prostatic hyperplasia: past, present and future. Differentiation 2011;82:184–99.

[78] Ho CK, Habib FK. Estrogen and androgen signaling in the pathogenesis of BPH. Nat Rev Urol 2011;8:29–41.

[79] Belanger A, Candas B, Dupont A, Cusan L, Diamond P, Gomez JL, et al. Changes in serum concentrations of conjugated and unconjugated steroids in 40- to 80-year-old men. J Clin Endocrinol Metab 1994;79:1086–90.

[80] Ellem SJ, Risbridger GP. The dual, opposing roles of estrogen in the prostate. Ann NY Acad Sci 2009;1155:174–86.

[81] Prins GS, Ho SM. Early-life estrogens and prostate cancer in an animal model. J Dev Orig Health Dis 2010;1:365–70.

[82] vom Saal FS, Timms BG, Montano MM, Palanza P, Thayer KA, Nagel SC, et al. Prostate enlargement in mice due to fetal exposure to low doses of estradiol or diethylstilbestrol and opposite effects at high doses. Proc Natl Acad Sci USA 1997;94:2056–61.

[83] Nagel SC, vom Saal FS, Thayer KA, Dhar MG, Boechler M, Welshons WV. Relative binding affinity-serum modified access (RBA-SMA) assay predicts the relative *in vivo* bioactivity of the xenoestrogens bisphenol A and octylphenol. Environ Health Perspect 1997;105:70–6.

[84] Prins GS, Hu WY, Shi GB, Hu DP, Majumdar S, Li G, et al. Bisphenol A promotes human prostate stem-progenitor cell self-renewal and increases *in vivo* carcinogenesis in human prostate epithelium. Endocrinology 2014;155:805–17.

[85] Hood E. Are EDCs blurring issues of gender? Environ Health Perspect 2005;113:A670–7.

[86] Zhou JN, Hofman MA, Gooren LJG, Swaab DF. A sex difference in the human brain and its relation to trans-sexuality. Nature 1995;378:68–70.

[87] Weiss B. Sexually dimorphic nonreproductive behaviors as indicators of endocrine disruption. Environ Health Perspect 2002;110(Suppl. 3):387–91.

[88] Weiss B. Endocrine disruptors as a threat to neurological function. J Neurol Sci 2011;305:11–21.

Endocrine Disruption and Cancer of Reproductive Tissues

Philippa D. Darbre and Graeme Williams

Endocrine Disruption and Human Health.
DOI: http://dx.doi.org/10.1016/B978-0-12-801139-3.00010-7

Abstract

This chapter discusses the potential for endocrine-disrupting chemicals (EDCs) to influence the development of cancer in female endocrine-sensitive tissues of the breast, endometrium, ovary, and cervix, and in male hormone-regulated tissues of the prostate, testis, and breast. Hanahan and Weinberg have established a framework for understanding the complexity of cancer development through their definition of hallmarks and enabling characteristics, and this offers the opportunity to explore the ability of complex environmental mixtures of EDCs to affect cancer. It is not necessary for each EDC to affect all the hallmarks, but if a mixture of EDCs can together affect all the hallmarks, and do so at environmentally relevant concentrations measurable in human tissues, then there is the potential for cancer development.

10.1 INTRODUCTION: HOW COULD ENDOCRINE DISRUPTION AFFECT CANCER?

Cancer is not a new problem; it has been documented in Egyptian papyrus scrolls dating back to 3000 BC, and it was recorded in the writings of ancient Greece by Hippocrates (460–375 BC) [1], but the worldwide rise in incidence over recent decades, particularly in endocrine-sensitive tissues is unprecedented. Breast cancer has become now the major cancer suffered by women and prostate cancer the major cancer suffered by men in many Westernized countries [2]. Although life expectancy may be greater in modern times than in ancient days and most cancer incidence tends to increase with age, some cancers with rising incidence, such as testicular cancer, affect young people [3]. Although the majority of breast cancer in the United Kingdom occurs over the age of 50 years, the 20% proportion of breast cancers under age 50 has remained constant despite a near doubling of incidence over the past 30 years, which demonstrates that the number of young-age breast cancer is also rising [4]. Development of cancer is a lengthy and complex process involving both genetic and environmental components, but the strong environmental link is demonstrated by studies of migrant populations who tend to take on cancer rates of the country to which they have moved, and this has been shown for breast and prostate cancers [5]. Twin studies have also highlighted the importance of environmental factors [6,7]. Serious questions need, therefore, to be posed about the potential for environmental chemicals with endocrine-disrupting properties to influence not only reproductive functions, but also the development of cancer in endocrine-sensitive tissues.

Cancer is a disease of cells that arises from a loss of normal cell growth control. It is a multistep process [8] (Figure 10.1) starting from initiating events that involve DNA damage, and specifically damage to DNA needed for expression of genes required for the normal processes of cell growth. Tumor promotion then enables the damaged cells to grow and further rounds of initiation/promotion may be required for carcinogenesis [8]. Subsequent steps of tumor growth cause the damaged cells to grow in an uncontrolled manner into a localized mass of cells that may begin to disrupt local tissue architecture and cause further changes to the microenvironment. Throughout this process, the uncontrolled cells become increasingly unstable, accumulating increasing numbers of genetic and phenotypic changes that result in what is then termed *tumor progression*. During progression, changes can also occur to cell adhesion and motility, enabling some cells to break away from the tumor mass. If these cells also acquire invasive properties, they then have the potential to move from the site of origin to distant sites around the body in a process termed *metastasis*. In endocrine-sensitive tissues where cell growth is under endocrine control, all of

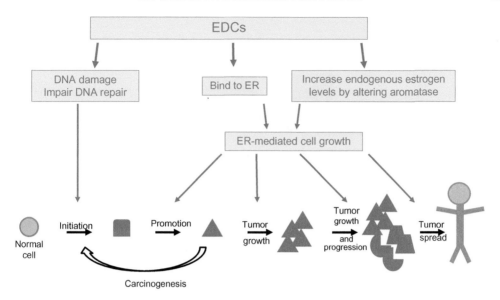

FIGURE 10.1 Schematic diagram of the stages in the development of cancer. EDCs may act at initiation through enabling DNA damage, impeding its repair, or both. EDCs may act at other stages by increasing cell growth through binding directly to ERs or through altering aromatase activity, and hence increasing levels of endogenous estrogens.

these steps of deregulation could be influenced by endocrine-disrupting chemicals (EDCs) through their ability to disrupt normal endocrine controls (Figure 10.1).

Hanahan and Weinberg have provided an alternative framework for understanding the complexity of cancer development in terms of a series of hallmarks [9,10] (Figure 10.2). The hallmarks and enabling characteristics describe a series of biological capabilities that result in the necessary changes for the cells to assume a transformed state and, ultimately, a fully malignant and metastatic state. The six basic hallmarks [9,10] are sustained proliferative signaling, evasion of growth suppressors, resistance to cell death, replicative immortality, induction of angiogenesis, and activation of invasion and metastasis. Two underlying enabling characteristics are genome instability and inflammation [10]. Two emerging hallmarks are evasion of immune destruction and reprogramming of energy metabolism [10]. This framework offers the opportunity to now explore the ability of complex environmental mixtures of EDCs to affect cancer. It is not necessary for each EDC to affect all the hallmarks but if a mixture of EDCs can together affect all the hallmarks, then there is the potential for cancer development (Figure 10.2). This will be discussed in this chapter for the female cancers of the breast, endometrium, ovary, and cervix, and for the male cancers of the prostate, testis, and breast (Figure 10.3).

10.2 CANCERS IN FEMALE REPRODUCTIVE TISSUES

Cancers in endocrine-responsive reproductive tissues comprised a total of 42.0% of all female cancers in England for 2012 as published in June 2014 [11], with breast cancer being

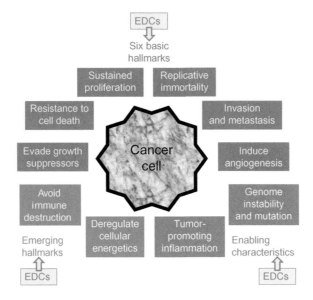

FIGURE 10.2   Schematic diagram showing the six basic hallmarks of cancer (red), two emerging hallmarks (orange), and two enabling characteristics (green), as defined by Hanahan and Weinberg [9,10]. EDCs may influence any of these hallmarks or characteristics.

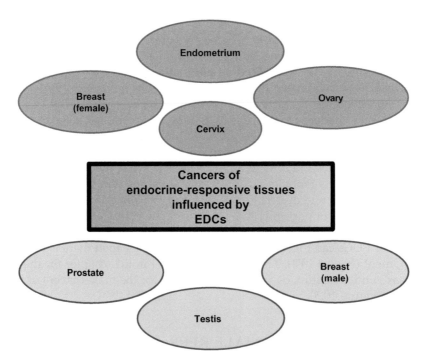

FIGURE 10.3   Cancers of endocrine-responsive tissues that may be influenced by EDCs. Female cancers are shown in pink, and male cancers in blue.

3. CONCERNS FOR HUMAN HEALTH

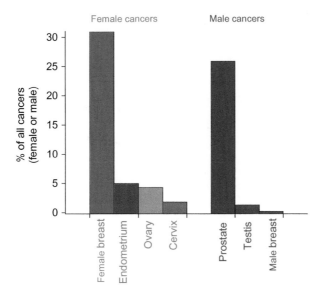

FIGURE 10.4   Percentage of total female cancer incidence in endocrine-responsive tissues (pink) and percentage of total male cancer incidence in endocrine-responsive tissues (blue) in England for 2012, as published in June 2014 [11].

the major cancer of women (30.9%) and cancers of endometrium (5.0%), ovary (4.3%), and cervix (1.8%) adding to the total (Figure 10.4).

10.2.1 Breast Cancer

10.2.1.1 Case for Involvement of EDCs in the Rising Incidence of Breast Cancer

The breast is an endocrine-responsive organ, and its development through puberty, pregnancy, and lactation is regulated by a complex network of coordinated hormonal controls. The anatomical structure shows a series of ducts and lobules lined with epithelial cells (which produce the milk) and surrounded by fatty stromal tissue (Figure 10.5). Although breast cancer comprises a wide range of pathologies, the majority of cancers now arise in the ductal epithelial cells. This has not always been so, because in the United Kingdom in the 1970s, fewer than 10% of breast cancers were ductal, lobular, or medullary, but by the end of the 1990s, this percentage had risen to 75%, with ductal carcinomas alone comprising 60% of all breast cancer cases [12]. Therefore, it must be acknowledged that along with the rising incidence is also a changing biology. One important anatomical feature of breast is the high fat content, and this is relevant in the context that many environmental EDCs are lipophilic and therefore can bioaccumulate in breast fat which surrounds the target cells for cancer (Figure 10.5).

Although loss of function of the DNA repair genes *BRCA1/2* [13,14], diet, radiation, and alcohol [15] have all been implicated as risk factors, the main influence in the development of breast cancer remains hormonal, particularly lifetime exposure to estrogen [15]. Pioneering experiments by Beatson in 1896 demonstrated that estrogen synthesized by the ovary in the premenopausal woman is a driving force for breast cancer growth [16] and subsequent clinical, epidemiological, animal, and cell culture studies have all confirmed this

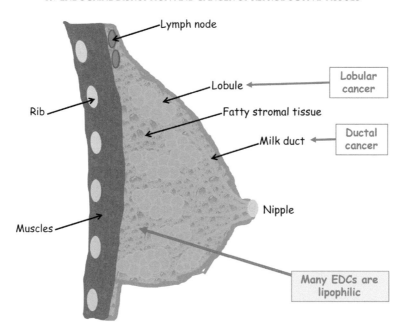

FIGURE 10.5   A diagram showing the anatomical structure of the human breast. Milk is produced in the epithelial cells lining the ducts and lobules and flows down the ducts to the nipple; these epithelial cells are also the main target cells for cancer. The ducts and lobules are embedded in fatty stromal tissue: since many EDCs are lipophilic, this concentrates them adjacent to the target cancer cells.

over the past century [17]. Epidemiological studies have confirmed a hormonal influence on breast cancer through enhanced risk resulting from early puberty, late menopause, nulliparity, late age of first pregnancy [15], use of oral contraceptives [18], and administration of hormone replacement therapy (HRT) [19–21]. The established role of estrogen in breast cancer is now the basis for the successful use of endocrine therapy using either antiestrogens to block estrogen receptors (ERs) or aromatase inhibitors to block estrogen synthesis [22]. It is this central role of estrogen in the development, progression, and treatment of breast cancer that then raises the question of whether environmental chemicals, which can enter human breast tissue and which possess estrogenic properties, could provide an environmental component in driving the increasing incidence of breast cancer [23,24]. Not all breast cancers are estrogen-responsive, but the majority of them are, and the proportion that are is increasing in the United Kingdom [25,26], in France [27], and in the United States [28,29]. It is, therefore, an unexplained paradox that 80% of breast cancers in the United Kingdom occur over the age of 50, at a time of life when endogenous estrogen levels have dropped with the onset of menopause [4], and this raises the possibility that it is environmental estrogenic chemicals that are driving this development of estrogen-responsive breast cancers in later life.

10.2.1.2 *Exposure to Exogenous Estrogens and Breast Cancer*

Diethylstilbestrol (DES) is a synthetic estrogen that was given to several million women to prevent threatened miscarriage between 1940 and 1971 until reported adverse effects resulted in cessation of further prescription (Section 8.4) [30]. Long-term follow-up studies have shown that women exposed to DES during pregnancy have an increased risk of breast cancer [31]. The incidence of breast cancer per 100,000 woman-years rose from 93 in the unexposed control group to 134 in the exposed group, giving a crude relative risk of 1.4 [31]. Early studies in the daughters born to DES-exposed mothers reported a strong association between DES and clear cell adenocarcinoma of the vagina and cervix [32], but longer-term studies have also found an increased breast cancer risk [33]. These studies provide evidence that breast cancer risk can be increased by exposure to a synthetic exogenous estrogen and that risk is increased irrespective of whether the exposure is confined to adult life or only in utero. This suggests that the breast may be sensitive to exposure to excess estrogen at multiple stages of life. However, since not all DES-exposed mothers or daughters have developed breast cancer, there must be further susceptibility factors that need to be identified.

Use of the contraceptive pill and HRT in adult life also involve the administration of synthetic estrogens (most notably ethinylestradiol) to millions of women worldwide. Breast cancer risk has been shown to be increased by long-term use of the contraceptive pill from a young age [18], but altered formulations of drugs with lower estrogen levels over time has reduced measurable risks [34,35]. This serves to demonstrate the importance of estrogen/progestin formulations and underlines the complexity of pharmaceutical exposures that now exist. HRT has been widely used for many years to relieve menopausal symptoms and also is associated with increased breast cancer risk [19–21]. Estrogen-only formulations are prescribed only after hysterectomy, and most users take an estrogen/progestin combination to minimize stimulatory effects of estrogen on endometrial tissue, but increased risk of breast cancer has to be weighed against the benefits of symptom relief. As for DES exposure, not everyone who is exposed to these synthetic hormones develops breast cancer, indicating that much still needs to be understood concerning individual susceptibility and interacting factors.

10.2.1.3 *Measurement of EDCs in Human Breast Tissue*

Many environmental chemicals with estrogenic properties have now been measured in human breast tissue or milk (itself a product of the breast epithelial cells), and although their presence alone cannot be taken to imply any adverse consequences, it does confirm that EDCs are ubiquitously present in human breast tissue. Estrogenic compounds can enter the human breast from many diverse oral, dermal, or respiratory exposure routes (Table 10.1) [23,24]. Organochlorine pesticides and herbicides with estrogenic properties enter the human breast ubiquitously from dietary consumption of residues on fruits and vegetables or of residues that have bioaccumulated and passed up the food chain in animal fat. Occupational or locational proximity to agricultural or domestic pesticide/herbicide spraying may lead to more direct inhalation. A range of pesticides and herbicides have now been measured as present in human breast tissue, including dichlorodiphenyltrichloroethane (DDT) and its metabolites, dieldrin, and hexachlorobenzene [36,37]. Pyrethroids have been measured in human breast milk in South Africa [38], the United States [39], Spain, and South America [40] and India [41]. Polychlorinated biphenyls (PCBs) from industrial use and dioxins from combustion of organochlorines enter human tissues mainly from dietary consumption of residues in animal fat, and many of the congeners are known to be present in human breast fat [42]. Phytoestrogens are consumed in relatively large amounts from

TABLE 10.1   Sources of Exposure of the Human Breast to EDCs

Source of exposure for the human breast	Use	Example compounds
Diet	Environmental contaminants of fruit and vegetables	Organochlorine agrochemicals
Diet	Environmental contaminants of meat	Organochlorine contaminants in animal fat, hormonally-active chemicals in meat production
Diet	Edible plant material	Phytoestrogens
Diet	Food additives	Parabens (preservatives); propylgallate (fats/oils); 4-hexylresorcinol (shellfish)
Diet	Food packaging	BPA, phthalates (plastics); aluminum (foil)
Pharmaceuticals	Oral contraceptive, HRT	Ethinylestradiol
Domestic environment	Plastics	BPA, phthalates
Domestic environment	Flame retardants on soft furnishings	Polybrominated diphenylethers
Domestic environment	Detergents	Alkyl phenols
Domestic environment	Stain repellant (furnishings and clothing)	Perfluorooctanoic acid/sulfonate/salts
Domestic environment	Antimicrobials	Triclosan (household cleaning products); Parabens (paper products)
Domestic environment	Household pesticides/herbicides	Pyrethroids, glyphosate
Domestic environment	Air fresheners	Volatile organic compounds (fragrance); limonene; phthalate esters
Total air environment	Toxic air emissions	Dioxins
Personal care products, including cosmetics	Lotions left on skin; rinse-off products; mouth pastes and lotions; impregnated clothing and sanitary products	See Figure 10.6
Occupational	Farming	Pesticides, herbicides

edible plant material, and although they are cleared mainly from the body within hours, they can have potent effects on breast epithelial cells [43]. Bisphenol A (BPA) can enter the human body from plastics in the domestic environment or in diet from its widespread use in plastic food packaging and has been measured in human breast milk [44]. Phthalates are also widely used in plastics and have been measured in human breast milk [45,46]. Alkyl phenols used in detergents have been measured in human breast milk [47]. Polybrominated diphenyl ethers are used as flame retardants on soft furnishings, and they are measurable in human breast milk [48–50].

Dermal application of personal care products provides another route of exposure to a range of estrogenic chemicals (Figure 10.6) [23,24]. Parabens, which are used as preservatives in personal care products as well as foods and pharmaceuticals, have been measured

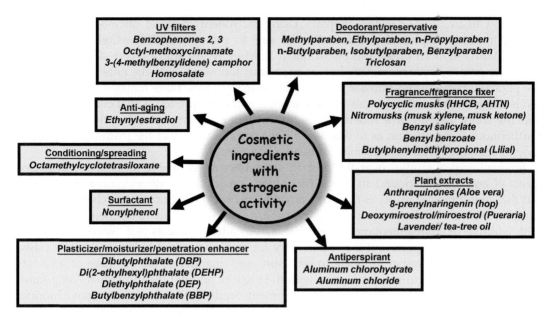

FIGURE 10.6   Chemical components of personal care products that have been shown to possess estrogenic activity using assay systems in vitro and in vivo. Chemicals are grouped according to their function in the product. References demonstrating their estrogenic activity have been collated previously [23,24]. HHCB, 1,3,4,6,7,8-hexahydro-4,6,6,7,8,8-hexamethylcyclopenta[g]-2-benzopyran; AHTN, 7-acetyl-1,1,3,4,4,6-hexamethyl-1,2,3,4-tetrahydronapthalene.

in human breast tissue [51,52]. Although aluminum is present in diet, its use as an active underarm antiperspirant agent provides high local exposure for the breast, and aluminum has been measured in human breast tissue [53], breast cyst fluid [54], and nipple aspirate fluid [55]. Triclosan [56,57], which is used as an antimicrobial agent, ultraviolet (UV) screens [58] and musk fragrance compounds [58,59], have been measured in human breast milk.

10.2.1.4 Functional Analysis of the Presence of EDCs in Human Breast Tissue

Since so many EDCs have been measured in human breast tissue, functional studies are needed to assess whether their presence in the long term at low doses, either alone or in combination as complex mixtures, can cause a number of adverse effects that might lead to cancer development. Approaches to assessing functionality have included the use of animal models and use of epidemiological studies that aim to correlate increased levels of chemicals in breast tissue with the presence of breast cancers. Both have their weaknesses and neither approaches have yielded conclusive results concerning the causation of human breast cancer.

Animal models of breast carcinogenesis have been used over the years to demonstrate effects of EDCs on breast cancer development in rodents. Based on animal models, 17β-estradiol has been classified as a class 1 carcinogen by the International Agency for Research on Cancer [60]. DES has been shown in animal models to cause breast carcinogenesis [30], supporting the findings of raised breast cancer risk in DES-exposed women (as discussed in Section 10.2.1.2 earlier in this chapter). Using the rodent chemical carcinogenesis model, 3,4,3′,4′-tetrachlorobiphenyl was found to be able to promote 7,12-dimethylbenz[a]anthracene (DMBA)-induced breast cancers in rats [61]. More recent studies have shown that BPA can cause preneoplastic mammary lesions in rodents following exposure either in utero or in the perinatal period from transfer in milk [62]. In many cases, there remains a gap between levels administered to the animals in these models and exposure levels that occur in humans, and the short lifespan of a rodent limits the modeling of long-term, low-dose exposures. Furthermore, it is uncertain as to whether differences in anatomy of the mammary glands in rodents compared with humans may influence outcomes.

Epidemiological studies over the past 15 years have been unable to associate increased levels of any one compound in breast tissue with breast cancer development consistently, but the environmental reality is that the human breast is exposed not to one chemical, but to complex mixtures of chemicals from different sources; and it is likely to be chemical mixtures with additive or complementary actions that lead to adverse effects [63]. Since many EDCs have overlapping properties, it is not necessary for each compound to be consistently raised in breast cancer, but rather for there to be a sufficient quantity of one or more of a variety of compounds with additive properties, with the mixture and not the individual compounds providing the stimulus to drive cancer development. Studies of 19 persistent organochlorines have shown that they were measurable at different levels in different people, but overall, 1 or more of the 19 was measurable at high levels in every sample [64]. Analogous results with five esters of parabens have shown that parabens were measurable also at varied levels in different human breast tissue samples, and tissues with high levels of one ester did not necessarily have high levels of another ester, but overall, at least one of the esters was measurable in 158 of 160 human breast tissue samples [52]. Further functional analysis showed that levels of parabens were at sufficient concentrations in many of these human breast tissue samples to stimulate growth of human breast cancer cells in culture, but it was different combinations of the esters that enabled the end-point response [65]. There is, therefore, now an urgent need to measure the concentrations of not just one, or one type, of compound in breast tissue, but rather to build a picture of the totality of EDCs in a single breast tissue sample.

Another major challenge in equating chemical concentrations in tissue samples with cancer development is that breast cancer may start many years before the symptoms appear [66], and in some cases, it is suggested even in utero [67]. Therefore, measurements of chemicals at the time of appearance of a tumor can be expected to reflect only recent tumor growth and progression and may not be reflective of the EDC loading during the early events of carcinogenesis, which emphasizes the need to understand more mechanistically how chemical mixtures in the human breast could act together over the long term to enable the many alterations needed to drive the complex and lengthy processes of cancer development (see Section 10.1).

10.2.1.5 EDCs and the Disproportionate Incidence of Breast Cancer in the Upper Outer Quadrant of the Breast

An evident anomaly of breast cancer incidence is the disproportionate number of tumors which start in the upper outer quadrant (UOQ) of the breast (Figure 10.7). This has been reported in clinical studies for several decades, but the published disproportionality appears to rise chronologically from 31% in the 1920s to 61% in the 1990s [68].

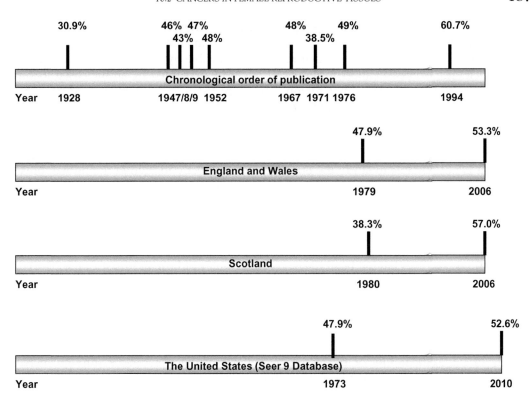

FIGURE 10.7 The relative incidence of breast cancer in the UOQ of the breast as reported in the scientific literature appears to increase chronologically with year of publication from 1928 to 1994 (for references, see [24,68]). Published incidence rates for England and Wales have shown a disproportionate increase in the UOQ from 1979 to 2006, and also from 1980 to 2006 for Scotland [24,68]. Incidence rates taken from the SEER9 database of the United States also show an increase from 1973 to 2010.

Single-population studies have shown that the disproportionality has risen in England and Wales from 47.9% in 1979 to 53.3% in 2006, and in Scotland from 38.3% in 1980 to 57.0% in 2006 on an annual basis [24]. Similar figures can be found on the SEER9 database of the United States (Figure 10.7).

The accepted explanation for more breast cancers starting in the UOQ is that this region contains a greater proportion of epithelial tissue [69], which is the target tissue for breast cancer, but this anatomical explanation cannot account for increasing incidence in that quadrant [24,68]. However, such an increase could be compatible with the increasing application of cosmetics such as antiperspirant/deodorant products to the adjacent underarm region if enough of the chemical components penetrate the skin to underlying breast tissue following long-term usage [70,71]. More recent studies have shown that some parabens [52] and aluminum [53] can be measured at higher levels in outer breast quadrants than inner breast quadrants, which could be compatible with a gradient from underarm application. However, although parabens and aluminum are used in cosmetic products under the arm, exposure can also occur through other routes, and so it is not possible to know whether such a gradient is due to dermal absorption from the underarm region or physiological mechanisms that result in higher levels of certain environmental chemicals being lodged in that region of the breast. Nevertheless, it remains a plausible hypothesis that the dispropor-tionate incidence of breast cancer in the UOQ might be explained by an increased loading of environmental chemicals in that region, and more tissue measurements are needed to explore the regional distribution of EDCs across the breast.

10.2.1.6 *Unraveling the Mechanisms of EDC Action in Relation to the Hallmarks of Cancer*

Since it is not possible to study the effects of EDCs directly in vivo in the human breast, one approach to investigating the implications of the presence of mixtures of EDCs in human breast tissue would be to study the effects of EDCs alone and in combination on human breast epithelial cells (transformed and nontransformed) in cell culture systems (especially those which recapitulate in vivo conditions through use of three-dimensional matrices and co-culture with stromal cells) and to do so using concentrations that have envi-ronmental relevance as having been measured in samples of human breast tissue. The con-ceptual framework of the hallmarks of cancer [9,10] then offers a focus on which to assess the overall ability of EDCs to influence processes leading to cancer development in breast cells (Figure 10.2). An example of such an approach has shown that parabens can enable multiple hallmarks of cancer to develop in human breast epithelial cells [72].

EDCs with estrogenic activity may act on breast epithelial cells either through binding directly to intracellular ERs or by increasing cellular estrogen synthesis through increas-ing aromatase activity (see Chapter 3). Since most estrogenic chemicals bind more weakly to ER than physiological estrogens [73], they have been termed *weak estrogens*. However, this simply means that higher concentrations of the compounds have to be present for an effect to be measurable, and most estrogenic chemicals are full agonists in in vitro assays when suffi-cient concentration of the compound is present. Most estrogenic chemicals do not have a weak efficacy, therefore, and what becomes important is not whether the chemicals bind with low affinity to ER, but how much chemical is present in the breast tissue. Furthermore, low doses of estrogenic chemicals have been shown capable in vitro of being added together to give responses at concentrations where each alone would have been ineffective, in the "something from nothing effect" [74,75], which demonstrates that dependency of response does not rest on the presence of single chemicals alone, but on the totality of chemical burden in a breast.

Through an ER-mediated mechanism, estrogenic EDCs (alone or in combination) may then enable the hallmark of sustained proliferation in ER+ breast cancer cells, which could drive processes of promotion and growth of the primary tumor together with growth of tumors at metastatic sites. The mechanisms by which estrogens increase the proliferation of human breast cancer cells remain incompletely understood but involves altered expression of thousands of genes on microarray analysis together with specific alterations to cell-cycle regulated proteins and interactions with growth factors and their receptor-signaling pathways [76]. Although mechanistic studies are lacking for EDCs, their estrogenic activity is primar-ily defined by their ability to drive the proliferation of estrogen-responsive human breast cancer cells in culture, most notably the MCF-7 cell line (see Chapter 3), and additive effects of mixtures of chemicals at low doses have been demonstrated on proliferation in this cell line [74,75]. This demonstrates the potential for a proliferative stimulus to be generated not only from individual chemicals if present at sufficient concentration in the breast, but also from complex mixtures of estrogenic chemicals that might be at concentrations too low to give a response individually. Since hundreds of estrogenic chemicals have been measured in human breast tissue (see Section 10.2.1.3 earlier in this chapter), it is plausible that an estrogenic stimulus could be generated from chemical mixtures in the breast; and this has been demonstrated for parabens at concentrations measurable in human breast tissue [65].

While estrogenic chemicals may influence sustained proliferation through their continuous and unregulated presence, it is likely that they will influence other estrogen-regulated hallmark processes such as apoptosis and evasion of growth suppressors [76]. It has also been shown that some EDCs such as phthalates [77,78], parabens [79], and aluminum [80] can increase migratory and invasive activity of human breast cancer cells in culture, which heralds the potential for driving the hallmark of invasion and metastasis. This is especially relevant for breast cancer, where mortality results primarily from growth of tumors at metastatic sites rather than from the tumor growth at the primary site in the breast.

Although it is clear that estrogens are necessary for growth of estrogen-responsive breast cancers, their involvement in the earlier stages of breast carcinogenesis have been suggested only more recently. The dominant theories of carcinogenesis invoke mutations as the initial cause of cancer, and this may be further exacerbated by increasing genetic instability and further mutational events, which are encompassed by the hallmark of genetic instability and mutation [9,10]. Two mechanisms have been proposed by which estrogen exposure could give rise to genetic alterations in cells (Figure 10.8) [81]. One mechanism may result from

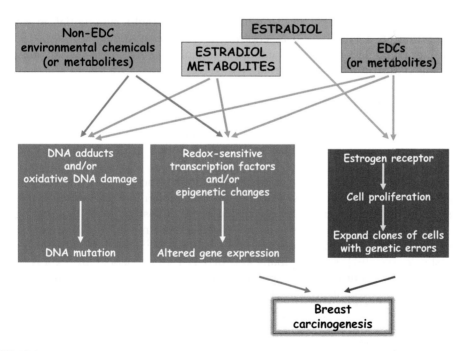

FIGURE 10.8   A diagram outlining potential mechanisms of estrogen-induced breast carcinogenesis.

the estrogen-driven sustained proliferation increasing the chance of multiplying genetically aberrant cells with unrepaired DNA alterations. A more direct mechanism could result from the ability of some catechol metabolites of estrogen to cause oxidative damage to DNA or to form adducts with DNA. While EDCs with estrogenic activity could also act through sustaining proliferation, some EDCs also possess DNA-damaging capabilities and might act more directly through damage to DNA. Furthermore, other DNA-damaging environmental chemicals that are not EDCs but can enter the human breast may also interact in the attack on the integrity of DNA. It is noteworthy that some studies have identified genomic instability in outer breast quadrants compared to inner breast quadrants [82,83], which might yet shed light on the disproportionate incidence of breast cancer in the UOQ of the breast. More recent theories of hormonal carcinogenesis have suggested that mistimed exposure of tissues to hormonally active compounds could act through epigenetic rather than mutational events. Alterations to DNA modifications such as methylation or acetylation could also influence gene expression patterns and lead to predisposition to cancer [84], and such epigenetic alterations are becoming apparent after exposure to EDCs in breast cells [85]. Furthermore, direct disruption to tissue architecture during development by EDCs may also serve to drive the later development of cancer [86].

10.2.2 Endometrial Cancer

The endometrium consists of inner basal and functional epithelial layers that line the thick myometrial muscle coat of the uterus, and most uterine cancers arise within the epithelial cells of the endometrium [87]. The endometrium is an endocrine-regulated tissue and in the normal premenopausal state, it undergoes cyclic growth, differentiation, shedding, and regeneration on a monthly basis, controlled by ovarian steroid synthesis. Estrogens have a proliferative effect on the endometrium, mainly during the follicular phase of the cycle, and this is balanced by progesterone, which can act to reduce the proliferative effects. Prolonged unopposed estrogen exposure is associated with most type 1 endometrial cancers [88], probably due to excessive mitotic activity [89]. Paradoxically, the selective ER modulator tamoxifen, which acts as an estrogen antagonist in the breast to reduce cell proliferation, acts as an agonist in uterine tissues and increases cancer risk by sixfold to eightfold [88], which serves as a reminder that different tissues may vary in their response to the same compound.

Since the uterotrophic assay is the gold standard animal model assay for estrogenic activity of an EDC (see Chapter 3), many EDCs have been shown to possess uterotrophic activity, but studies relating to cancer are fewer. Neonatal exposure of the developing rodent reproductive tract to xenoestrogens is a well-characterized model of tumorigenesis in the uterus involving ERα-dependent mechanisms [90], and DES has been shown to lead to preneoplastic lesions [91]. Greater than 90% of CD-1 pups neonatally exposed to DES or the phytoestrogen genistein developed endometrial cancer by 18 months of age, while C57BL/6 mice were resistant, which serves as a reminder of individual susceptibilities [92]. Epidemiological studies have investigated the association of exposure to DDT, dioxins, and BPA, but the significance was weak [93]. Some evidence suggests that long-term cadmium intake may increase endometrial cancer risk [94]. In vitro studies have shown that BPA can act as an estrogen agonist in Ishikawa human endometrial adenocarcinoma cells [95].

10.2.3 Ovarian Cancer

Ovarian cancers originate predominantly from the ovarian surface epithelium [96]. In the majority of cases, ovarian cancer is detected at a late stage due to a lack of specific symptoms or screening tests, and so the disease has often disseminated outside the pelvic cavity before clinical detection, which results in a poor prognosis and low 5-year survival rate [96]. Risk factors are similar to those for breast cancer [97] and include exposure to exogenous hormones such as in HRT [98]. Ovarian cancers are known to possess ER and have been associated with a reduced expression of ERβ relative to ERα [99]. ERβ acts as a tumor suppressor, and overexpression of ERβ has been shown to reduce proliferation of ovarian epithelial cells [100]. The known role of estrogens in ovarian cancer then suggests that EDCs might also affect risk. There are very few published studies of EDCs, but one epidemiological study has reported an association between exposure to triazine pesticides such as atrazine and risk of ovarian cancer [101].

10.2.4 Cervical Cancer

Cervical cancer has long been known to have a viral etiology associated with sexually transmitted high-risk human papillomavirus (HPV) infection [102]. The disease progresses through precancerous stages of intraepithelial neoplasia over at least a decade, offering the option for early detection using the Pap smear, and the viral etiology offers the opportunity for vaccine development [103]. Cervical tissue is, however, hormone-sensitive and highly responsive to estrogen. During the menstrual cycle, cervical epithelial cells proliferate and differentiate as estrogen levels increase [103]. Long-term (i.e., 5 years) oral contraceptive use is known to increase cervical cancer risk by 1.9-fold [104]. Exposure to DES in utero is known to increase risk of developing grade 2 or greater cervical intraepithelial neoplasia in the DES-exposed daughters (see Table 8.1). The strongest evidence that estrogen directly contributes to cervical carcinogenesis comes from studies in HPV-transgenic mice where development of cervical cancer has been demonstrated to be estrogen-dependent [103,105,106]. In vitro studies have shown that estrogen can also increase expression of the E6 and E7 oncogenes, which is the major driving force behind HPV-mediated cervical cancer development [103,107]. Although there are currently no reported studies in the literature concerning EDCs and cervical cancer, the role of estrogen in cervical cancer development suggests that this should be an area for future research.

10.3 CANCERS IN MALE REPRODUCTIVE TISSUES

Cancers in endocrine-responsive reproductive tissues comprised a total of 27.4% of all male cancers in England for 2012 as reported in June 2014 [4], with prostate cancer being the major cancer in men (25.9%) and cancers of testis (1.3%) and breast (0.2%) adding to the total (Figure 10.4).

10.3.1 Prostate Cancer

Prostate cancer is an endocrine-regulated cancer, and androgens play a central role in the development and growth of the tumors [108]. The androgen receptor is, therefore, a target for therapy, and many patients can undergo a period of remission with androgen ablation therapy either through inhibiting androgen synthesis or through use of antiandrogens to antagonize androgen action at the receptor [109] until androgen-resistant tumor growth develops [110]. However, paradoxically, the incidence of prostate cancer increases with age when men have declining testosterone levels, which raises the question of whether testosterone is the only driving force. In addition to androgens, estrogens are now known to be involved in prostate carcinogenesis and progression, although the mechanisms are not fully understood [111–116]. In humans, chronically elevated estrogens have been associated with increased risk of prostate cancer [117], and in rodent models, estrogens in combination with androgens induce prostate cancer [118]. Although age, race, family history, and diet are risk factors for prostate cancer, environmental factors are also known to be involved [119], and EDCs with estrogenic activity have been implicated [120].

Epidemiological studies of farming communities have shown a link between chronic exposure to agrochemicals and increased prostate cancer risk [120], especially the fungicide methyl bromide, and in men with a familial history, the pesticides chlorpyrifos, fonofos, coumaphos, phorate, permethrin, and butylate also increased risk [121]. Interestingly, the first five of these pesticides strongly inhibit the cytochrome P450 enzymes CYP1A2 and CYP3A4, which metabolize estradiol, estrone, and testosterone [122,123]. This fact raises the possibility that these agrochemicals may act to increase prostate cancer risk by interfering with steroid metabolism. Animal models, studies using human prostate cancer cell lines, and prostate stem/progenitor cell models have shown that BPA, PCBs, dioxins, and cadmium can all interfere with the normal cellular and molecular functions of prostate cells [120]. Animal models have demonstrated that estrogen reprogramming of the prostate gland following developmental exposures to EDCs can result in permanent epigenetic alterations, which can lead to increased prostatic lesions with aging [120].

10.3.2 Testicular Cancer

Testicular cancer has a much lower overall incidence compared to prostate cancer (Figure 10.4) and has a high 5-year survival rate [124]. However, incidence has increased sharply, with an estimated doubling in the last 40 years in some populations [125]. The increasing trends seem to be influenced by birth cohort [126] and with striking geographical variations, most notably between Denmark and Finland (Figure 10.9) [127]. This marked difference between two Baltic countries has raised speculation that the rising incidence might be environmental in origin and in particular relate to exposure to EDCs [127].

Testicular cancers are 98% germ cell tumors, although histologically, they can be divided into classic seminomas (from germ cells) and nonseminomas (e.g., embryonal carcinomas, teratomas, yolk sac tumors, and choriocarcinomas). There are three broad categories of testicular germ cell tumors (TGCTs), with type I found primarily in neonatal and young boys, type II affecting men aged 20–40 years, and type III affecting older men more than 50 years of age. It is only the type II TGCTs that have increased over recent decades, and this finding has led again to speculation that environmental factors may be responsible [128]. Since the type II TGCTs develop from a dysfunctional fetal germ cell, this indicates that risk factors would need to be identified during early male fetal development [128]. One hypothesis attributes risk to an increase in endogenous estrogen levels during prenatal life, exposure to EDCs with estrogenic activity, or both [129].

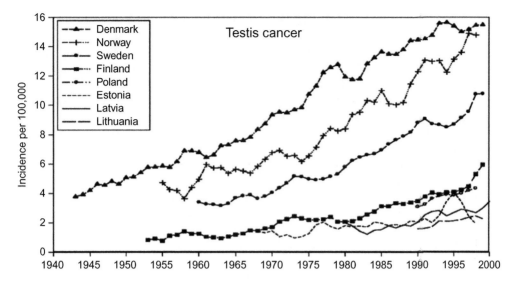

FIGURE 10.9 Incidence of testicular cancer in eight northern European countries. *Source: Taken from Bay and colleagues [127] with permission.*

A consistent risk factor for testicular cancer is cryptorchidism (undescended testes; see Section 9.6), which increases risk by fivefold [130], but common epidemiological trends and clinical experience also suggest a coincidence with hypospadias and poor semen quality (see Chapter 9). These associations led Skakkebaek and colleagues to propose in 2001 that they were all symptoms of a common underlying entity termed *testicular dysgenesis syndrome* (TDS; see Section 9.8) with a common origin in fetal life [131]. Disrupted embryonic programming and gonadal development in fetal life was suspected to be caused by environmental factors (most probably EDCs) acting in the context of genetic determinants that altered susceptibility. In an attempt to test this hypothesis, rodent models of phthalate exposure have been developed and have shown that phthalate-exposed rats can develop dysgenetic focal areas in the testes that are similar to those seen in an adult human with testicular cancer [132]. However, it remains uncertain as to whether the doses of phthalates given to the rats would be reached in the human body.

10.3.3 Male Breast Cancer

Although breast cancer occurs in men with only about 1/100th of the frequency in women, the incidence in men is increasing. Risk factors are similar to female breast cancer, including genetic susceptibility from loss of function of BRCA genes and exposure to excess estrogen [133]. What is especially intriguing is that the frequency of ER positivity in male breast cancer is even higher than in female breast cancer with more than 90% of cancers containing ER [133]. There are no studies on EDCs and male breast cancer, but given the high degree of estrogen responsiveness of male breast cancer, research is justified.

10.4 FINAL COMMENTS

Initial research aimed at understanding whether EDCs can affect human cancer has rightly started by monitoring the ability of EDCs to enter human tissue. If EDCs were not retained in the human body, there would be no questions over any resulting consequences, whatever the effects after exposures in culture systems or animal models may be. However, since many hundreds of EDCs have now been measured in various human tissues, and many of these were found rather ubiquitously across the population in human blood or urine, questions have to be raised as to whether there are functional consequences to their presence. Due to feasibility of sampling, most large studies (e.g., in the National Health and Nutrition Examination Survey in the United States) have used urine or blood, and they enable valuable long-term biomonitoring of EDC concentrations over time. However, the levels of the EDCs may not necessarily be the same in every target organ as they are in blood or urine. For example, due to their lipophilic properties, many persistent organic pollutants (POPs) can distribute differently in fatty breast adipose tissue and in milk with high fat content compared to blood [134]. This may explain why higher levels of some POPs have been reported in breast adipose tissue from people with breast cancer than those without [51]. Unfortunately, due to availability of material, studies of breast adipose tissue tend to have smaller sample sizes (and therefore lower statistical power), and this tends to dwarf their findings compared to the larger blood/urine studies with higher statistical power, which tend to report inconsistent associations [23]. Aluminum, with more hydrophilic properties, has been surprisingly measured in breast fat as well as in breast tissue, but it has different regional distribution in the tissue than in the fat [53]. More specific measurements, therefore, are now urgently needed in breast tissue to define variations in regional distribution of EDCs (not least in relation to understanding the disproportionate incidence of breast cancer in the UOQ) and to identify variations between multiple EDCs in single breasts. While more measurements in female breast tissue are needed, studies are severely lacking for the other female and male reproductive tissues, and measurements are urgently needed for endometrium, ovary, prostate, and testis.

Functional analysis of the presence of EDCs in human tissues remains an outstanding challenge and is in need of a paradigm shift in experimental and epidemiological strategy from studying single chemicals to assessing long-term, low-dose mixtures. It is no longer sufficient to dismiss one chemical as insignificant on the basis that it is not at higher levels in the tissues of every cancer case. Overlapping functions and complementary actions of different chemicals mean that a single chemical can contribute different weightings to each EDC load but still remain functionally significant. The detailed content of each load will reflect lifestyle; therefore, it inevitably differs in the exact chemical composition, but all that is needed is for the entirety of each load to enable the hallmarks of cancer to develop. The reversibility of some reproductive problems (see Chapters 8 and 9) are more likely to reveal specific culprit environmental exposures, simply because if they can be reversed upon ceasing exposure, functionality can be demonstrated. The challenge of identifying causation is much greater for cancer, not just because of the complexity of the development stages and the length of time it takes, but also because it is not reversible. For this reason, more heed should be paid to exposures causing reproductive problems as a warning sign. Most animal models report some form of tissue disorganization or hyperplasia prior to cancer. If these warning signs could then be used to invoke a precautionary principle, then some progress possibly could be made toward preventative strategies for cancer.

The challenge for the future, then, will not be to question whether EDCs can affect cancer development, but rather to identify the specific exposures that may be most significant in causing EDC loading in the different body tissues in order to inform priorities for preventative action. Clearly, different lifestyles will give rise to different EDC loadings, and since multiple chemicals may have overlapping functions, one lifestyle factor is unlikely to be a sole cause. For example, for breast cancer, it has been suggested that underarm cosmetic use might be one causative factor due to the proximity of application to the UOQ of the breast that is the major site of breast cancer development [23,24,70,71]. Other studies have reported increased risk of ER+ breast cancers as related to the percentage of agricultural land and therefore pesticide exposure [135], and yet others increased breast cancer risk for those working in automotive plastics or food canning industries [136]. These are not mutually exclusive risks but may rather reflect simply different sources of EDC exposures with overlapping functions to be added to already known risks associated with exogenous hormones in contraceptives and HRT. Meaningful outcomes of such studies, however, will depend on the design of control groupings such that the controls could not have been exposed to an alternative source of EDCs. One major obstacle will be the ill-defined nature of individual susceptibilities, which encompass a multitude of genetic and epigenetic differences between individuals and give rise to a spectrum of variations in how each individual absorbs, transports, and eliminates different chemicals and then in how those chemicals may affect the tissues at different life stages. The increasing penetrance of breast cancer susceptibility genes demonstrates an increasing environmental component combined with individual susceptibility [137]. In view of the near-ubiquitous claim that obesity is a risk factor for all the cancers described in this chapter, and in view of the lipophilic nature of many EDCs, more effort needs to be invested in how variations in dietary fat consumption (not only amount but type) and variations in metabolic processing of dietary fat can result in variations in the amount and type of chemicals that are retained in fatty tissues. Furthermore, since adipose tissue contains high levels of aromatase that converts androgens to estrogens, variations in individual responses to obesity could also relate to varied increase in estrogen synthesis [138], which may be further exacerbated by the presence of EDCs that can alter aromatase activity (see Chapter 3). If the paradigm shift to long-term low-dose exposure to complex mixtures of chemicals set in a background of individual susceptibility and differing lifestyle settings can be fully embraced, at that point, then maybe strategies for prevention could be developed.

References

[1] Donegan WL. History of breast cancer. In: Winchester DJ, Winchester DP, Hudis CA, Norton L, editors. Breast cancer. Ontario, BC: Marcel Dekker; 2006. p. 1–14.
[2] Ferlay J, Shin HR, Bray F, Forman D, Mathers C, Parkin DM. Estimates of worldwide burden of cancer in 2008: GLOBOCAN 2008. Int J Cancer 2010;127:2893–917.
[3] Shanmugalingam T, Soultati A, Chowdhury S, Rudman S, Hemelrijck MV. Global incidence and outcome of testicular cancer. Clin Epidemiol 2013;5:417–27.
[4] Office of National Statistics, England. Series MB1, Published Crown Copyright, London. From 1979 to 2014 (MB series 1 numbered to 43).

[5]   Shimizu H, Ross RK, Bernstein L, Yatani R, Henderson BE, Mack TM. Cancers of the prostate and breast among Japanese and white immigrants in Los Angeles County. Br J Cancer 1991;63:963–6.

[6]   Lichtenstein P, Holm NV, Verkasalo PK, Iliadou A, Kaprio J, Koskenvuo M, et al. Environmental and heritable factors in the causation of cancer—analyses of cohorts of twins from Sweden, Denmark and Finland. N Engl J Med 2000;343:78–85.

[7]   Luke B, Hediger M, Min SJ, Brown MB, Misiunas RB, Gonzalez-Quintero VH, et al. Gender mix in twins and fetal growth, length of gestation and adult cancer risk. Paediatr Perinat Epidemiol 2005;19:41–7.

[8]   Weinberg RA. The biology of cancer, 2nd ed. New York: Garland Science; 2014. ISBN 978-0-8153-4220-5.

[9]   Hanahan D, Weinberg RA. The hallmarks of cancer. Cell 2000;100:57–70.

[10] Hanahan D, Weinberg RA. Hallmarks of cancer: the next generation. Cell 2011;144:646–74.

[11] Office of National Statistics, England. Series MB1 number 43, Published Crown Copyright, London, 2014.

[12] Quinn MJ, Cooper N, Rachet B, Mitry E, Coleman MP. Survival from cancer of the breast in women in England and Wales up to 2001. Br J Cancer 2008;99:S53–5.

[13] Roy R, Chun J, Powell SN. BRCA1 and BRCA2: different roles in a common pathway of genome protection. Nat Rev Cancer 2011;12:68–78.

[14] Apostolou P, Fostira F. Hereditary breast cancer: the era of new susceptibility genes. Biomed Res Int 2013:1–11. Article ID 747318.

[15] Key TJ, Verkasalo PK, Banks E. Epidemiology of breast cancer. Lancet Oncol 2001;2:133–40.

[16] Beatson GT. On the treatment of inoperable cases of carcinoma of the mamma: suggestions for a new method of treatment, with illustrative cases. Lancet 1896;148:162–5.

[17] Miller WR. Estrogen and breast cancer. London: Chapman & Hall; 1996.

[18] Collaborative Group on Hormonal Factors in Breast Cancer Breast cancer and hormonal contraceptives: collaborative reanalysis of individual data on 53,297 with breast cancer and 100,239 women without breast cancer from 54 epidemiological studies. Lancet 1996;347:1713–27.

[19] Beral V, Million Women Study Collaborators Breast cancer and hormone replacement in the Million Women Study. Lancet 2003;362:419–27.

[20] Cuzick J. Hormone replacement therapy and the risk of breast cancer. Eur J Cancer 2008;44:2344–9.

[21] Santen RJ, Allred DC, Ardoin SP, Archer DF, Boyd N, Braunstein GD, Endocrine Society Postmenopausal hormone therapy: an Endocrine Society scientific statement. J Clin Endocrinol Metab 2010;95(Suppl. 1):S1–S66.

[22] Lonning PE. Endocrinology and treatment of breast cancer. Best Pract Res Clin Endocrinol Metab 2004;18: 1–130.

[23] Darbre PD. Environmental oestrogens, cosmetics and breast cancer. Best Pract Res Clin Endocrinol Metab 2006;20:121–43.

[24] Darbre PD, Charles AK. Environmental oestrogens and breast cancer: evidence for a combined involvement of dietary, household and cosmetic xenoestrogens. Anticancer Res 2010;30:815–28.

[25] Bradburn MJ, Altman DG, Smith P, Fentiman IS, Rubens RD. Time trends in breast cancer survival: experience in a single centre, 1975–89. Br J Cancer 1998;77:1944–9.

[26] Brown SBF, Mallon EA, Edwards J, Campbell FM, McGlynn LM, Elsberger B, et al. Is the biology of breast cancer changing? A study of hormone receptor status 1984–1986 and 1996–1997. Br J Cancer 2009;100:807–10.

[27] Pujol P, Hilsenbeck SG, Chamness GC, Elledge RM. Rising levels of estrogen receptor in breast cancer over 2 decades. Cancer 1994;74:1601–6.

[28] Li CI, Daling JR, Malone KE. Incidence of invasive breast cancer by hormone receptor status from 1992 to 1998. J Clin Oncol 2003;21:28–34.

[29] Glass AG, Lacey JV, Carreon JD, Hoover RN. Breast cancer incidence 1980–2006: combined roles of menopausal hormone therapy, screening, mammography and estrogen receptor status. J Natl Cancer Inst 2007;99:1152–61.

[30] Harris RM, Waring RH. Diethylstilboestrol—a long-term legacy. Maturitas 2012;72:108–12.

[31] Greenberg ER, Barnes AB, Resseguie L, Barrett JA, Burnside S, Lanza LL, et al. Breast cancer in mothers given diethylstilbestrol in pregnancy. N Engl J Med 1984;311:1393–8.

[32] Herbst AL, Ulfelder H, Poskanzer DC. Adenocarcinoma of the vagina: association of maternal stilboestrol therapy with tumor appearance in young women. N Engl J Med 1971;284:878–81.

[33] Troisi R, Hatch EE, Titus-Ernstoff L, Hyer M, Palmer JR, Robboy SJ, et al. Cancer risk in women prenatally exposed to diethylstilbestrol. Int J Cancer 2007;121:356–60.

[34] Nelson HD, Zakher B, Cantor A, et al. Risk factors for breast cancer for women aged 40 to 49 years: a systematic review and meta-analysis. Ann Intern Med 2012;156:635–48.

[35] Marchbanks PA, Curtis KM, Mandel MG, Wilson HG, Jeng G, Folger SG, et al. Oral contraceptive formulation and risk of breast cancer. Contraception 2012;85:342–50.

[36] Snedeker SM. Pesticides and breast cancer risk: a review of DDT, DDE, and dieldrin. Environ Health Perspect 2001;109:35–47.

[37] Brody JG, Moysich KB, Humblet O, Attfield KR, Beehler GP, Rudel RA. Environmental pollutants and breast cancer: epidemiologic studies. Cancer 2007;109:2667–711.

[38] Bouwman H, Sereda B, Meinhardt HM. Simultaneous presence of DDT and pyrethroid residues in human breast milk from a malaria endemic area in South Africa. Environ Pollut 2006;144:902–17.

[39] Weldon RH, Barr DB, Trujillo C, Bradman A, Holland N, Eskenazi B. A pilot study of pesticides and PCBs in the breast milk of women residing in urban and agricultural communities of California. J Environ Monit 2011;13:3136–44.

[40] Corcellas C, Feo ML, Torres JP, Malm O, Ocampo-Duque W, Eljarrat E, et al. Pyrethroids in human breast milk: occurrence and nursing daily intake estimation. Environ Int 2012;47:17–22.

[41] Bedi JS, Gill JP, Aulakh RS, Kaur P, Sharma A, Pooni PA. Pesticide residues in human breast milk: risk assessment for infants from Punjab, India. Sci Total Environ 2013;463–4:720–6.

[42] Furst P. Dioxins, polychlorinated biphenyls and other organohalogen compounds in human milk. Mol Nutr Food Res 2006;50:922–33.

[43] Woods HF (Chairman). Phytoestrogens and health. London: Food Standards Agency. Crown copyright UK, <http://cot.food.gov.uk/pdfs/phytoreport0503>; 2003.

[44] Zimmers SM, Browne EP, O'Keefe PW, Anderton DL, Kramer L, Reckhow DA, et al. Determination of free bisphenol A (BPA) concentrations in breast milk of U.S. women using a sensitive LC/MS/MS method. Chemosphere 2014;104:237–43.

[45] Calafat AM, Slakman AR, Silva MJ, Herbert AR, Needham LL. Automated solid-phase extraction and quantitative analysis of human milk for 13 phthalate metabolites. J Chromatogr B Analyt Technol Biomed Life Sci 2004;805:49–56.

[46] Hines EP, Calafat AM, Silva MJ, Mendola P, Fenton SE. Concentrations of phthalate metabolites in milk, urine, saliva, and serum of lactating North Carolina women. Environ Health Perspect 2009;117:86–92.

[47] Ademollo N, Ferrera F, Delise M, Fabietti F, Funari E. Nonylphenol and octylphenol in human breast milk. Environ Int 2008;34:984–7.

[48] Schecter A, Pavuk M, Papke O, Ryan JJ, Birnbaum L, Rosen R. Polybrominated diphenylethers (PBDEs) in US mother's milk. Environ Health Perspect 2003;111:1723–9.

[49] Kalantzi OI, Martin FL, Thomas GO, Alcock RE, Tang HR, Drury SC, et al. Different levels of polybrominated diphenyl ethers (PBDEs) and chlorinated compounds in breast milk from two UK regions. Environ Health Perspect 2004;112:1085–91.

[50] Costa LG, Giordano G, Tagliaferri S, Caglieri A, Mutti A. Polybrominated diphenyl ethers (PBDE) flame retardants: environmental contamination, human body burden and potential adverse health effects. Acta Biomed 2008;79:172–83.

[51] Darbre PD, Aljarrah A, Miller WR, Coldham NG, Sauer MJ, Pope GS. Concentrations of parabens in human breast tumours. J Appl Toxicol 2004;24:5–13.

[52] Barr L, Metaxas G, Harbach CAJ, Savoy LA, Darbre PD. Measurement of paraben concentrations in human breast tissue at serial locations across the breast from axilla to sternum. J Appl Toxicol 2012;32:219–32.

[53] Exley C, Charles LM, Barr L, Martin C, Polwart A, Darbre PD. Aluminium in human breast tissue. J Inorg Biochem 2007;101:1344–6.

[54] Mannello F, Tonti GA, Darbre PD. Concentration of aluminium in breast cyst fluids collected from women affected by gross cystic breast disease. J Appl Toxicol 2009;29:1–6.

[55] Mannello F, Tonti GA, Medda V, Simone P, Darbre PD. Analysis of aluminium content and iron homeostasis in nipple aspirate fluids from healthy women and breast cancer-affected patients. J Appl Toxicol 2011;31:262–9.

[56] Adolfsson-Erici M, Petersson M, Parkkonen J, Sturve J. Triclosan, a commonly used bacteriocide found in human milk and in the aquatic environment in Sweden. Chemosphere 2002;46:1485–9.

[57] Allmyr M, Adolfsson-Erici M, McLachlan MS, Sandborgh-Englund G. Triclosan in plasma and milk from Swedish nursing mothers and their exposure *via* personal care products. Sci Total Environ 2006;372:87–93.

[58] Schlumpf M, Kypke K, Wittassek M, Angerer J, Mascher H, Mascher D, et al. Exposure patterns of UV filters, fragrances, parabens, phthalates, organochlorpesticides, PBDEs and PCBs in human milk: correlation of UV filters with use in cosmetics. Chemosphere 2010;81:1171–83.

[59] Reiner JL, Wong CM, Arcaro KF, Kannan K. Synthetic musk fragrances in human milk from the United States. Environ Sci Technol 2007;41:3815–20.

[60] International Agency for Research on Cancer (IACR) Monographs vol 6: p. 99 (1974); vol 21: p. 279 (1979); Suppl. 7: p. 284 (1987); vol 72: p. 399 (1999).

[61] Nesaretnam K, Hales E, Sohail M, Krausz T, Darbre P. 3,3′,4,4′-Tetrachlorobiphenyl (TCB) can enhance DMBA-induced mammary carcinogenesis in the rat. Eur J Cancer 1998;34:389–93.

[62] Rochester JR. Bisphenol A and human health: a review of the literature. Reprod Toxicol 2013;42:132–55.

[63] Darbre PD, Fernandez MF. Environmental oestrogens and breast cancer: long-term low-dose effects of mixtures of various chemical combinations. J Epidemiol Community Health 2013;67:203–5.

[64] Porta M, Pumarega J, Gasull M. Number of persistent organic pollutants detected at high concentrations in a general population. Environ Int 2012;44:106–11.

[65] Charles AK, Darbre PD. Combinations of parabens at concentrations measured in human breast tissue can increase proliferation of MCF-7 human breast cancer cells. J Appl Toxicol 2013;33:390–8.

[66] Russo J, Russo IH. Biology of disease. Biological and molecular bases of mammary carcinogenesis. Lab Invest 1987;57:112–37.

[67] Soto AM, Brisken C, Schaeberle C, Sonnenschein C. Does cancer start in the womb? Altered mammary gland development and predisposition to breast cancer due to *in utero* exposure to endocrine disruptors. J Mammary Gland Biol Neoplasia 2013;18:199–208.

[68] Darbre PD. Recorded quadrant incidence of female breast cancer in Great Britain suggests a disproportionate increase in the upper outer quadrant of the breast. Anticancer Res 2005;25:2543–50.

[69] Haagensen CD. Diseases of the breast, 2nd ed. Philadelphia, PA: WB Saunders; 1971.

[70] Darbre PD. Underarm cosmetics are a cause of breast cancer. Eur J Cancer Prev 2001;10:389–93.

[71] Darbre PD. Underarm cosmetics and breast cancer. J Appl Toxicol 2003;23:89–95.

[72] Darbre PD, Harvey PW. Parabens can enable hallmarks and characteristics of cancer in human breast epithelial cells: a review of the literature with reference to new exposure data and regulatory status. J Appl Toxicol 2014;34:925–38.

[73] Blair RM, Fang H, Branham WS, Hass BS, Dial SL, Moland CL, et al. The estrogen receptor binding affinities of 188 natural and xenochemicals: structural diversity of ligands. Toxicol Sci 2000;54:138–53.

[74] Rajapakse N, Silva E, Kortenkamp A. Combining xenoestrogens at levels below individual no-observed-effect concentrations dramatically enhances steroid hormone action. Environ Health Perspect 2002;110:917–21.

[75] Kortenkamp A. Ten years of mixing cocktails: a review of combination effects of endocrine-disrupting chemicals. Environ Health Perspect 2007;115(Suppl. 1):98–105.

[76] Darbre PD. Molecular mechanisms of oestrogen action on growth of human breast epithelial cells in culture. Horm Mol Biol Clin Invest 2012;9:65–85.

[77] Hsieh TH, Tsai CF, Hsu CY, Kuo PL, Hsi E, Suen JL, et al. *n*-Butyl benzyl phthalate promotes breast cancer progression by inducing expression of lymphoid enhancer factor 1. PLoS One 2012;7:e42750.

[78] Hsieh TH, Tsai CF, Hsu CY, Kuo PL, Lee JN, Chai CY, et al. Phthalates induce proliferation and invasiveness of estrogen receptor-negative breast cancer through the AhR/HDAC6/c-Myc signaling pathway. FASEB J 2012;26:778–87.

[79] Khanna S, Dash PR, Darbre PD. Exposure to parabens at the concentration of maximal proliferative response increases migratory and invasive activity of human breast cancer cells *in vitro*. J Appl Toxicol 2014;34:1051–9.

[80] Darbre PD, Bakir A, Iskakova E. Effect of aluminium on migratory and invasive properties of MCF-7 human breast cancer cells in culture. J Inorg Biochem 2013;128:245–9.

[81] Chang M. Dual roles of estrogen metabolism in mammary carcinogenesis. BMB Rep 2011;44:423–34.

[82] Ellsworth DL, Ellsworth RE, Love B, Deyarmin B, Lubert SM, Mittal MD, et al. Outer breast quadrants demonstrate increased levels of genomic instability. Ann Surg Oncol 2004;11:861–8.

[83] Ellsworth DL, Ellsworth RE, Liebman MN, Hooke JA, Shriver CD. Genomic instability in histologically normal breast tissues: implications for carcinogenesis. Lancet Oncol 2004;5:753–8.

[84] Zhang XA, Ho SM. Epigenetics meets endocrinology. J Mol Endocrinol 2011;46:R11–32.

[85] Knower KC, To SQ, Leung YK, Ho SM, Clyne CD. Endocrine disruption of the epigenome: a breast cancer link. Endocr Relat Cancer 2014;21:T33–55.

[86] Soto AM, Sonnenschein C. Environmental causes of cancer: endocrine disruptors as carcinogens. Nat Rev Endocrinol 2010;6:364–71.

[87] Colombo N, Preti E, Landoni F, Carinelli S, Colombo A, Marini C, ESMO Guidelines Working Group Endometrial cancer: ESMO clinical practice guidelines for diagnosis, treatment and follow-up. Ann Oncol 2011;22(Suppl. 6):vi35–9.

[88] SGO Clinical Practice Endometrial Cancer Working Group Endometrial cancer: a review and current management strategies: Part 1. Gynecol Oncol 2014;134:385–92.

[89] Akhmedkhanov A, Zeleniuch-Jacquotte A, Toniolo P. Role of exogenous and endogenous hormones in endometrial cancer: review of the evidence and research perspectives. Ann NY Acad Sci 2001;943:296–315.

[90] Couse JF, Dixon D, Yates M, Moore AB, Ma L, Maas R, et al. Estrogen receptor-alpha knockout mice exhibit resistance to the developmental effects of neonatal diethylstilbestrol exposure on the female reproductive tract. Dev Biol 2001;238:224–38.

[91] Cook JD, Davis BJ, Goewey JA, Berry TD, Walker CL. Identification of a sensitive period for developmental programming that increases risk for uterine leiomyoma in Eker rats. Reprod Sci 2007;14:121–36.

[92] Kabbarah O, Sotelo AK, Mallon MA, Winkeler EL, Fan MY, Pfeifer JD, et al. Diethylstilbestrol effects and lymphomagenesis in Mlh1-deficient mice. Int J Cancer 2005;115:666–9.

[93] Gibson DA, Saunders PTK. Endocrine disruption of oestrogen action and female reproductive tract cancers. Endocr Relat Cancer 2014;21:T13–31.

[94] Åkesson A, Julin B, Wolk A. Long-term dietary cadmium intake and postmenopausal endometrial cancer incidence: a population-based prospective cohort study. Cancer Res 2008;68:6435–41.

[95] Li Y, Burns KA, Arao Y, Luh CJ, Korach KS. Differential estrogenic actions of endocrine-disrupting chemicals bisphenol A, bisphenol AF, and zearalenone through estrogen receptor α and β in vitro. Environ Health Perspect 2012;120:1029–35.

[96] Cho KR, Shih IeM. Ovarian cancer. Ann Rev Pathol 2009;4:287–313.

[97] Doufekas K, Olaitan A. Clinical epidemiology of epithelial ovarian cancer in the UK. Int J Women's Health 2014;6:537–45.

[98] Beral V, Bull D, Green J, Reeves G. Ovarian cancer and hormone replacement therapy in the Million Women Study. Lancet 2007;369:1703–10.

[99] Pujol P, Rey JM, Nirde P, Roger P, Gastaldi M, Laffargue F, et al. Differential expression of estrogen receptor-α and -β messenger RNAs as a potential marker of ovarian carcinogenesis. Cancer Res 1998;58:5367–73.

[100] Bossard C, Busson M, Vindrieux D, Gaudin F, Machelon V, Brigitte M, et al. Potential role of estrogen receptor beat as a tumor suppressor of epithelial ovarian cancer. PLoS One 2013;7:e44787.

[101] Young HA, Mills PK, Riordan DG, Cress RD. Triazine herbicides and epithelial ovarian cancer risk in central California. J Occup Environ Med 2005;47:1148–56.

[102] Zur Hausen H. Papillomaviruses in the causation of human cancers—a brief historical account. Virology 2009;384:260–5.

[103] Chung SH, Franceschi S, Lambert PF. Estrogen and ERα: culprits in cervical cancer? Trends Endocrinol Metab 2010;21:504–11.

[104] Appleby P, Beral V, Berrington de Gonzales A, et al. Cervical cancer and hormonal contraceptives: collaborative reanalysis of individual data for 16,573 women with cervical cancer. Lancet 2007;370:1609–21.

[105] Brake T, Lambert P. Estrogen contributes to the onset, persistence, and malignant progression of cervical cancer in human papillomavirus-transgenic mouse model. Proc Natl Acad Sci USA 2005;102:2490–5.

[106] Chung S, Wiedmeyer K, Shai A, Korach K, Lambert P. Requirement for estrogen receptor alpha in a mouse model for human papillomavirus-associated cervical cancer. Cancer Res 2008;68:9928–34.

[107] Kim CJ, Um SJ, Kim TY, Kim EJ, Park TC, Kim SJ, et al. Regulation of cell growth and HPV genes by exogenous estrogens in cervical cancer cells. Int J Gynecol Cancer 2000;10:157–64.

[108] Trapman J, Brinkmann OA. The androgen receptor in prostate cancer. Pathol Res Pract 1996;192:752–60.

[109] Helsen C, Van den Broeck T, Voet A, Prekovic S, Van Poppel H, Joniau S, et al. Androgen receptor antagonists for prostate cancer therapy. Endocr Relat Cancer 2014;21:T105–18.

[110] Feldman BJ, Feldman D. The development of androgen independent prostate cancer. Nat Rev Cancer 2001;1:34–45.

[111] Ellem SJ, Risbridger GP. Treating prostate cancer: a rationale for targeting local oestrogens. Nat Rev Cancer 2007;7:621–7.

[112] Prins GS, Birch L, Tang WY, Ho SM. Developmental estrogen exposures predispose to prostate carcinogenesis with aging. Reprod Toxicol 2007;23:374–82.

[113] Prins GS, Korach KS. The role of estrogens and estrogen receptors in normal prostate growth and disease. Steroids 2008;73:233–44.

[114] Leung YK, Lam HM, Wu S, Song D, Levin L, Cheng L, et al. Estrogen receptor beta2 and beta5 are associated with poor prognosis in prostate cancer, and promote cancer cell migration and invasion. Endocr Relat Cancer 2010;17:675–89.

[115] Hu WY, Shi GB, Lam HM, Hu DP, Ho SM, Madueke IC, et al. Estrogen-initiated transformation of prostate epithelium derived from normal human prostate stem-progenitor cells. Endocrinology 2011;152:2150–63.

[116] Nelles JL, Hu WY, Prins GS. Estrogen action and prostate cancer. Expert Rev Endocrinol Metab 2011;6:437–51.

[117] Modugno F, Weissfeld JLW, Trump DL, Zmuda JM, Shea P, Cauley JA, et al. Allelic variants of aromatase and androgen and estrogen receptors: toward a multigenic model of prostate cancer risk. Clin Cancer Res 2001;7:3092–6.

[118] Bosland MC. Chemical and hormonal induction of prostate cancer in animal models. Urol Oncol 1996;2:103–10.

[119] Reuben SH, LaSalle Jr. DL, Kripke ML. Reducing environmental cancer risk: what we can do now. The President's Cancer Panel. Bethesda, MD: National Institutes of Health; 2010; p. 1–147

[120] Hu WY, Shi GB, Hu DP, Nelles JL, Prins GS. Actions of estrogens and endocrine disrupting chemicals on human prostate stem/progenitor cells and prostate cancer risk. Mol Cell Endocrinol 2012;354:63–73.

[121] Alavanja MC, Samanic C, Dosemeci M, Lubin J, Tarone R, Lynch CF, et al. Use of agricultural pesticides and prostate cancer risk in the Agricultural Health Study cohort. Am J Epidemiol 2003;157:800–14.

[122] Usmani KA, Rose RL, Hodgson E. Inhibition and activation of the human liver microsomal and human cytochrome P450 3A4 metabolism of testosterone by deployment-related chemicals. Drug Metab Dispos 2003;31:384–91.

[123] Usmani KA, Cho TM, Rose RL, Hodgson E. Inhibition of the human liver microsomal and human cytochrome P450 1A2 and 3A4 metabolism of estradiol by deployment-related and other chemicals. Drug Metab Dispos 2006;34:1606–14.

[124] Horwich A, Shipley J, Huddart R. Testicular germ-cell cancer. Lancet 2006;367:754–65.

[125] Bray F, Richiardi L, Ekbom A, Pukkala E, Cuninova M, Moller H. Trends in testicular cancer incidence and mortality in 22 European countries: continuing increases in incidence and declines in mortality. Int J Cancer 2006;118:3099–111.

[126] Richiardi L, Bellocco R, Adami HO, et al. Testicular cancer incidence in eight northern European countries: secular and recent trends. Cancer Epidemiol Biomarkers Prev 2004;13:2157–66.

[127] Bay K, Asklund C, Skakkebaek NE, Andersson AM. Testicular dysgenesis syndrome: possible role of endocrine disrupters. Best Pract Res Clin Endocrinol Metab 2006;20:77–90.

[128] McIver SC, Roman SD, Nixon B, Loveland KL, McLaughlin EA. The rise of testicular germ cell tumours: the search for causes, risk factors and novel therapeutic targets. F1000Res 2013;2:55.

[129] Giannandrea F, Paoli D, Figa-Talamanca I, Lombardo F, Lenzi A, Gandini L. Effect of endogenous and exogenous hormones on testicular cancer: the epidemiological evidence. Int J Dev Biol 2013;57:255–63.

[130] Dieckmann KP, Pichlmeier U. Clinical epidemiology of testicular germ cell tumors. World J Urol 2004;22:2–14.

[131] Skakkebaek NE, Rajpert-De Meyts E, Main KM. Testicular dysgenesis syndrome: an increasingly common developmental disorder with environmental aspects. Hum Reprod 2001;16:972–8.

[132] Sharpe RM. Pathways of endocrine disruption during male sexual differentiation and masculinisation. Best Pract Res Clin Endocrinol Metab 2006;20:91–110.

[133] Sousa B, Moser E, Fatima C. An update on male breast cancer and future directions for research and treatment. Eur J Pharmacol 2013;717:71–83.

[134] Darbre PD. Environmental contaminants in milk: the problem of organochlorine xenobiotics. Biochem Soc Trans 1998;26:106–12.

[135] St-Hilaire S, Mandal R, Commendador A, Mannel S, Derryberry D. Estrogen receptor positive breast cancers and their association with environmental factors. Int J Health Geogr 2011;10(32):1–8.

[136] Brophy JT, Keith MM, Watterson A, Park R, Gilbertson M, Tyndale EM, et al. Breast cancer risk in relation to occupations with exposure to carcinogens and endocrine disruptors: a Canadian case-control study. Environ Health 2012;11(87):1–17.

[137] Tryggvadottir L, Sigvaldason H, Olafsdottir H, Jonasson JG, Jonsson T, Tulinius H, et al. Population-based study of changing breast cancer risk in Icelandic BRCA2 mutation carriers, 1920–2000. J Natl Cancer Inst 2006;98:116–22.

[138] Cleary MP, Grossman ME. Minireview: obesity and breast cancer: the estrogen connection. Endocrinology 2009;150:2537–42.

11

Endocrine Disruption of Thyroid Function: Chemicals, Mechanisms, and Toxicopathology

Catherine Sutcliffe and Philip W. Harvey

Endocrine Disruption and Human Health.
DOI: http://dx.doi.org/10.1016/B978-0-12-801139-3.00011-9

Abstract

The endocrine disruption of thyroid function is reviewed with reference to chemicals, mechanisms, and toxicopathology. Following a review of hypothalamo-pituitary-thyroid (HPT) endocrinology, consideration is given to the mechanisms of thyroid chemical disruption delineating direct toxicity (e.g., neuropharmacological effects on control of the thyroid, thyroid peroxidase inhibition, and thyroglobulin inhibition) from indirect or secondary responses on HPT function (accelerated hepatic clearance of thyroid hormones, effects on circulatory thyroid hormone transport, or effects on peripheral tissue deiodinases). The occurrence of more than one mechanism is discussed, and examples of drugs and chemicals that are both enzyme inducers and thyroid inhibitors are provided. Distinguishing features of the mechanisms of thyroid dysfunction typically seen in toxicology studies [endocrinology profiles and thyroid hypertrophy mediated by thyroid-stimulating hormone (TSH) excess] are described. Finally, the emerging evidence that TSH plays a role in human thyroid tumor promotion and of environmental chemical exposures in human hypothyroidism and cancer, both conditions associated with excess TSH, are considered.

The consequences of thyroid follicular cell dysfunction, either hyperthyroidism or hypothyroidism, on human health are well recognized in clinical medicine. Conditions of thyroid follicular cell secretory excess, such as Graves' disease, result in morbidity and occasional mortality secondary to the powerful physiological action of the thyroid hormones: hyperthyroidism can result in oversensitization of the heart to the action of catecholamines. Conditions resulting in the loss of thyroid follicular cell hormone production/secretion, such as Hashimoto's thyroiditis or iodine deficiency, are equally debilitating, and hypothyroidism occurring early in life can result in significant developmental neurological retardation. The thyroid also contains parafollicular or C-cells that secrete calcitonin in response to high blood calcium, and calcitonin acts on bone, intestine, and kidneys to reduce blood calcium levels, effectively antagonizing the effects of parathyroid hormone. In the context of toxicology and endocrine disruption, the focus has been on pituitary-thyroid follicular cell function and reviews of parafollicular (C-cell) toxicity and toxicopathology can be found elsewhere [1,2], as can reviews of parathyroid toxicology [1–3].

The two active hormones of the human/mammalian thyroid follicular cells are thyroxine (tetra-iodothyronine, T4) and triiodothyronine (T3) which, as their names suggest, differ in the iodine atoms on a common tyrosine skeleton. Thyroperoxidase (TPO) is an essential enzyme in the synthesis of thyroid hormones. Drugs such as carbimazole, methimazole (MMI), and propylthiouracil (PTU) are used to control thyroid function in human medicine and act as inhibitors of thyroid peroxidase, and consequently thyroid hormone production. The fact that drugs influence thyroid function demonstrates that thyroid dysfunction can be modulated chemically and raises the question of whether the thyroid may be a target for endocrine disruption by other chemicals at environmentally relevant chemical exposure.

This chapter will consider the evidence and mechanisms of thyroid endocrine disruption. The endocrinology of the hypothalamo-pituitary-thyroid (HPT) axis and physiological actions of thyroid hormones are briefly reviewed to appreciate the impact that functional disruption can have. The common in vivo manifestations and mechanisms of thyroid toxicity are discussed, including thyroid hypertrophy as a marker of toxicity, and illustrated with characteristic histopathological changes. A strategy for assessing and distinguishing mechanisms of thyroid functional disruption is presented. Finally, evidence that environmental chemical exposure is affecting thyroid function in humans is considered.

11.1 ENDOCRINOLOGY OF THE HPT AXIS

Figure 11.1 illustrates the control of the HPT axis. Thyrotropin-releasing hormone (TRH) produced in the hypothalamus stimulates the production and secretion of thyroid-stimulating hormone (TSH; thyrotropin) from the pituitary gland. Somatostatin, also released by the hypothalamus, has an inhibitory action on TSH secretion. TSH is carried in the blood to the thyroid gland, where it stimulates the production and secretion of the thyroid hormones T4 and T3, which in turn feedback to both the pituitary and the hypothalamus to attenuate TSH secretion.

Thyroglobulin stored in the lumen of thyroid follicles forms the substrate for thyroid hormone assembly. TPO, an essential enzyme in the synthesis of thyroid hormones, acts to bind iodide to tyrosyl residues in the thyroglobulin and monoiodothyronine (MIT) and diiodothyronine are intermediate molecules in hormone synthesis [2]. Figure 11.2 shows immunohistochemical staining of TPO in the cytoplasm of thyroid follicular epithelial cells. T4 is considered functionally a prohormone for T3 (which can be derived from the deiodination of T4 by deiodinase in a variety of tissues), with T3 prominent in exerting physiological effects (primarily basal metabolic rate and cellular oxygen consumption) and regulating the endocrine axis by negative feedback control of the secretion of TSH. Full details of thyroid hormone synthesis can be found in Refs. [1,2]. The functions of thyroid hormones are shown in Figure 11.1, and as well as maintaining basal metabolic rate, they are involved in bone growth, neural maturation, and erythropoiesis. Holt and Hanley [4] review clinical endocrinology of the thyroid including axis control, hormone synthesis and actions and the consequences of dysfunction.

The thyroid is unusual as an endocrine gland because it has a relatively large functional reserve capacity due to the storage of preformed hormone in the thyroid follicles

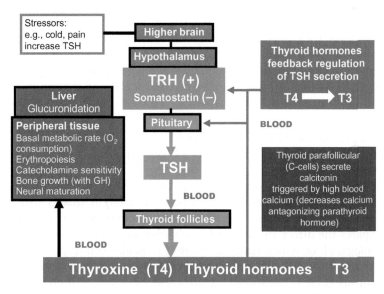

FIGURE 11.1   Control of the HPT axis and functions of thyroid hormones. Abbreviations: TRH, thyrotropin-releasing hormone; TSH, thyroid-stimulating hormone (thyrotropin); T4, thyroxine (tetraiodothyronine); T3, triiodothyronine; GH, growth hormone.

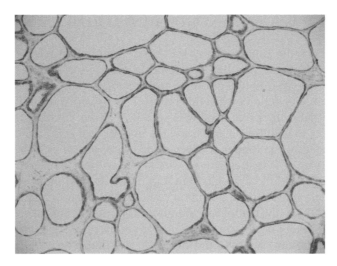

FIGURE 11.2   Immunohistochemical staining for TPO. Staining seen in the follicular epithelial cell cytoplasm—cynomolgus monkey (×20).

(thyroglobulin in the colloid within the follicular lumen) prior to release into the bloodstream. This reservoir also attenuates large acute variations in blood hormone concentrations, but prolonged excess TSH secretion will eventually deplete these reserves and produce characteristic histopathological changes in the thyroid (reviewed later in this chapter). As with other endocrine organs that are part of a negative feedback–controlled endocrine axis (e.g., the adrenal), many of the changes seen histopathologically in the thyroid gland are secondary to the effects of the trophic hormone, TSH, which both stimulates hormone production/secretion and stimulates growth of the gland as a whole. Thyroid follicular cell hypertrophy is a common finding in toxicology studies and is usually caused by excess TSH. The challenge in toxicology and endocrine disruption research is to establish the mechanism behind the excess TSH secretion.

11.2 EXAMPLES OF CHEMICAL DISRUPTERS OF THYROID FUNCTION

There are a number of mechanisms by which HPT function can be disturbed, and examples of direct and indirect mechanisms are discussed later in this chapter (these examples are not intended to be exhaustive but provide principles of the various mechanisms). Figure 11.3 compares the direct and indirect mechanisms of toxicity most commonly seen in endocrine toxicology, all of which result in thyroid follicular cell hypertrophy mediated by excess TSH secretion. Boas et al. [5] provide a recent review of thyroid effects of endocrine-disrupting chemicals (EDCs) organized by chemical class rather than toxicological target and mechanism [e.g., polychlorinated biphenyls (PCBs) and dioxins, polybrominated flame retardants, polyfluorinated chemicals, phthalates, bisphenol A (BPA), ultraviolet (UV) filters, and the pesticides dichlorodiphenyltrichloroethane (DDT), hexachlorobenzene, and

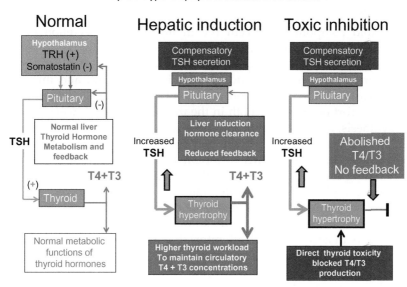

FIGURE 11.3 Mechanisms of direct and indirect thyroid toxicity producing thyroid hypertrophy.

methoxychlor]. It is interesting to see in these examples the number of halogenated compounds; and of course, iodine is also a halogen essential for thyroid hormone synthesis and incorporation. Capen [6] reviews mechanistic data and risk assessment of selected toxic end points for the thyroid gland, covering direct and indirect mechanisms.

11.2.1 Direct Mechanisms

11.2.1.1 Neuroendocrine and Neuropharmacological Effects on the HPT Axis

There are examples of drugs and chemicals that act on the HPT axis at the neuroendocrine level. Caffeine and theophylline have been reported to decrease TSH secretion when administered to rats at doses of 40–50 mg/kg [7]. The mechanism was independent of corticosterone (which can inhibit TSH), and TSH suppression was observed in adrenalectomized and ovariectomized rats. In a study in humans, caffeine administered at 4 mg/kg had no effect on TSH or thyroid hormones [8]. Amphetamine is reported to reduce TSH secretion [9]. Dopamine agonists such as bromocriptine and apomorphine are reported to reduce TSH in humans, and dopamine antagonists such as metoclopramide, domperidone, and sulpiride increase TSH [10,11] indicating the role of neurotransmitters in central neuroendocrine control. Clofibrate (antihyperlipidemic) also directly reduces TSH [clofibrate also has other effects on deiodinase, thyroid-binding globulin (TBG), and liver function affecting the HPT axis; see later in this chapter] and a number of drugs are known to increase TRH-stimulated TSH secretion (e.g., cimetidine and spironolactone) or decrease TRH-stimulated TSH secretion (e.g., phentolamine, fenclofenac) [10,11] as off-target effects unrelated to their pharmacological use.

11.2.1.2 Antithyroid Effects: Inhibition of Iodide Uptake, Thyroid Peroxidase, and Thyroglobulin

Direct antithyroid compounds prevent the manufacture or secretion of thyroid hormones, which typically results in elevated TSH (see Figure 11.3). The initial step in thyroid hormone biosynthesis is the uptake of iodide, and a number of anions are competitive inhibitors of the transport system, including perchlorate [2,11,12] and thiocyanate [2]. In addition, nitrate, carbutamide, amiodarone, and acetazolamide [11] are reported to inhibit iodide uptake, transport of iodide, or both in the thyroid follicle. However, the second step in thyroid biosynthesis, the action of thyroid peroxidase in catalyzing the binding of iodide to tyrosyl residues in thyroglobulin, shows particular vulnerability to chemical inhibition. Whole classes of chemicals are known to inhibit thyroid peroxidase action (reviewed in Refs. [2,11]) including the thionamides (e.g., thiourea, thiouracil, PTU, MMI, carbimazole, and goitrin); aniline derivatives (e.g., sulfonamides, *para*-aminobenzoic acid, *para*-aminosalicylic acid, and amphenone); substituted phenols (e.g., resorcinol, phloroglucinol, and 2,4-hydroxybenzoic acid). Other compounds known to inhibit thyroid peroxidase are aminoglutethimide (also an adrenocortical inhibitor), the antimicrobials cotrimoxazole and cotrifamole, the diuretic acetazolamide, and the polybrominated biphenyl congeners (see Ref. [11]). Polybrominated and polychlorinated biphenyls have particular relevance to environmental chemical exposure and have been consistently detected in human tissues. PCB blood concentrations have also been clinically correlated with reduced thyroid hormone levels in humans [12]. Indeed, Jugan et al. [12] present correlational evidence of the human thyroid effects (e.g., comparing human blood or urine chemical levels with effects on thyroid hormones) of a range of chemicals of environmental significance, including perchlorates (which occur naturally, are used in industry, and are detectable in drinking water supplies), brominated flame retardants, and phthalate plasticizers. Miller et al. [13] review human epidemiological and animal toxicological evidence to extrapolate population risk for thyroid disrupting chemicals, and Capen [6] reviews the mechanistic and risk assessment considerations, including species differences in physiology, for direct-acting thyrotoxic chemicals.

Propranolol, the β-adrenoceptor antagonist that is used to slow the heart rate, is reported to inhibit thyroglobulin synthesis [14], representing another target of direct-acting thyroid follicular functional inhibition.

11.2.2 Indirect Mechanisms

Following the secretion of thyroid hormones into the circulation, the activity in target tissues is determined by the proportion of T4:T3, the proportion of hormone bound to carrier molecules (TBG and albumin) where it is the free unbound fraction that is available to exert physiological activity, the action of peripheral deiodinase enzymes, and finally hepatic metabolism and the clearance of thyroid hormones. There are examples of compounds affecting each of these targets or processes. Effects on the induction of the hepatic phase II conjugating enzyme uridine diphosphate glucuronyltransferase (UDP-GT) presents a common proposed mechanism of thyroid dysfunction in regulatory toxicology studies, resulting in increased clearance of thyroid hormones, compensatory increases in pituitary TSH secretion, and characteristic histopathological changes in the thyroid (see later in this chapter).

11.2.2.1 Peripheral Deiodinase Effects

Deiodinases expressed in peripheral tissues remove iodine from thyroid hormones, converting T4 to T3, an important action in increasing hormone potency, and further removing iodine to inactivate the hormones completely. Thus, interference with this system can have far-reaching effects on thyroid physiology and on the action of thyroid hormones in target tissues. Atterwill et al. [11] present a literature survey of compounds known to affect deiodinases, including omeprazole, PTU, cimetidine, amphetamine, and glucocorticoids, which decrease 5-deiodinase activity; propranolol, which is a competitive inhibitor of 5-deiodiase; and ranitidine, 2, 4-dinitrophenol, and growth hormone, which increase 5-deiodinase activity. Clofibrate, phenobarbitone, and estrogens are also reported to affect deiodination rates of T4. The fact that hormones (growth hormone, glucocorticoids, and estrogens in these examples) affect the deiodination of thyroid hormones illustrates how effects in one endocrine axis can influence another. Glucocorticoids and estrogens also directly influence TSH secretion (see Ref. [7]).

11.2.2.2 Thyroid Hormone Binding to Plasma Proteins

There are species differences in thyroid hormone transport in the blood. Rats and mice do not have TBG, but thyroid hormones are transported loosely bound to albumins in the plasma [2]. Humans, monkeys, and dogs have specific thyroid hormone-binding globulins [2]. Generally, it is the free unbound fraction of a hormone in the blood that is available to exert its physiological effect on a target tissue, and many hormones have binding globulins, which serve an important function in buffering against large acute variations in hormone concentrations in the blood. In thyroid function tests, two measurements are usually conducted, and a free T4 and total T4 or T3 measurements can be assessed. Numerous compounds known to affect plasma binding include salicylates, fenclofenac, heparin, phenytoin, and propranolol, which reduce binding, and diamorphine, methadone, clofibrate, and 5-fluorouracil, which increase TBG, together with a wide variety of other compounds shown to have effects in various species or in vitro [11].

11.2.2.3 Hepatic Metabolism and Conjugation

Thyroid hormones are ultimately metabolized in the liver and an important metabolic pathway is via the phase II glucuronidation by UDP-GT. The rate of this process can be increased as a function of the induction of this enzyme, which in turn can affect the homeostatic balance of the entire HPT axis. Increased clearance of thyroid hormone ultimately results in loss of negative feedback regulation within the HPT axis, and this leads to compensatory increase in TSH secretion to maintain a euthyroid state. The increase in TSH further stimulates the thyroid, which can result in growth and characteristic histopathological changes in the gland, which is discussed later in this chapter. Essentially, the thyroid is working at an increased rate to maintain normal blood T4 and T3 levels. Measurement of thyroid hormones will often show a normal profile of T4 and T3 at the expense of elevated TSH, and different blood profiles are considered later in this chapter.

A great deal of work was conducted in the 1980s on liver enzyme inducers that also altered thyroid function in rats because the end-point pathology of lifetime elevations in TSH was thyroid gland neoplasia [15]. Many new drugs and chemicals were found to result in thyroid neoplasia secondary to liver enzyme induction (with increased clearance of thyroid hormones and elevated TSH), and the relevance of this to humans became the focus of debate (see Ref. [16]). Classifications evolved of phenobarbitone-like inducers, which were characterized by a profile of induction in the liver and subsequent thyroid effects. This mechanism of UDP-GT induction, increased clearance of thyroid hormones, excess compensatory TSH, and subsequent thyroid pathology, remains one of the most common findings in rodent regulatory toxicology studies; and a large number of compounds from a variety of chemical classes demonstrate these actions, including phenobarbitone and analogs, clofibrate, carbamazepine, methylphenidate, polychlorinated and polybrominated biphenyls, dioxin, methylcholanthrene, and benzpyrene [11]. Detailed and robust study has been made of PCBs, compounds of relevance in an environmental exposure context [e.g., PCB 105 (2,3,3′,4,4′-pentachlorobiphenyl) and PCB 153 (2,2′,4,4′,5,5′-hexachlorobiphenyl)], in subchronic rodent toxicity studies where elevations in liver UDP-GT activity were associated with thyroid histopathology in the rat [17,18]. Indeed, it became recognizable that not only potent enzyme inducers, but virtually any low toxicity compound, when administered at relatively high dose levels, could increase metabolic burden in the liver and consequently the induction of various metabolic enzymes, often including UDP-GT, which results in increased conjugation of thyroid hormones. Typical changes in the liver are marked increases in liver weights and hypertrophy of hepatocytes, which is first noticeable in the centrilobular areas, and these changes are correlated with increased enzyme induction and increased activity of enzymes. This mechanism has received considerable regulatory interest, which is discussed later in this chapter in the context of extrapolation to human risk assessment and toxicology strategy. The use of toxicogenomics has been applied to thyroid toxicity assessments and perfluorooctanoic acid and perfluorooctane sulfonate have been shown to perturb thyroid hormone metabolism genes matched by depletion of serum thyroid hormones in vivo in the rat [19].

11.2.2.4 *Consideration of More Than One Mechanism: Thyroid Blocker and Coincident Liver Enzyme Inducer*

It is an important point to note that chemicals may act as both direct-acting thyroid toxicants (e.g., hormone synthesis blockers) and as hepatic enzyme inducers. In such a case, a direct thyrotoxic agent (although it is likely its potency will be relatively weak) may be missed if the changes observed in the thyroid are misattributed to liver enzyme induction alone. The question must be raised on the level of evidence required to claim that thyroid changes are secondary to liver enzyme induction and increased thyroid hormone conjugation and clearance. Regulatory toxicology studies can only show an association between thyroid histopathological changes and changes in the liver that are then considered as evidence of enzyme induction (e.g., increased liver weight or hepatocyte hypertrophy indicative of increased metabolic activity). The two findings must be recognized as correlative only, not proof of causation. Additional evidence is required to both show normal functionality of the thyroid, and that liver enzymes, particularly UDP-GT, are indeed induced to support the secondary indirect mechanism of hepatic disturbance of thyroid function with any certainty, and this is discussed later in toxicology strategies.

Examples of compounds with effects on liver enzyme induction-mediated thyroid hormone clearance, which also have other direct effects on thyroid function, are PTU (increases biliary clearance of T4, a process indicative of increases in UDP-GT conjugation and excretion, and prevents the organification of iodide via inhibition of thyroid peroxidase [20]), polybrominated biphenyls (increase hepatic UDP-GT activity and also inhibit thyroid peroxidase [21]), and phenobarbitone (a potent liver enzyme inducer that also increases the deiodination of T4 via peripheral 5-deiodinase [20]). Similarly, clofibrate is a well-known hepatic inducer that increases biliary clearance of T4 [20], decreases the peripheral deiodination of T4 by deiodinases [20], and is also reported to increase TBG in humans [10]. Interestingly, clofibrate decreases plasma binding in rats [20]. Rats do not have TBG, but thyroid hormones bind loosely to albumins, which results in a shorter half-life of T4 in the rat than in the human (see Refs. [6,11]).

11.2.2.5 Consideration of Pituitary–Thyroid Blood Hormone Profiles Related to Type of Disruption Mechanism

The profile of TSH, T4, and T3 varies with the mechanism of toxicity affecting the thyroid. If the thyroid remains functional, T3 and T4 are capable of being manufactured and secreted to maintain some negative feedback regulation of TSH. Typically with enzyme inducers, the HPT axis is destabilized by increased clearance of thyroid hormone, the blood profiles of T3 and T4 are relatively normal, but TSH is moderately higher than normal. In this case, the magnitude of TSH elevation depends on the rate of thyroid hormone clearance and varies by chemical inducer. Essentially, the thyroid is being moderately overstimulated by TSH to maintain normal homeostatic relationships between pituitary and thyroid (i.e., a euthyroid state).

The profile with a direct thyroid-blocking agent is for markedly depleted T3 and T4, which can be undetectable in blood (personal observation of unpublished data) and markedly elevated TSH. In this case, T3 and T4 production and secretion is abolished, there is unopposed TSH secretion (i.e., no negative feedback control), and TSH is elevated far in excess of normal range, often showing 3 to 5+ fold differences, dependent on species, pituitary capacity, and duration of response (personal observation of unpublished data). The magnitude of TSH elevation, together with the presence of T3 and T4, can assist in distinguishing between mechanisms.

11.3 CHARACTERISTIC TOXICOPATHOLOGY OF THE THYROID GLAND

The common factor in the direct thyroid toxicity mechanisms so far outlined is the reduction of thyroid hormone production and secretion. The reduction of thyroid hormones (T4 or T3) results in compensatory increased secretion of TSH due to the concomitant diminution of feedback control (see Figure 11.3). It is important to note that increased TSH stimulation of the thyroid produces the same histopathological effects irrespective of the mechanism by which TSH is increased, including thyroid growth evidenced by increased size and weight. As previously discussed, the magnitude of increased TSH is often the distinguishing diagnostic feature of thyroid endocrine disruption (since chemicals may be only partial inhibitors of thyroid function and the ability is retained to produce some thyroid hormone at the expense of greater stimulation by TSH). Indeed, the hepatic induction

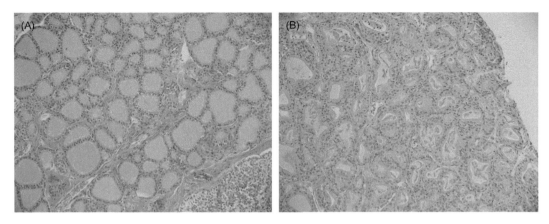

FIGURE 11.4   (A) Normal thyroid—Han Wistar rat (H&E staining ×20). (B) Thyroid follicular cell hypertrophy—Han Wistar rat (×20).

mechanism often results in a resetting of the homeostatic balance within the HPT axis, such that a steady state is achieved of normal circulatory thyroid hormone concentrations despite increased UDP-GT conjugation and clearance, maintained by higher TSH. It is therefore important to illustrate the range of histopathological changes seen in the thyroid as a result of TSH overstimulation. Toxicological pathology reviews of the thyroid can also be found in Refs. [1,22].

A progression of changes in the thyroid can be seen as a function of the duration and severity of the increased TSH stimulation. Early changes comprise depletion of colloid in the lumen of the follicle as it is released. The colloid contains the thyroglobulin and the action of TSH is to stimulate the manufacture and secretion of thyroid hormone. Characteristic adaptive changes can then be observed in the follicular epithelium correlating with the increased stimulus to secrete hormone.

There are only a limited number of morphological changes that the thyroid can undergo in response to either overstimulation or understimulation of the gland. In the rat, follicular cell hypertrophy is seen following TSH stimulation (Figure 11.4). An increase in liver weight, associated with liver enzyme induction and seen as centrilobular hypertrophy in some cases, is commonly observed, along with thyroid follicular cell hypertrophy, and is a physiological response, as mentioned previously. Follicular cell hypertrophy is characterized by an increase in the height of the follicular cells diffusely throughout the thyroid gland. The cells become more columnar in shape, while maintaining a basally located nucleus. There is a reduction in the staining intensity of colloid associated with the utilization of thyroglobulin.

With persistent TSH stimulation, follicular cell hyperplasia is seen, especially in long-term toxicity studies as a background finding, especially in older rodents. This is probably related to the lack of the TBG "buffer" in rodents (shorter half-life and increased clearance of thyroid hormones), making the rodent more susceptible to greater variations in TSH levels. Male rats also have higher circulating levels of TSH than females. Follicular cell hyperplasia is seen either as a diffuse or as a focal change. Diffuse, bilateral hyperplasia as the result of continued

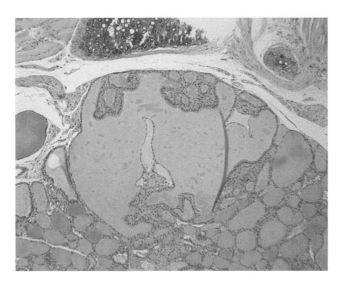

FIGURE 11.5   Follicular cell hyperplasia (cystic form) B6C3F1 mouse, 104-week study (×6).

TSH stimulation is seen macroscopically as enlarged thyroid glands. Microscopically, the epithelial cells are often cuboidal or even flattened, and there is an increase in the number of cells as they become stratified or develop papillary infoldings. There can be some compression of, but little architectural distinction from, the adjacent parenchyma, making these lesions poorly demarcated. These areas are not encapsulated. The hyperplastic foci often arise within cystic follicles due to the increase in colloid produced (Figure 11.5). These hyperplastic lesions can regress after the removal of the TSH stimulus.

Prolonged TSH stimulation can progress to adenomas and carcinomas. Adenomas can appear very similar to areas of focal hyperplasia. However, they are well demarcated from the surrounding parenchyma, occasionally they are minimally encapsulated, and are usually compressive, which is often the criterion for diagnosing adenoma over follicular cell hyperplasia. The architecture is different from the normal follicular epithelium as the cells lose their polarity; however, the morphology within the adenoma can be homogenous. The growth pattern within the tumor can be papillary, solid (macrofollicular or microfollicular types), or cystic. Adenomas can be single or multiple within one or both thyroid glands. Cells are usually seen to be in a single layer, cuboidal to columnar with a low mitotic index, but have an increased nuclear to cytoplasmic ratio. This change is irreversible (Figure 11.6).

Follicular cell carcinomas can be unilateral or bilateral, with papillary, solid, follicular, cystic, scirrhous, or a mixture of patterns within one mass. Cells may form multiple layers with areas of necrosis, and the mitotic index can be high. Invasion through the capsule is a recommended finding in order to diagnose carcinoma. This may progress into adjacent tissues and via the blood or lymph, resulting in distant metastasis, which indicates malignancy (Figure 11.7).

Follicular epithelial cell atrophy, secondary to reduced TSH levels reaching or acting on the thyroid, is seen microscopically as a flattening of the follicular epithelial cells throughout

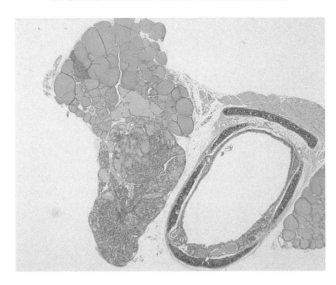

FIGURE 11.6   Thyroid follicular cell adenoma B6C3F1 mouse, 104-week study (×2).

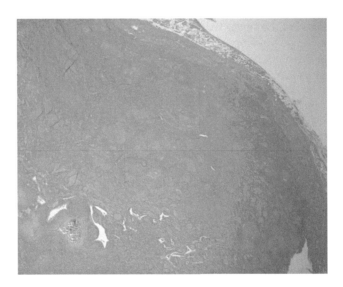

FIGURE 11.7   Follicular cell carcinoma Sprague Dawley rat, 104-week study (×2).

the thyroid, with pale homogenous colloid in often distended follicles [23]. This can also be seen as the result of a primary degenerative condition of follicular cells (Figure 11.8).

In the case of a TSH receptor blocking agent, pale and vacuolated hypertrophic cells considered to be thyrotrophs in the pars distalis of the pituitary can be seen, as they are distended with TSH [23] (Figure 11.9).

3. CONCERNS FOR HUMAN HEALTH

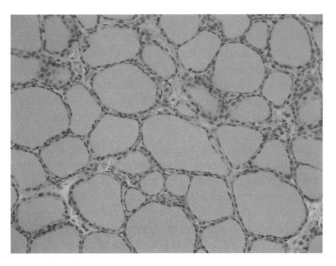

FIGURE 11.8   Follicular cell atrophy Han Wistar rat, 28-day study (×40). *Source: By permission of the copyright holders.*

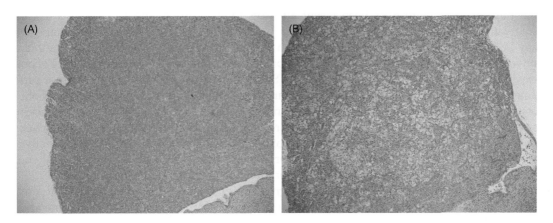

FIGURE 11.9   Pars distalis Han Wistar rat (×10): (A) normal pituitary and (B) pituitary cell hypertrophy with pallor and vacuolation. *Source: By permission of the copyright holders.*

11.4 REGULATORY CONSIDERATIONS AND TOXICOLOGY STRATEGY FOR EXAMINING THYROID FUNCTIONAL DISRUPTION

There is a tendency among regulatory toxicologists and pathologists to disregard thyroid pathology consistent with TSH stimulation in rats when there is coincident evidence of hepatic enzyme induction. In addition, the changes induced in the rat, ultimately including thyroid tumors, have generally been considered species specific [6,15,16,24]. Rationales include species-specific physiology, such as the absence of TBG in rats; differences in T4 half-life, which is much shorter in rats [6]; and that there was little evidence in humans that TSH was a tumor promoter (see Refs. [15,16]). Indeed, it was commonly considered that the rat thyroid was more sensitive and the human thyroid more resistant to the tumorigenic effects of TSH [2,15,24], but this view may now be challenged [25]. A more pragmatic argument, however, could be made based on risk assessment principles, in that thyroid changes secondary to liver enzyme induction often occur in rodent studies at chemical doses, causing a metabolic burden, which are commonly orders of magnitude above realistic human exposures.

Consequently, regulatory strategy has focused on excluding direct effects on the thyroid as the mechanism of elevated TSH. Direct effects are generally considered to apply across all species, and findings in rodents (for example) are considered relevant to humans. Indirect elevation of TSH was generally considered not to have such relevance to human risk assessment, even in cases of TSH-mediated thyroid tumorigenesis. To this end, regulatory agencies such as the US Environmental Protection Agency (EPA) typically requested endocrine function studies (measuring TSH, T3, and T4) coupled with liver enzyme assessment to provide evidence that the mechanism was not direct thyrotoxicity. The use of the perchlorate discharge test to detect thyroid iodide accumulation and organification (essentially assessing thyroid peroxidase activity) was also used to distinguish direct from indirect effects on thyroid function, and there have been recent attempts to standardize and validate this test in a regulatory toxicology context [26]. However, the recent reemergence of evidence that TSH may be involved in the progression of human thyroid tumors [25] may challenge assumed conventional toxicology wisdom that thyroid pathology in the rat due to elevated TSH is not relevant to human risk assessment. Clearly, if TSH is found to be a human thyroid tumor promoter, compounds causing increased TSH by any mechanism in rats (or indeed other laboratory species) may be directly relevant to human risk assessment. Thus the balance of concern may shift from whether the compound is a direct thyroid blocker (relevant to humans) versus liver enzyme inducer (usually considered of minimal toxicological relevance), to whether any elevation in TSH is of toxicological (tumorigenic) concern. As with all toxicological end points, exposure and margins of safety considerations are fundamental to risk analyses.

A recent attempt has been made to assign a weighted ranking to the endocrine end points, including thyroid effects, in the regulatory screening battery for endocrine disruption [27]. The analysis is restricted to the tests used in the Tier 1 Endocrine Screening Battery set forward by the EPA, and thus only considers the relevance of end points from the Amphibian Metamorphosis Assay and the Male and Female Pubertal Assay protocols, but the relevance and ranking of the types of finding (e.g., thyroid histopathology and thyroid endocrinology), together with limitations, confounding factors, and surrogate data indicative of thyroid disruption (e.g., growth and pubertal milestones), are critically discussed in a regulatory data context.

11.5 EVIDENCE OF ENVIRONMENTALLY MEDIATED THYROID ENDOCRINE DISRUPTION: RELEVANCE TO HUMAN HEALTH

Studies conducted on laboratory animal species, or in vitro on tissues and cell lines, form the core of toxicological hazard assessment. The significance and extrapolation of findings to humans forms the basis for risk assessment. A large number of drugs and chemicals have been shown in toxicity tests to disturb the function of the thyroid via a variety of mechanisms. The question of whether these chemicals pose a risk to human health hinges on the potential for human exposure. This is usually estimated as part of the risk analysis process in the absence of actual human data. When human exposure data does exist, including measurement of chemicals in human blood, serum, or urine, this is often not related to biomarkers of biological effects. However, there are studies available correlating human tissue concentrations of environmental chemicals, particularly PCBs, with altered thyroid function [12,13]. Such studies are correlational by nature and do not provide proof of causation, and other factors may be involved, but when added to other data, the weight of evidence can accumulate. It is now generally considered that there is enough evidence that PCBs are thyroid-disrupting chemicals also affecting humans [5]. Miller et al. [13] reviews the literature with regard to thyroid-disrupting chemicals, including the evidence of causality and sensitive populations. As with many areas of endocrine disruption research, there is a lack of robust controlled human data on the potential thyroid effects of environmental chemical exposures.

It is interesting to refer to the incidence rates of thyroid conditions in the medical epidemiology literature. The primary cause of hypothyroidism worldwide is iodine deficiency, and one-third of the world's population lives in iodine-deficient areas [28]. However, the incidence of hypothyroidism appears to be increasing in iodine-replete areas and populations [28,29]. Leese et al. [29] report on increasing prevalence and incidence of hypothyroidism (reduced thyroid hormone secretion and concomitant elevated TSH) in Scotland (the Thyroid Epidemiology Audit and Research Study), and the overall prevalence of thyroid dysfunction has increased from 2.3% to 3.8% (1994–2001), with the standardized incidence of hyperthyroidism increased from 0.68 to 0.87 per 1000 females/year (representing a 6.3% annual increase) and incidence of hypothyroidism in males increased from 0.65 to 1.01 per 1000 males/year. The underlying reasons and mechanisms are unknown but are likely to include environmental factors. Similarly, in a US cross-sectional study (Colorado 9 Health Fair screening), a total of 33,661 people were randomly screened for thyroid function by hormone measurements, and of 24,337 not already diagnosed with thyroid disorders or taking thyroid medication, 103 were diagnosed as clinically hypothyroid and 2067 were subclinically hypothyroid, giving a prevalence of 9.9% previously undiagnosed hypothyroidism [30]. Thyroid dysfunction, particularly hypothyroidism, is therefore considered to be common. It may be suggested from these studies collectively that the thyroid is vulnerable to dysfunction and that rising incidences over relatively short time scales (i.e., a few decades) suggest that lifestyle or environmental factors are exerting additional adverse effects. Further, the fact that thyrotoxic chemicals are known to be present in human tissues raises the possibility of chemical involvement in rising incidences of subclinical hypothyroidism.

There are also reports that the incidence of thyroid cancer is increasing [31,32], and although some of the increase has been attributed to earlier and increased detection of the disease, other reports conclude that medical surveillance and more sensitive diagnostic techniques "cannot completely explain the increased incidences of thyroid cancer and other factors may be involved" [32]. It is again worth restating that hypothyroidism results in elevated TSH and that elevated TSH is now suggested to play a central role in the development and/or progression of human thyroid carcinomas [25]. Thus, there is biological plausibility in the suggestion that thyrotoxic chemicals [reducing thyroid hormones and increasing TSH, as has been shown for PCBs (e.g., [5,12,13])] may also play a role in thyroid cancer via the tumor-promoting action of elevated TSH. Finally, the current state of endocrine disruption research policy (which after two decades is still focused on basic chemical hazard assessment in the laboratory) will not allow for progress in this area unless a fully integrated research strategy incorporating human studies, at the very least correlating chemical exposures with thyroid function and epidemiology monitoring, is developed and undertaken.

References

[1] Rosol TJ, DeLellis RA, Harvey PW, Sutcliffe C. Endocrine system Haschek WM, Rousseaux CG, Wallig MA, editors. Haschek and Rousseaux's handbook of toxicologic pathology: Elsevier Inc., Academic Press, New York; 2013. pp. 2391–492.

[2] Capen CC. Thyroid and parathyroid toxicology. In: Harvey PW, Rush KC, Cockburn A, editors. Endocrine and hormonal toxicology. Chichester: Wiley; 1999. pp. 33–66.

[3] Capen CC. Pathophysiology and xenobiotic toxicity of parathyroid glands in animals Atterwill CK, Flack JD, editors. Endocrine toxicology. Cambridge University Press, Cambridge; 1992. pp. 183–240.

[4] Holt RIG, Hanley NA. Essential endocrinology and diabetes, 6th ed. Chichester: Wiley Blackwell; 2012.

[5] Boas M, Feldt-Rasmussen U, Main KM. Thyroid effects of endocrine disrupting chemicals. Mol Cell Endocrinol 2012;355:240–8.

[6] Capen CC. Mechanistic data and risk assessment of selected toxic endpoints of the thyroid gland. Toxicol Pathol 1997;25:39–48.

[7] Spindel E, Griffith L, Wurtman RJ. Neuroendocrine effects of caffeine. II. Effects on thyrotropin and corticosterone secretion. J Pharmacol Exp Ther 1983;225:346–50.

[8] Spindel E, Wurtmann RJ, McCall A, Carr DB, Conlay L, Griffith L, et al. Neuroendocrine effects of caffeine in normal subjects. Clin Pharmacol Ther 1984;36:402–7.

[9] Spindel E. Action of methylxanthines on the pituitary and pituitary dependent hormones. Prog Clin Biol Res 1984;158:355–63.

[10] Wenzel KW. Pharmacological interference with in vitro tests of thyroid function. Metabolism 1981;30:717–32.

[11] Atterwill CK, Jones C, Brown CG. Thyroid gland II—mechanisms of species-dependent thyroid toxicity, hyperplasia and neoplasia induced by xenobiotics. Atterwill CK, Flack JD, editors. Endocrine toxicology. Cambridge University Press, Cambridge; 1992. pp. 137–82.

[12] Jugan M-L, Levi Y, Blondeau J-P. Endocrine disruptors and thyroid hormone physiology. Biochem Pharmacol 2010;79:939–47.

[13] Miller MD, Croftom KM, Rice DC, Zoeller RT. Thyroid-disrupting chemicals: interpreting upstream biomarkers of adverse outcomes. Environ Health Perspect 2009;117:1033–41.

[14] Monaco F, Pontecorvi A, de Luca M, de Pirro RD, Armiento M, Roche J. Inhibition of the biosynthesis of thyroglobulin with propranolol in the rat. C R Soc Biol (Paris) 1982;176:607–12.

[15] McCLain RM. The significance of hepatic microsomal enzyme induction and altered thyroid function in rats: implications for thyroid gland neoplasia. Toxicol Pathol 1989;17:294–306.

[16] Thomas GA, Williams ED. Thyroid gland I—physiologic control and mechanisms of carcinogenesis Atterwill CK, Flack JD, editors. Endocrine toxicology. Cambridge University Press, Cambridge; 1992. pp. 117–36.

[17] Chu I, Poon R, Yagminas A, Lecavalier P, Hakansson H, Valli VE, et al. Subchronic toxicity of PCB 105 (2,3,3',4,4'-pentachlorobiphenyl) in rats. J Appl Toxicol 1998;18:285–92.

[18] Chu I, Villeneuve DC, Yagminas A, Lecavalier P, Poon R, Feeley M, et al. Toxicity of 2,2',4,4',5,5'-hexachlorobiphenyl in rats: effects following 90-day oral exposure. J Appl Toxicol 1996;16:121–8.

[19] Martin MT, Brennan RJ, Hu W, Ayanoglu E, Lau C, Ren H, et al. Toxicogenomic study of triazole fungicides and perfluoroalkyl acids in rat livers predicts toxicity and categorizes chemicals based on mechanisms of toxicity. Toxicol Sci 2007;97:595–613.

[20] Cavalieri RR, Pitt-Rivers R. The effects of drugs on the distribution and metabolism of thyroid hormones. Pharmacol Rev 1981;33:55–80.

[21] Akoso BT, Sleight SD, Nachreiner RF, Aust SD. Effects of purified polybrominated biphenyl congeners on the thyroid and pituitary gland of rats. J Am Coll Toxicol 1982;3:23–36.

[22] Capen CC. Mechanisms and manifestations of endocrine organ toxicity and carcinogenicity. Toxicol Pathol 2001;29:8–33.

[23] Greaves P. Histopathology of preclinical toxicity studies: interpretation and relevance in drug safety evaluation, 4th ed. Academic Press, New York; 2012. pp. 733 & 767.

[24] Gopinath C. Comparative endocrine carcinogenesis. In: Harvey PW, Rush KC, Cockburn A, editors. Endocrine and hormonal toxicology. Chichester: Wiley; 1999. pp. 155–67.

[25] Boelaert K. The association between serum TSH concentration and thyroid cancer. Endocr Relat Cancer 2009;16:1065–72.

[26] Coelho-Palermo Cuhna G, van Ravenzwaay B. Standardization of the perchlorate discharge assay for thyroid toxicity testing in rats. Regul Toxicol Pharmacol 2007;48:270–8.

[27] Borgert CJ, Stuchal LD, Mihaich EM, Becker RA, Bentley KS, Brausch JM, et al. Relevance weighting of tier 1 endocrine screening endpoints by rank order. Birth Defects Res (Part B) 2014;101:90–113.

[28] Vanderpump MPJ. The epidemiology of thyroid disease. Br Med Bull 2011;99:39–51.

[29] Leese GP, Flynn RV, Jung RT, MacDonald TM, Murphy MJ, Morris AD. Increasing prevalence and incidence of thyroid disease in Tayside, Scotland: the Thyroid Epidemiology, Audit and Research Study (TEARS). Clin Endocrinol (Oxf) 2008;68:311–6.

[30] Canaris GJ, Manowitz NR, Mayor G, Ridgway EC. The Colorado thyroid disease prevalence study. Arch Intern Med 2000;160:526–34.

[31] Davies L, Welch HG. Increasing incidence of thyroid cancer in the United States, 1973–2002. JAMA 2006;295:2164–7.

[32] Enewold L, Zhu K, Ron E, Marrogi AJ, Stojadinovic A, Peoples GE, et al. Rising thyroid cancer incidence in the United States by demographic and tumor characteristics, 1980–2005. Cancer Epidemiol Biomarkers Prev 2009;18:784–91.

Endocrine Disruption of Adrenocortical Function

Philip W. Harvey

Abstract

Endocrine disruption of the adrenal gland is a neglected area. This is surprising, given its role as a vital organ, knowledge of its dysfunction in disease, and the fact that medical experience records mortality due to side effects of drugs on adrenocortical steroidogenesis and that the adrenal is the most common toxicological target organ in the endocrine system. This review outlines the endocrinology of the hypothalamo-pituitary-adrenocortical (HPA) axis, physiological actions of adrenocortical steroids, common manifestations of adrenocortical toxicity (particularly adrenal hypertrophy in adrenocortical insufficiency), and a strategy for distinguishing the mechanisms of adrenal functional disruption. Factors predisposing the adrenal to toxic insult are identified and adrenocortical steroidogenesis reviewed in the context of the range of targets that this presents: this is illustrated with examples of chemicals affecting every step and enzyme in the steroidogenic pathway. Finally, environmental chemicals affect adrenal function in wildlife sentinels and similar human susceptibility to environmental adrenal endocrine disruption is considered.

Endocrine Disruption and Human Health.
DOI: http://dx.doi.org/10.1016/B978-0-12-801139-3.00012-0

219

The consequences of adrenal dysfunction, either medulla or cortex, on human health are well recognized in clinical medicine. The adrenal gland is a vital organ, and abnormal function causes significant morbidity and mortality. Conditions of adrenal secretory excess, such as pheochromocytoma (an adrenomedullary catecholamine secreting tumor), Conn's disease (excess production of the adrenocortical mineralocorticoid aldosterone), Cushing's disease (excess production of the adrenocortical glucocorticoid cortisol), and adrenogenital syndrome (excess production of adrenocortical androgens during development), all result in profound morbidity secondary to the powerful physiological action of the respective adrenal hormone, which is secreted in abnormally high concentrations. However, conditions resulting in the loss of adrenal hormone production and secretion (generally termed *adrenocortical insufficiency*), such as the salt-wasting syndromes in neonates and Addison's disease and its phenotypic variants [1,2], are more serious and acute, life-threatening conditions.

The two main hormones of the human adrenal cortex are the glucocorticoid cortisol and the mineralocorticoid aldosterone. Adrenocortical insufficiency can result in an Addisonian crisis. The loss of glucocorticoid reduces anti-inflammatory defense and glucose metabolism, both of which are important for stress tolerance. The loss of mineralocorticoid causes reduced vascular volume, renal sodium loss, bowel water and electrolyte loss, loss of potassium excretion, and ultimately cardiovascular collapse. Although the etiology of Addison's disease in adulthood is commonly autoimmune destruction of adrenocortical cells or infection (the English physician Thomas Addison originally described tuberculosis, which was common in Victorian England, as a cause), which in turn compromises the steroidogenic capacity of the adrenal cortex, a number of drugs have been shown to chemically induce adrenocortical insufficiency (including Addisonian crisis) by a highly selective inhibition of critical enzymes in the steroid biosynthetic pathway. Drugs such as aminoglutethimide (a sedative used as an antidepressant) and etomidate (an anesthetic induction agent) resulted in patient deaths, and only later was it recognized that this was due to inhibition of cytochrome P450 11β-hydroxylase (CYP11B1), which is essential for cortisol production [2–6]. Other drugs known to affect adrenocortical function through off-target side effects or toxicity include ketoconazole (an antifungal), which is known to inhibit a number of steroidogenic enzymes (e.g., CYP 17, 21, and 11B1; see later in this chapter), and suramin (anti-helminthic), which can cause frank adrenal pathology and cellular destruction (see Ref. [2]). In addition, drugs such as phenytoin, barbiturates, and rifampin are reported to accelerate cortisol metabolism [2], potentially reducing the physiological effectiveness of endogenously secreted hormone and illustrating that effects on adrenal function at the whole body level can be influenced by factors outside the endocrine axis. Similarly, nonsteroidal anti-inflammatory drugs have been reported to decrease the binding capacity of corticosteroid-binding globulin (CBG), apparently by a mechanism other than simple competitive displacement of the bound glucocorticoid (see Ref. [7]).

The fact that drugs can influence adrenocortical function and produce adrenal insufficiency through steroidogenic enzyme inhibition (or indeed other mechanisms) raises the question of whether the adrenal may be a target for endocrine disruption by other chemicals. This certainly seems to be the case, and Harvey et al. [8–10] have documented over 70 chemicals that impair adrenocortical function and steroidogenic capability in vivo, in vitro, or both, and the targets in the pathway that they affect. There are examples of chemicals adversely affecting every molecular-functional site, ranging from the adrenocorticotrophic hormone (ACTH) receptor and steroid acute regulatory protein (StAR) cholesterol transporter to every enzyme in the pathway, from cholesterol to cortisol and aldosterone production. The question, then, is not whether such chemicals can influence human adrenocortical function, but *can human adrenal endocrine disruption occur at environmentally relevant chemical exposures?* Further, the adrenal cortex as a steroidogenic tissue is unique in possessing universal steroidogenic capability (i.e., it is able to synthesize and secrete all naturally occurring steroids to a greater or lesser degree by virtue of the range of enzymes that it expresses); thus it has a comparatively large number of molecular targets for disruption, which is considered a major factor that conveys vulnerability of the gland to toxic insult [11]. This may explain why the adrenal gland is the most common toxicological target organ in the endocrine system [12].

This chapter will consider the evidence and mechanisms of adrenal endocrine disruption. Almost all work has focused on the adrenal cortex, and the reader is referred to general toxicology and toxicopathology reviews for information on adrenomedullary toxicity [13,14]. The endocrinology of the hypothalamo-pituitary-adrenocortical (HPA) axis and physiological actions of adrenocortical steroids is briefly reviewed to appreciate the impact that functional disruption can have. The common in vivo manifestations of adrenocortical toxicity are discussed, including adrenal hypertrophy as a marker of adrenocortical insufficiency, and a strategy for assessing and distinguishing mechanisms of adrenal functional disruption is presented. The process of adrenocortical steroidogenesis is reviewed in the context of the large range of targets that this presents, and this is illustrated with examples of chemical inhibitors from a wide range of chemical classes. As the adrenal is the most common target organ in toxicology studies, the factors predisposing the adrenal to toxic insult are identified. Finally, the evidence that environmental chemical exposures are affecting adrenal function in wildlife sentinel species is considered in the context of whether low-level exposures may also pose a risk to human health.

12.1 ENDOCRINOLOGY OF THE HPA AXIS AND PHYSIOLOGICAL ACTIONS OF ADRENOCORTICAL STEROIDS

The adrenal cortex is comprised of three distinct layers or zones of cells (see Ref. [15] and Figure 12.1). The outermost zone is the zona glomerulosa, comprising 15% of cortical volume and the primary steroid hormone produced is the mineralocorticoid aldosterone. The zona glomerulosa is part of the renin–angiotensin system (Figure 12.2). Renin is secreted from the kidney in response to a fall in blood pressure and converts angiotensinogen to angiotensin I, which is in turn converted to angiotensin II, which then stimulates production and release of aldosterone from the zona glomerulosa cells of the adrenal cortex. High potassium also provokes aldosterone secretion and the action of aldosterone back on the kidney is to assist with potassium excretion, promote retention of sodium and water, increase vascular volume, and hence maintain blood pressure. Further details of the renin–angiotensin system can be found in Ref. [1]. In addition, vasopressin [arginine vasopressin (AVP); anti-diuretic hormone] also acts to regulate reabsorption of water in the kidney. This hormone also promotes secretion of ACTH [16], thereby promoting secretion of glucocorticoids which also have mineralocorticoid effects, as discussed later in this chapter.

The middle layer is the zona fasciculata (Figure 12.1) and comprises approximately 70% of the cortex. This zone is under the influence of pituitary ACTH (corticotropin), which is in

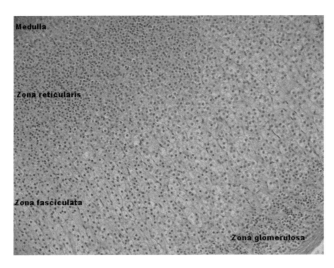

FIGURE 12.1   The normal structure of the adrenal cortex in the cynomolgus monkey (*Macaca fascicularis*). *Source: Reproduced from Harvey and Sutcliffe [15] with permission from John Wiley & Sons.*

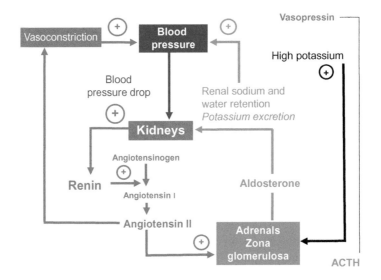

FIGURE 12.2   The renin-angiotensin system controlling aldosterone secretion.

turn controlled by corticotrophin-releasing hormone (CRH) and directly transported to the pituitary down neurons from the hypothalamus and AVP. ACTH is secreted into the blood-stream to provoke the secretion of glucocorticoid (cortisol in humans, but rats and mice produce corticosterone as they lack CYP17) from the cells of the zona fasciculata of the adrenal cortex. Excess ACTH (e.g., persistently secreted in the stress response) causes adrenal

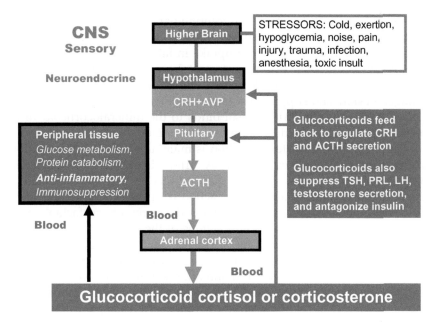

FIGURE 12.3   The HPA axis. Abbreviations: CRH, corticotrophin-releasing hormone; AVP, arginine vasopressin; ACTH, adrenocorticotrophic hormone (corticotrophin); TSH, thyroid-stimulating hormone; PRL, prolactin; LH, luteinizing hormone; CNS, central nervous system.

size growth (hypertrophy), increased adrenal weight, and increase in the thickness of the zona fasciculata. The glucocorticoid is secreted in the blood to mediate its effects on glucose and protein metabolism, but it also plays a central role in the stress response via anti-inflammatory action, which is considered vital under conditions of stress, injury, and illness [16]. Most glucocorticoid is bound to CBG during circulatory transit, with only the free fraction available to modulate effects; it is the proportion of unbound free steroid that increases dramatically during stress activation of the HPA axis. The glucocorticoids maintain a negative feedback action on the hypothalamus and pituitary to regulate their secretion (Figure 12.3). A full review of the endocrinology of the HPA axis is provided by Buckingham [16].

An important point is that loss of glucocorticoid (e.g., by chemical inhibition of steroidogenesis) results in loss of negative feedback control of ACTH secretion and persistent ACTH secretion, which in turn overstimulates the adrenal cortex and can also cause hypertrophy, which is indistinguishable from that induced by stress, since both result from ACTH overstimulation. This mechanism is designed to compensate for falling steroidogenic capability. Thus, it is not possible to distinguish the mechanism of adrenal hypertrophy when an increase in gland size is the only finding. The distinguishing features of both mechanisms and the need to confirm functionality of the adrenal cortex in all cases of adrenal hypertrophy (see Ref. [15]) is discussed later in this chapter.

The glucocorticoids have numerous fundamental actions affecting every cell and tissue in the body, but certain actions are more prominent. Full details of glucocorticoid pharmacological actions are provided elsewhere [1,16,17]. The glucocorticoids were originally named because of their effects on intermediary metabolism and specifically glucose. They tend to increase blood glucose levels by promoting gluconeogenesis (increasing hepatic glucose output), inhibiting glucose uptake in fat and muscle and antagonizing the effects of insulin. Glucocorticoids also increase protein catabolism and lipolysis. The effects on protein synthesis can reduce muscle mass, and glucocorticoids also inhibit keratinocytes and collagen in skin, and suppress osteoblast action (bone manufacture) and stimulate osteoclast action (bone breakdown). Cortisol binds to the mineralocorticoid receptor with approximately equal affinity to aldosterone and has mineralocorticoid activity: in normal situations, the specificity for aldosterone action is maintained by the deactivation of cortisol by conversion to cortisone peripherally by 11β-hydroxysteroid dehydrogenase type II (HSD11B2). The glucocorticoids have profound effects on fetal development, especially growth [1,2,16,18], but one important specific action is in the differentiation of certain cell types to adult phenotypes such as the lung, where they promote surfactant secretion neonatally. However, one of the most important actions of the glucocorticoids is in quenching the inflammatory response [16] via actions on cells of the immune system: glucocorticoids suppress T-lymphocytes and eosinophils, increase neutrophils (collectively known as the stress leukogram), and rapidly suppress inflammation within tissues by inhibiting cytokine production and macrophage activity. The effects of glucocorticoids on immune function and inflammation (see Refs. [17,19]) have been known for many years, and this is the basis for the use of these steroids in medicine.

The innermost zone of the adrenal cortex, bordering the medulla, is the zona reticularis, which comprises the final 15% of cortical volume. This zone produces weak androgens such as dehydroepiandrosterone (DHEA) and androstenedione, which can then form substrates for conversion to estrone, testosterone, dihydrotestosterone (DHT), and estradiol peripherally. This zone is absent in some species, such as the marmoset [20], and thus is not a vital zone in mammals. The loss of functionality in this zone is not life-threatening, but inborn errors of metabolism affecting this zone in humans can produce adrenogenital syndrome, characterized by excess androgen production and masculinization of the female fetus, which is most obvious in the ambiguous appearance of external genitalia.

12.2 STEROIDOGENIC PATHWAY AND EXAMPLES OF CHEMICAL DISRUPTERS

A schematic diagram of human steroidogenesis is given in Figure 12.4. The cells of each zone differentially express specific cytochrome P450 (CYP) and hydroxysteroid dehydrogenase (HSD) enzymes, which convey the ability to synthesize specific steroids. For example, only the zona glomerulosa expresses CYP11B2 to catalyze the conversion of corticosterone to aldosterone. In humans, CYP17 converts pregnenolone and progesterone to their 17-α forms, which are then converted in the zona fasciculata to 11-deoxycortisol and ultimately cortisol. Full details of adrenal steroidogenesis are provided in Refs. [21] and [22] with discussions and comparisons between normal human adrenal cells and the H295R cell line (discussed later in this chapter) and between humans and rodents (see also Refs. [10,11]), where the latter lacks expression of CYP17 and hence cannot produce cortisol.

HUMAN ADRENOCORTICAL STEROIDOGENESIS

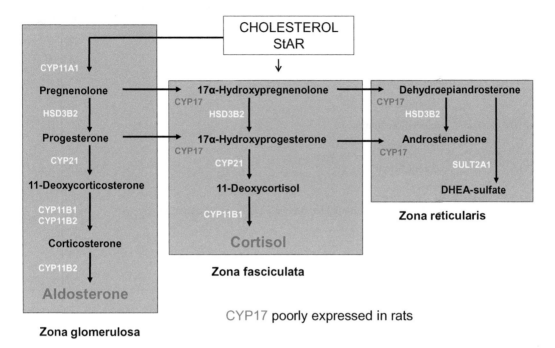

FIGURE 12.4 Adrenocortical steroidogenesis pathway in human and rat. Abbreviations: StAR, steroidogenic acute regulatory protein; CYP, cytochrome P450 enzyme (different enzymes are identified by the numerical nomenclature: synonyms include CYP11A1 = cholesterol side chain cleavage; CYP11B1 = 11β-hydroxylase; CYP11B2 = aldosterone synthase; CYP21 = 21-hydroxylase; CYP17 = 17α-hydroxylase 17,20-lyase); HSD, hydroxysteroid dehydrogenase (3β-hydroxysteroid dehydrogenase type II); SULT 2A1, dehydroepiandrosterone-sulfotransferase. The rat is deficient in CYP17. *Source: Adapted from Harvey and Sutcliffe [15] with permission from John Wiley & Sons.*

It can be seen in Figure 12.4 that there are a large number of potential targets that can be affected in the adrenocortical steroidogenic pathway. The adrenal cortex expresses the ACTH receptor, and aminoglutethimide is reported to downregulate this receptor [23]. StAR functions as a cholesterol transporter across the mitochondrial membrane (a rate-limiting step for steroidogenesis), and numerous compounds have been reported to affect this protein at least in vitro, such as econazole, miconazole, lindane, glyphosate, dimethoate, carbachol, ethanol, arsenite, anisomycin, bromocriptine, and spironolactone (reviewed in Ref. [9]). Of note is that these compounds come from a variety of chemical classes and applications, including crop protection herbicides, fungicides, centrally active drugs with primary pharmacology unrelated to adrenal function, and simple, natural products such as alcohol. This makes structure activity predictions difficult on the current data set. A single compound may also have multiple targets and aminoglutethimide, and as well as downregulating the ACTH receptor [23] also inhibits CYP11A1 cholesterol side chain cleavage [24] and CYP11B1 [25]. In fact, there are numerous examples of chemicals affecting the expression of every enzyme in the steroidogenic pathway, selected examples of which are presented in Table 12.1. Clearly, when

TABLE 12.1   Examples of Chemicals Inducing Adrenocortical Toxicity and Targets in The Steroidogenic Pathway

Target	Compound	Reference(s)
ACTH receptor	Aminoglutethimide	[23]
StAR protein	Econazole, miconazole, lindane	[26–28]
	Bromocriptine	[29]
	Spironolactone	[30]
CYP11A1 (CYPscc)	Aminoglutethimide	[25,31]
	Bromocripitine	[29]
CYP17	Spironolactone	[32]
	PCB126	[33]
	Penta, octa, deca-brominated diphenyl ethers, tetrabromobisphenol-A	[34]
	Ketoconazole	[25]
3-Hydroxysteroid dehydrogenase Δ -4,5 Isomerase	Cyanoketone	[35]
	Trilostane	[36]
	PCBs (101, 110, 126, 149)	[37]
	PAHs/PCBs	[38]
	Bromophenols, polybrominated biphenyls, 2,3,7,8-tetrabromodibenzo-p-dioxin, 2,3,7,8-terabromodibenzofuran	[39]
	Pioglitazone	[40]
17β-Hydroxysteroid dehydrogenase	PCBs (101, 110, 126, 149)	[37]
CYP21	RU486	[41]
	Ketoconazole	[25]
	Flavonoids	[42]
	PCB126	[33]
	PAHs/PCBs	[38]
CYP11B1 (CYP11β/18)	Metyrapone	[25,43]
	Mitotane (o,p-DDD); MeSO$_2$-DDE	[25,44,45]
	Etomidate	[6,7]
	Ketoconazole; aminoglutethimide	[25]
	Flavonoids	[42]
	PCB126	[33]
	PCBs (101, 110, 126, 149)	[37]
	Efonidipine, mibefradil	[46]

(Continued)

3. CONCERNS FOR HUMAN HEALTH

TABLE 12.1   (Continued)

Target	Compound	Reference(s)
CYP19 (aromatase)	Prochloraz, imazalil	[47]
	Triazines—atrazine, simazine, propazine	[48]
	Dibutyl, tributyl, and phenyltin chlorides	[49]
	Fadrozole	[50]
	PCBs (101, 110, 126, 149)	[37]
	Amoxicillin	[51]
CYP11B2 (aldosterone synthase)	PCB126	[33]
	Fadrozole	[50]
	PCBs (101, 110, 126, 149)	[37]
	Efonidipine, mibefradil	[46]
	PAHs/PCBs	[38]
	Amoxicillin, erythromycin	[51]

Adapted from Harvey et al. [9] with permission from John Wiley & Sons.

investigated in specific test systems such as the H295R cell line, or in vivo, there is ample evidence that adrenal steroidogenesis is a common and major target for endocrine disruption.

The H295R cell line represents the best available in vitro tool to study the effects of chemicals on adrenocortical function. The derivation and properties of this cell line have been fully described elsewhere (see Refs. [21,22]), but it is worth briefly providing an overview here. The H295R cell line is derived from a human adrenocortical tumor that is considered to have originated on the border between the zona glomerulosa and zona fasciculata. Consequently, it is able to synthesize and secrete both cortisol and aldosterone. Indeed, it has full steroidogenic capability and has very similar properties, expression profiles, and steroidogenic secretion profiles to normal human adrenocortical tissue [28]. It does have a lower concentration of ACTH receptors [22], and usually forskolin is used to stimulate cortisol production (this activates the cAMP signal transduction pathway in a similar manner to the downstream actions of ACTH). Angiotensin II is used to challenge the cell line for aldosterone secretion. Typical protocols involve incubating the cells with a range of concentrations of a test compound; challenging with forskolin, angiotensin II, or both; and examining the response by measuring secreted steroids or the expression of various steroidogenic enzymes. The retention of universal steroidogenic enzyme expression, and in turn steroidogenic capability, gives this cell line the distinct advantage over any rodent cell lines because they lack full steroidogenic capability (e.g., Y1 cells, discussed in Ref. [22]). In addition, the cell line has been used in cell and molecular endocrinology studies for the past two decades, only more recently being utilized in toxicology endocrine disrupter research, and thus it is extremely well characterized. To this end, the U.S. Environmental Protection Agency (EPA) has added the use of this cell line to its in vitro endocrine disruption panel to investigate effects on steroidogenesis. Unfortunately, the assay in this context is forced to produce, and is only validated for, sex steroid production, so an opportunity was missed for the evaluation of adrenocortical specific steroidogenesis, namely aldosterone or cortisol production, which are far more important to health.

12.3 TOXICOLOGY STRATEGY FOR EXAMINING ADRENOCORTICAL FUNCTIONAL DISRUPTION

A strategy for the investigation of adrenocortical endocrine disruption has been suggested by Harvey et al. [8–10,15,52] and involves both the use of in vivo and in vitro studies depending on what is required. Central to the strategy is providing empirical evidence of adequate (if not entirely normal) adrenocortical competence; that is, that the adrenal is capable of steroidogenic functionality under the influence of a chemical. It was suggested that the use of the H295R cell line, as the most reliable currently available in vitro model, forms one arm of this strategy. As an in vitro system, it lends itself to high-throughput screening; and as a human-derived cell line with high functional concordance with normal human cells [28], it also lends itself to extrapolation for relevant hazard assessment and risk analysis. Certainly for drug candidates, detailed information on pharmacokinetics and drug concentrations exist in the preclinical and clinical packages upon which to base relevant dose concentrations for risk comparisons.

The second arm of the strategy comprises endocrinology assessments in vivo, and several options exist (see Refs. [9,15]). The first is to take blood samples under controlled conditions from the animal model, treated with a range of dose levels of the drug or chemical, and measure the key adrenal products of interest (e.g., corticosterone or cortisol). There can be substantial variability in these parameters across the common laboratory species, and obtaining good-quality blood samples rapidly to avoid the influence of stress can be problematic. However, in most circumstances, stress should not be considered a serious confounding factor since the primary aim of the study is to prove that the adrenal can produce adequate steroid even if this is stress-provoked—i.e., impaired adrenals from animals treated with an adrenocortical inhibitor will probably still be deficient compared with stressed control comparators. A more controlled study to evaluate adrenocortical competency is to conduct an ACTH challenge study that removes the variability of stress influences on the HPA axis. This is a common test in human and veterinary medicine; a standard dose of ACTH (Synacthen challenge) is administered to subjects also receiving the test compound, and a blood sample is taken some time later and resultant glucocorticoid concentrations measured. Results are compared with a concurrent control or with data previously obtained from the same subjects not receiving the test drug or chemical.

Of course, the main advantage of performing in vivo endocrinology assessments is that the function of the entire HPA axis can be assessed. For example, a recent study on perflurooctane sulfonate [53] showed that oral administration reduced corticosterone secretion in male rats. However, it was also shown that ACTH and CRH secretion was inhibited, indicating that the hypothalamo-pituitary control of the adrenal was also suppressed (a finding that would be missed if only H295R cells were used). Further, relative expressions of ACTH receptors and proopiomelanocortin genes were increased in adrenal and pituitary glands, respectively (which was probably a secondary adaptive/compensatory response to the inhibition of hormone production throughout the HPA axis). This illustrates the functional dependence of the adrenal cortex on the hypothalamus and pituitary in a toxicological context and the importance of studying the entire endocrine axis. Another point is that change in the adrenal can be mediated by general toxicity, whereby a drug or chemical may not directly affect the hypothalamus, pituitary, or adrenal, but does so indirectly by general toxicity, extra endocrine targets (e.g., liver, CBG, or peripheral enzymes such as HSD11B2), or activation of the stress response, which can only be evaluated in vivo.

In toxicology studies, distinguishing direct adrenocortical toxicity from indirect, stress-related changes in the adrenal is crucial, and Harvey and Sutcliffe [15] have described the evidence and distinguishing features of both mechanisms. This is particularly important as stress (e.g., [54]), ACTH administration (e.g., [55]), and chemical inhibition of adrenocortical steroidogenesis (e.g., [56]) all produce adrenocortical hypertrophy, which is histopathologically indistinguishable microscopically. This is because they all commonly result in elevated ACTH, and the trophic action of this hormone causes adrenal hypertrophy. It is the reason for the elevation of ACTH that is of critical importance to establish to distinguish the underlying mechanism and relevance. Stress is a benign adaptive and reversible response that is considered nonadverse in the toxicological sense, while adrenocortical toxicity is certainly adverse. The mechanism by which stress or adrenocortical toxicity (steroidogenesis inhibition) result in adrenal hypertrophy is illustrated in Figure 12.5, and the use of the in vitro

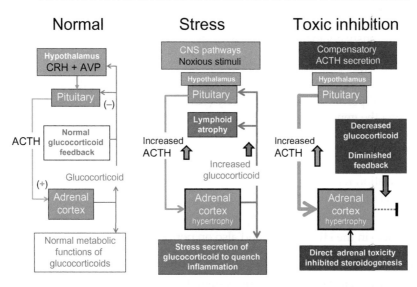

FIGURE 12.5 Adrenocortical hypertrophy: comparison of stress and adrenocortical toxicity. Adrenocortical hypertrophy is invariably caused by excess ACTH stimulation. In stress, ACTH secretion is provoked by noxious stimuli transduced through the CNS. In toxic inhibition, a drug or chemical blocks steroidogenesis and glucocorticoid synthesis/secretion and the loss of negative feedback inhibition to both hypothalamus and pituitary results in ACTH secretion. *Source: Adapted from Harvey and Sutcliffe [15] with permission from John Wiley & Sons.*

and in vivo studies described previously are required to establish the actual mechanism of adrenocortical effects. A detailed review of interpreting the stress response in routine toxicology studies illustrates the diverse effects of stress on a number of parameters [54], and these should be used to build the case for either mechanism [15].

It is worth noting that adrenal atrophy (manifesting as reduced size or weight of the adrenal and/or reduction in the width of the cortical zones, typically the zona fasciculata) is also an adverse effect indicating loss of function of the adrenal cortex. As excess ACTH causes adrenal hypertrophy, ACTH deficiency results in adrenal atrophy. The deficiency in ACTH may be due to an effect of the drug or chemical at the pituitary or at the hypothalamus (inhibiting CRH), and perflurooctane sulfonate is reported to affect both [53]. The net result of loss of stimulation of the adrenal cortex by ACTH is loss of glucocorticoid secretion and adrenal insufficiency results.

12.4 FACTORS PREDISPOSING THE ADRENAL CORTEX TO TOXICITY

The adrenal gland is the most commonly affected endocrine organ in toxicology studies [12]. In terms of the expression of toxicity, the adrenal gland is particularly predisposed to insult because of a number of physiological and anatomical features (see Refs. [11,57]). These are listed here:

Features affecting toxicant exposure

- Lipophilicity due to rich cholesterol and steroid content favoring the local deposition of lipophilic compounds
- High vascularity; disproportionately large blood volume received per unit mass of adrenal tissue, ensuring exposures to toxicants

Features mediating toxicity

- High content of unsaturated fatty acids in adrenocortical cell membranes susceptible to damage by lipid peroxidation both directly (via parent compound or its metabolites) and indirectly (via the generation of reactive species such as free radicals due to high content of enzymes, as discussed next)
- High content of cytochrome P450 (CYP) enzymes present in the adrenal cortex, which can produce reactive metabolites of parent compound toxicants, which then mediate toxicity; and hydroxylation reactions, which may generate free radicals, which in turn damage adrenocortical cells and membrane

In addition, as previously mentioned, the adrenal cortex depends on upstream endocrine function elsewhere in the HPA system and also on peripheral functional mediators as follows:

General endocrine, nonendocrine factors, and collective number of potential targets

- Functional dependence on the nervous system, hypothalamus, and pituitary
- Functional dependence on peripheral hormone carrier molecules (e.g., CBG) and peripheral enzymes (e.g., the conversion of cortisol to relatively inactive cortisone in tissues)
- Influenced by hepatic metabolism of steroids (drugs such as phenytoin, barbiturates, and rifampin accelerate cortisol metabolism)

- Overall, there are a large number of potential toxicological targets such as enzymes (both within the adrenal and systemically), receptors, and biochemical functional mediators (e.g., adrenomedullin) increasing the probability of functional insult; glucocorticoid and mineralocorticoid production are at the end of pathways of sequentially dependent steroidogenic synthesis steps and are vulnerable to upstream toxicity [e.g., from the inhibition of any of the steroidogenic enzymes or StAR, or indeed trophic hormone (ACTH or angiotensin II) receptors]

12.5 EVIDENCE OF ENVIRONMENTALLY MEDIATED ADRENAL ENDOCRINE DISRUPTION: RELEVANCE TO HUMAN HEALTH

As with other endocrine disruption modalities, environmental species can act as sentinels and provide evidence of toxicity. There are reports that fish and other aquatic species are showing evidence of the impairment of adrenal function as a result of chemical exposures (reviewed in Ref. [58]). Aquatic species, especially fish, are considered particularly sensitive because of their constant exposure to pollutant compounds in water (especially for constant absorption via gills), as well as the effect of food chain accumulation. Of particular concern is the recent report of adrenal impairment in dolphins attributed to the Deepwater Horizon oil spill in 2010 [59]. Birds are also reported to experience effects on adrenal function [60], and a recent study has correlated reduced adrenal competency in Arctic black-legged kittiwakes with tissue concentrations of organic pollutants such as polychlorinated biphenyls (PCBs) and selected pesticides [61]. In considering many of the chemicals in Table 12.1, these are recognized to be pervasive pollutants, and there is a large body of literature reporting the detection of such chemicals in human tissues. Diesel exhaust fumes are reported to impair adrenocortical function in mice following inhalational exposure to filtered atmospheres [62], and nitrophenols isolated from diesel have been shown to suppress cortisol secretion in H295R cells in vitro [63] together, indicating that ubiquitous products of industrialization, to which all but the most isolated human communities are exposed, have the potential to induce adrenocortical functional disruption.

It is unlikely that ambient exposures to a single compound present in the environment at typical low levels would have a significant impact on human adrenal function. But the human population is not exposed to a single compound at any given time, and the effects of low-level exposures to a multitude of chemicals, with potentially cumulative actions and different targets in the steroidogenic pathway combining to influence end products such as cortisol or aldosterone, should be considered. It has previously been discussed that a reason that the adrenal is vulnerable to toxic insult is the relatively large number of targets in the steroidogenic pathway (such as receptors, transporter proteins, and enzymes); and as each of these targets has been shown to be affected by different chemicals (see Table 12.1), the plausibility of the risk of combined action at different sites in the steroidogenic pathway can be visualized. Just as no single culprit chemical has been categorically confirmed in the debate about declining semen quality, an overview "bigger picture" position must be considered that environmental chemical residues may be having an occult detrimental effect on human adrenocortical function. As with all areas of endocrine disruption research, evidence is lacking of human health effects because the epidemiological and biological research has not been conducted: however, *absence of evidence is not evidence of absence*. Chemical exposure is recognized as a potential factor in human adrenal insufficiency [64] in the medical literature. The fact that the major mechanism of human adrenal insufficiency is currently autoimmune disease (e.g., [1,2,64]) does not detract from chemical involvement indirectly (i.e., contributing to autoimmune responses). A further consideration is the potential contribution of chemical insults on adrenals that already have been functionally compromised through disease or other reasons for reduced capacity: there may be vulnerable subpopulations of individuals susceptible to adrenal functional disruption that would otherwise not experience harmful effects. There is a clear case to address the gap in evaluation of adrenal function testing in regulatory endocrine disruption strategy [65]. Finally, there is evidence that the incidence of adrenal insufficiency (frank clinical autoimmune Addison's disease) is increasing [66], and the immediate questions to be addressed by further research are, what are the underlying factors in this finding, and is there a hidden subclinical effect on human adrenocortical function mediated by environmental endocrine-disrupting chemicals.

References

[1] Holt RIG, Hanley NA. An overview of human adrenal dysfunction. In: Harvey PW, Everett DJ, Springall CJ, editors. Adrenal toxicology. New York, NY: Informa Healthcare; 2009. p. 39–75.
[2] Ten S, New M, Maclaren N. Clinical review 130. Addison's disease 2001. J Clin Endocrinol Metab 2001; 86:2909–22.
[3] Vermeulen A, Paridaens R, Heuson JC. Effects of aminoglutethimide on adrenal steroid secretion. Clin Endocrinol 1983;19:673–82.
[4] Wagner RL, White PF, Kan PB, et al. Inhibition of adrenal steroidogenesis by the anaesthetic etomidate. N Engl J Med 1984;310:1415–21.
[5] Lundy JB, Slane ML, Frizzi JD. Acute adrenal insufficiency after a single dose of etomidate. J Intensive Care Med 2007;22:111–7.
[6] Leddingham IM, Watt I. Influence of sedation on mortality in multiple trauma patients. Lancet 1983;1:1270.
[7] Raven PW, Hinson JP. Transport, actions and metabolism of adrenal hormones and pathology and pharmacology of the adrenal gland. In: Harvey PW, editor. The adrenal in toxicology: target organ and modulator of toxicity. London: Taylor & Francis; 1996. pp. 53–79.
[8] Harvey PW, Everett D. The adrenal cortex and steroidogenesis as cellular and molecular targets for toxicity: critical omissions from regulatory endocrine disrupter screening strategies for human health. J Appl Toxicol 2003;23:81–7.
[9] Harvey PW, Everett DJ, Springall CJ. Adrenal toxicology: a strategy for assessment of functional toxicity to the adrenal cortex and steroidogenesis. J Appl Toxicol 2007;27:103–15.
[10] Harvey PW, Everett DJ, Springall CJ. Adrenal toxicology: molecular targets, endocrine mechanisms, hormonal interactions, assessment models and species differences in toxicity. In: Harvey PW, Everett DJ, Springall CJ, editors. Adrenal toxicology. New York, NY: Informa Healthcare; 2009. pp. 3–35.
[11] Harvey PW. Toxic responses of the adrenal cortex. In: McQueen CA, editor. Comprehensive toxicology, vol. 11. Oxford: Academic Press; 2010. pp. 265–89.
[12] Ribelin WE. The effects of drugs and chemicals upon the structure of the adrenal gland. Fund Appl Toxicol 1984;4:105–19.
[13] Elmore SA, Nyska A, Tischler AS. The adrenal medulla as a target organ in toxicologic studies of rats and mice. In: Harvey PW, Everett DJ, Springall CJ, editors. Adrenal toxicology. New York, NY: Informa Healthcare; 2009. pp. 111–38.
[14] Rosol TJ, DeLellis RA, Harvey PW, Sutcliffe C. Endocrine system. In: Haschek WM, Rousseaux CG, Wallig MA, editors. Haschek and Rousseaux's handbook of toxicologic pathology. Elsevier Inc., Academic Press, New York, NY; 2013. pp. 2391–492.
[15] Harvey PW, Sutcliffe C. Adrenocortical hypertrophy: establishing cause and toxicological significance. J Appl Toxicol 2010;30:617–26.

[16] Buckingham JC. The hypothalamo–pituitary–adrenocortical axis: endocrinology, pharmacology, pathophysiology and developmental effects. In: Harvey PW, Everett DJ, Springall CJ, editors. Adrenal toxicology. New York, NY: Informa Healthcare; 2009. pp. 77–107.

[17] Gumbleton M, Nicholls PJ. Molecular and systems pharmacology of glucocorticosteroids. In: Harvey PW, editor. The adrenal in toxicology: target organ and modulator of toxicity. London: Taylor & Francis; 1996. pp. 81–128.

[18] Baldwin JA. Glucocorticosteroids, stress and developmental toxicology. In: Harvey PW, editor. The adrenal in toxicology: target organ and modulator of toxicity. London: Taylor & Francis; 1996. pp. 223–42.

[19] Kimber I. Glucocorticosteroids and immunotoxicity. In: Harvey PW, editor. The adrenal in toxicology: target organ and modulator of toxicity. London: Taylor & Francis; 1996. pp. 243–57.

[20] Kaspareit J. Adrenal gland background pathology of primates in toxicological studies. In: Harvey PW, Everett DJ, Springall CJ, editors. Adrenal toxicology. New York, NY: Informa Healthcare; 2009. pp. 139–59.

[21] Sanderson T. Adrenocortical toxicology *in vitro*: assessment of steroidogenic enzyme expression and steroid production in H295R cells. In: Harvey PW, Everett DJ, Springall CJ, editors. Adrenal toxicology. New York, NY: Informa Healthcare; 2009. pp. 175–82.

[22] Parmar J, Rainey W. Comparisons of adrenocortical cell lines as *in vitro* test systems. In: Harvey PW, Everett DJ, Springall CJ, editors. Adrenal toxicology. New York, NY: Informa Healthcare; 2009. pp. 183–204.

[23] Fassnacht M, Beuschlein F, Vay S, et al. Aminoglutethimide suppresses adrenocorticotrophin receptor expression in the NCI-h295 adrenocortical tumor cell line. J Endocrinol 1998;159:35–42.

[24] Camacho AM, Cash R, Brough AJ, Wilroy RS. Inhibition of adrenal steroidogenesis by aminoglutethimide and the mechanism of action. J Am Chem Soc 1967;202:114–20.

[25] Johansson MK, Sanderson JT, Lund BO. Effects of 3-MeSO$_2$-DDE and some CYP inhibitors on glucocorticoid steroidogenesis in the H295R human adrenocortical carcinoma cell line. Toxicol In Vitro 2002;16:113–21.

[26] Walsh LP, Kuratko CN, Stocco DM. Econazole and miconazole inhibit steroidogenesis and disrupt steroidogenic acute regulatory (StAR) protein expression post-transcriptionally. J Steroid Biochem Mol Biol 2000;75:229–36.

[27] Walsh LP, Stocco DM. Effects of lindane on steroidogenesis and steroidogenic acute regulatory protein expression. Biol Reprod 2000;63:1024–33.

[28] Oskarsson A, Ulleras E, Plant KE, Hinson JP, Goldfarb PS. Steroidogenic gene expression in H295R cells and the human adrenal gland: adrenotoxic effects of lindane *in vitro*. J Appl Toxicol 2006;26:484–92.

[29] Kan SF, Kau MM, Low-Tone Ho L, Wang PS. Inhibitory effects of bromocriptine on corticosterone secretion in male rats. Eur J Pharmacol 2003;468:141–9.

[30] Hilscherova K, Jones PD, Gracia T, Newsted JL, Zhang X, Sanderson JT, et al. Assessment of the effects of chemicals on the expression of ten steroidogenic genes in theH295R cell line using real-time PCR. Toxicol Sci 2004;81:78–89.

[31] Hecker M, Newsted JL, Murphy MB, Higley EB, Jones PD, Wu R, et al. Human adrenocarcinoma (H295R) cells for rapid *in vitro* determination of effects on steroidogenesis: hormone production. Toxicol Appl Pharmacol 2006;217:114–24.

[32] Kossor DC, Kominami S, Takemori S, Colby HD. Role of the steroid 17 a-hydroxylase in spironolactone-mediated destruction of adrenal cytochrome P-450. Mol Pharmacol 1991;40:321–5.

[33] Li LA, Wang PW. PCB126 induces differential changes in androgen, cortisol and aldosterone biosynthesis in human adrenocortical H295R cells. Toxicol Sci 2005;85:530–40.

[34] Canton RF, Sanderson JT, Nijmeijer S, Bergman A, Letcher RJ, van den Berg M. *In vitro* effects of brominated flame retardants and metabolites on CYP17 catalytic activity: a novel mechanism of action. Toxicol Appl Pharmacol 2006;216:274–81.

[35] McCarthy JL, Reitz CW, Wesson LK. Inhibition of adrenal corticosteroidogenesis in the rat by cyanotrimethylandrostenolone, a synthetic androstane. Endocrinology 1966;79:1123–39.

[36] Potts GO, Creange JE, Harding HR, Schane HP. Trilostane, an orally active inhibitor of steroid biosynthesis. Steroids 1978;32:257–67.

[37] Xu Y, Yu RM, Zhang X, Murphy MB, Giesy JP, Lam MH, et al. Effects of PCBs and MeSO$_2$-PCBs on adrenocortical steroidogenesis in H295R human adrenocortical carcinoma cells. Chemosphere 2006;63:772–84.

[38] Blaha L, Hilscherova K, Mazurova E, Hecker M, Jones PD, Newsted JL, et al. Alteration of steroidogenesis in H295R cells by organic sediment contaminants and relationships to other endocrine disrupting effects. Environ Int 2006;32:749–57.

3. CONCERNS FOR HUMAN HEALTH

[39] Ding L, Murphy MB, He Y, Xu Y, Yeung LWY, Wang J, et al. Effects of brominated flame retardants and brominated dioxins on steroidogenesis in H295R human adrenocortical carcinoma cell line. Environ Toxicol Chem 2007;26:764–72.

[40] Kempna P, Hofer G, Mullis PE, Fluck CE. Pioglitazone inhibits androgen production in NCIH295R cells by regulating gene expression of CYP17 and HSD3 B2. Mol Pharmacol 2007;71:787–98.

[41] Albertson BD, Hill RB, Sprague KA, Wood KE, Nieman LK, Loriaux DL. Effects of the antiglucocorticoid RU486 on adrenal steroidogenic enzyme activity and steroidogenesis. Eur J Endocrinol 1994;130:195–200.

[42] Ohno S, Shinoda S, Toyoshima S, Nakazawa H, Makino T, Nakajin S. Effects of flavonoid phytochemicals on cortisol production and on activities of steroidogenic enzymes in human adrenocortical H295R cells. J Steroid Biochem Mol Biol 2002;80:355–63.

[43] Liddle GW, Island DP, Lance EM, Harris AP. Alterations in adrenal steroid patterns in man resulting from treatment with a chemical inhibitor of 11-hydroxylase. J Clin Endocrinol 1958;18:906–12.

[44] Hornsby PJ. Steroid and xenobiotic effects on the adrenal cortex: mediation by oxidation and other mechanisms. Free Radical Biol Med 1989;6:103–15.

[45] Lindhe O, Skoseid B, Brandt I. Cytochrome P450-catalysed binding of 3-methylsulfonyl-DDE and o,p-DDD in human adrenal zona fasciculata/reticularis. J Clin Endocrinol Metab 2002;87:1319–26.

[46] Imagawa K, Okayama S, Takaoka M, Kawata H, Naya N, Nakajima T, et al. Inhibitory effect of efonidipine on aldosterone synthesis and secretion in human adrenocarcinoma (H295R) cells. J Cardiovasc Pharmacol 2006;47:133–8.

[47] Andersen HR, Vingaard AM, Rasmusse TH, Gjerdmansen IM, Bonefeld-Jorgensen EC. Effects of currently used pesticides in assays for estrogenicity and aromatase activity in vitro. Toxicol Appl Pharmacol 2000;179:1–12.

[48] Sanderson JT, Letcher RJ, Heneweer M, Giesy JP, van den Berg M. Effects of chloro-s-triazine herbicides and metabolites on aromatase activity in various human cell lines and on vitellogenin production in male carp hepatocytes. Environ Health Perspect 2001;109:1027–31.

[49] Sanderson JT, Boerma J, Lansbergen GW, van den Berg M. Induction and inhibition of aromatase (CYP19) activity by various classes of pesticides in H295R human adrenocortical carcinoma cells. Toxicol Appl Pharmacol 2002;82:44–54.

[50] Muller-Vieira U, Angotti M, Hartman RW. The adrenocortical tumor cell line NCI-H295R as an in vitro screening system for the evaluation of CYP11 B2 (aldosterone synthase) and CYP11B1 (steroid-11beta-hydroxylase) inhibitors. J Steroid Biochem Mol Biol 2005;96:259–70.

[51] Gracia T, Hilscherova K, Jones PD, Newsted JL, Zhang X, Hecker M, et al. Modulation of steroidogenic gene expression and hormone production of H295R cells by pharmaceuticals and other environmentally active compounds. Toxicol Appl Pharmacol 2007;225:142–53.

[52] Harvey PW, Johnson I. Approaches to the assessment of toxicity data with endpoints related to endocrine disruption. J Appl Toxicol 2002;22:241–7.

[53] Pereiro N, Moyano R, Blanco A, Lafuente A. Regulation of corticosterone secretion is modified by PFOS exposure at different levels of the hypothalamic–pituitary–adrenal axis in adult male rats. Toxicol Lett 2014;230: 252–62. doi: 10.1016/j.toxlet.2014.01.003.

[54] Everds NE, Snyder PW, Bailey KL, Bolon B, Creasy DM, Foley GL, et al. Interpreting stress responses during routine toxicity studies a review of the biology, impact, and assessment. Toxicol Pathol 2013;41:560–614.

[55] Pudney J, Price GM, Whitehouse BJ, Vinson GP. Effects of chronic ACTH stimulation on the morphology of the rat adrenal cortex. Anat Rec 1984;210:603–15.

[56] Akana SF, Shinsako J, Dallman MF. Drug-induced adrenal hypertrophy provides evidence for reset in the adrenocortical system. Endocrinology 1983;113:2232–7.

[57] Hinson JP, Raven PW. Effects of endocrine-disrupting chemicals on adrenal function. Best Pract Res Clin Endocrinol Metab 2006;20:111–20.

[58] Hontela A, Vijayan MM. Adrenocortical toxicology in fishes. In: Harvey PW, Everett DJ, Springall CJ, editors. Adrenal toxicology. New York, NY: Informa Healthcare; 2009. pp. 233–56.

[59] Schwake LH, Smith CR, Townsend FI, et al. Health of common Bottlenose Dolphins (Tursiops truncatus) in Barataria Bay, Louisiana, following the Deepwater Horizon oil spill. Environ Sci Technol 2014;48:93–103.

[60] Baos R, Blas J. Adrenal toxicology in birds: environmental contaminants and the avian response to stress. In: Harvey PW, Everett DJ, Springall CJ, editors. Adrenal toxicology. New York, NY: Informa Healthcare; 2009. pp. 257–93.

3. CONCERNS FOR HUMAN HEALTH

[61] Tartu S, Angelier F, Herzke D, Moe B, Bech C, Gabrielsen GW, et al. The stress of being contaminated? Adrenocortical function and reproduction in relation to persistent organic pollutants in female black legged kittiwakes. Sci Total Environ 2014;476–477:553–60.

[62] Li CM, Li X, Suzuki AK, Fujitani Y, Jigami J, Nagaoka K, et al. Effects of exposure to nanoparticle-rich diesel exhaust on adrenocortical function in adult male mice. Toxicol Lett 2012;209:277–81.

[63] Furuta C, Noda S, Li CM, Suzuki AK, Taneda S, Watanabe G, et al. Nitrophenols isolated from diesel exhaust particles regulate steroidogenic gene expression and steroid synthesis in the human H295R adrenocortical cell line. Toxicol Appl Pharmacol 2008;229:109–20.

[64] Bornstein SR. Predisposing factors for adrenal insufficiency. N Engl J Med 2009;360:2328–39.

[65] Harvey PW, Everett DJ. Regulation of endocrine-disrupting chemicals: critical overview and deficiencies in toxicology and risk assessment for human health. Best Pract Res Clin Endocrinol Metab 2006;20:145–65.

[66] Løvås K, Husebye ES. High prevalence and increasing incidence of Addison's disease in western Norway. Clin Endocrinol 2002;56:787–91.

Endocrine Disruption of Developmental Pathways and Children's Health

Monica K. Silver and John D. Meeker

Abstract

Widespread human exposure to known or suspected endocrine-disrupting chemicals (EDCs) has been documented worldwide, while rates of endocrine-related diseases and disorders among children are increasing. This chapter provides an overview of the current state of the epidemiological evidence for the adverse impacts of common persistent and nonpersistent EDCs on child development. The selected health end points discussed here include fetal growth, early reproductive tract development, pubertal development, obesity, and neurodevelopment. Despite their limitations, the studies mentioned here add to a growing body of evidence that exposure to chemicals commonly found in consumer goods, personal care products, food, drinking water, and other sources may adversely affect child development through altered endocrine function in a variety of pathways. Given the range of these potential serious developmental effects, efforts to reduce EDC exposure as a precaution among pregnant women and children are warranted.

13.1 OVERVIEW

Exposure to exogenous chemicals can affect endocrine function at multiple sites and through numerous specific modes of action, which may have far-reaching impacts on human health and development. Widespread human exposure to known or suspected endocrine-disrupting chemicals (EDCs) has been documented in the United States and worldwide, as have trends for increased rates of endocrine-related diseases and disorders among children. While human epidemiology studies of exposure to EDCs and children's health remain limited, there is a growing body of evidence showing that exposure to a number of chemicals commonly found in consumer goods, personal care products, food, drinking water, and other sources may adversely affect child development through altered endocrine function. This chapter provides an overview of the state of the evidence for the adverse impacts of some of the most common persistent and nonpersistent EDCs on child development, focusing specifically on fetal growth, early reproductive tract development, pubertal development, obesity, and neurodevelopment as the health end points of interest. Contemporary review and primary research articles are referenced here, and the interested reader is directed toward those for additional details.

13.1.1 General Concerns for Health Effects of EDCs

EDCs can affect the endocrine system through a multitude of specific mechanisms that can target different levels of the hypothalamic-pituitary-gonad/thyroid/adrenal axes, ranging from effects on hormone receptors to effects on hormone synthesis, secretion, or metabolism; therefore, they can have far-reaching health implications throughout the life course [1,2]. Transgenerational effects are also possible, as is now being observed in the offspring of women who had been exposed to diethylstilbestrol (DES) in utero decades ago [3]. The realization that exposure to many environmental EDCs is now ubiquitous, coupled with proven or suggested trends for increased rates of certain endocrine-related diseases and disorders among children, has resulted in growing concern regarding potential links between the two among scientists, governments, physicians, and patients. Several scientific bodies, including the Endocrine Society of the United States, now support the idea that EDCs can affect human health [1,2]. However, human studies investigating possible adverse health effects of EDCs, especially among children, are limited for many EDCs.

13.1.2 Specific Concerns for Infants and Children

There is widespread exposure to EDCs among men, women, and children throughout the world. Exposure can occur via multiple routes, including the diet, drinking water, air, soil and house dust, or through direct contact with various household materials or consumer products. High exposures and increased susceptibility in children are likely for a number of reasons (Table 13.1). First, children have unique behavior and activity patterns that may contribute to increased exposures. Children are more likely to have contact with potentially contaminated soil and dust because they tend to spend large amounts of time sitting, crawling, and playing either on or close to the ground. In addition, they often put their hands, toys, and other items into their mouths. The toys may contain contaminated dust or be shedding EDCs. Children also have differences in their physiology and metabolism that will

TABLE 13.1   Factors, Unique to Children, That Contribute to Increased Exposure and Susceptibility to EDCs

Increased exposure	Increased susceptibility
Sit, crawl, and play on the ground	Blood–brain barrier not fully developed
Put hands, toys, and other items into their mouths	Undergoing periods of rapid growth
Eat, drink, and breathe more, relative to their body weight, than adults	Inefficient liver and kidneys
EDCs can accumulate in breast milk	Lack of metabolizing/detoxifying enzymes
EDCs can pass through the placenta	Permeable skin

likely increase their susceptibility to EDCs. Children eat, drink, and breathe more, relative to their body weight, than adults do. They also have fewer metabolizing enzymes that are capable of breaking down toxicants into less toxic forms, and a less efficient liver and kidneys. Their blood-brain barrier is still developing and their skin is more permeable, thereby increasing their risk for exposure. Finally, the timing of exposure to EDCs may be critical in determining the severity of the effects. Children are rapidly developing, especially during the fetal period, the first several years of life, and puberty. EDC exposure, even in small doses, that occurs during one of these highly sensitive periods of rapid growth may have the potential to lead to long-term health effects [4]. Fetal and infant exposures are particularly worrisome since many EDCs have the ability to pass through the placenta and accumulate in breast milk, thereby passing from mother to infant. Recent concerns have also arisen surrounding the high levels of EDCs in hospital tubing and other medical equipment. Premature infants who are placed in the neonatal intensive care unit have been shown to have elevated levels of phthalates [5] and BPA [6].

Childhood or prenatal exposure to EDCs can lead to perturbations in a number of important developmental end points. EDC exposures occurring during these critical periods of growth have been found to be associated with reduced fetal growth and length of gestation, altered male reproductive tract development, shifts in age of onset of puberty, increases in obesity, and deficits in neurodevelopment and neurological function. While most of the early work surrounding children's health and EDC exposure was focused on persistent organic pollutants (POPs), more recently researchers have also begun to examine the health effects of some highly ubiquitous, nonpersistent chemicals.

13.1.3 Persistent Organic Pollutants

POPs are lipophilic chemicals with long half-lives that can bioaccumulate up the food chain. These include polychlorinated biphenyls (PCBs), organochlorine (OC) pesticides, such as dichlorodiphenyltrichloroethane (DDT), chlordane, hexachlorobenzene, polybrominated diphenyl ethers (PBDEs) and other brominated flame retardants, and perfluorinated compounds (PFCs), such as perfluorooctanesulphonic acid (PFOS) and perfluorooctanoic acid (PFOA), among others. Due to concerns about the effects on wildlife and the potential to harm human health, PCBs and some of the more heavily used OC pesticides were banned in many nations in the 1970s. More recently, a number of PBDEs have also been banned or phased out of use. Due to their environmental ubiquity and persistence, human exposure to POPs can continue for decades after their use ceases.

POPs have been associated with a wide range of adverse health effects in studies of adults, including male and female reproductive problems, thyroid effects, obesity, diabetes, and endocrine-related cancers [7–9].

13.1.4 Nonpersistent Chemicals

The nonpersistent EDCs of concern include high- and low-molecular-weight phthalates, bisphenol A (BPA), and contemporary-use pesticides. These chemicals all have relatively short half-lives and had largely been thought to be safer because of it, though recent research has shed doubt on this assumption. Exposure to phthalates and BPA is nearly ubiquitous due to their widespread use in industry and their presence in a wide range of products. Urinary metabolites of these chemicals have been detected in virtually everyone [10]. Most pesticides in use today are nonpersistent and designed to break down quickly. However, it has been shown that even nonpersistent pesticides can remain for years after application in homes and other indoor environments where they are protected from moisture, sunlight, and other degradation mechanisms.

Studies have revealed a wide range of health effects as a result of exposure to these nonpersistent EDCs. Some phthalates are antiandrogenic, and these substances have demonstrated significant adverse impacts on male reproductive development and numerous other end points in rodents at high doses [11]. In studies of adult humans, phthalates have been related to decreases in sex steroid and thyroid hormone levels, poor sperm quality, endometriosis, insulin resistance, obesity, and possibly breast cancer [12,13]. BPA is known to be weakly estrogenic, and recent animal studies have reported a variety of developmental problems following early life exposure, such as altered reproductive organ development and neurobehavioral effects [14]. In human adults, there have also been suggestive relationships with male and female reproductive end points, altered thyroid hormones and liver function, cardiovascular disease, and diabetes [15]. Contemporary-use pesticides, particularly the insecticides [organophosphates (OPs), carbamates, and pyrethroids], are neurotoxic, especially in high doses, and many are also known or suspected EDCs, though studies of potential endocrine effects are still lacking.

13.1.5 Other Chemicals of Concern

There are many other types of known or suspected EDCs for which widespread human exposure has been documented. There is a large body of evidence showing that a number of heavy metals, such as lead, cadmium, and mercury, may affect endocrine function in addition to their other modes of toxicity. There is also a growing list of newly emerging EDCs of concern, which include, among others, parabens, triclosan, perchlorate, and alternative brominated and chlorinated flame retardants. A handful of studies suggest that these emerging compounds may be associated with endocrine-related end points in animals and humans. However, the number of human studies that have been conducted for any one chemical or class of chemicals is sparse. Thus, the remainder of this chapter will focus on developmental end points associated with the persistent and nonpersistent EDCs introduced previously.

13.2 DEVELOPMENTAL END POINTS OF CONCERN (FIGURE 13.1)

13.2.1 Fetal Growth and Length of Gestation

Low birth weight (LBW) and preterm birth, both of which have increased significantly since 1990, are the leading causes of infant mortality and precursors of future morbidity in the United States [16]. Numerous studies have assessed relationships between a large number of chemical exposures and birth weight [17,18]; however, studies of EDCs lag behind those of air pollutants.

A number of recent studies have investigated associations between maternal exposure during pregnancy to POPs (as a proxy for fetal exposure) and birth weight or other parameters of fetal growth. The available literature provides some evidence of restricted growth as a result of prenatal PBDE exposure (LBW) [19], prenatal PCB exposure (decreased birth weight and gestational length) [20], prenatal PFOS exposure (infant weight at 20 months, LBW, head circumference being small for gestational age) [21–24], and prenatal PFOA exposure (LBW) [23,25]. However, other studies reported no association [20] and positive associations [26] between PCBs and birth weight and no association between PFCs and birth weight [27]. Meta-analyses report significant associations between prenatal PCBs [28] and prenatal PFOA [29] and birth weight.

There are also many new studies of the associations between nonpersistent EDCs and reduced fetal growth. Several studies provide evidence that prenatal BPA [30–32] or phthalates [33] may increase the risk of LBW, decreased head circumference [30], and being small for gestational age [31]. Two additional studies have reported reduced birth weights with higher maternal occupational exposure to contemporary pesticides during early pregnancy [34] and with the total number of nonpersistent pesticides detected in umbilical cord blood [35].

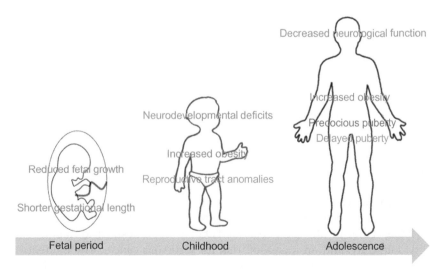

FIGURE 13.1   Child health effects observed following prenatal or childhood EDC exposures. Green signifies effects reported in both boys and girls; blue, effects reported in boys; and pink, effects reported in girls.

Comprehensive review studies have also reported evidence for a relationship between maternal exposure to POPs during pregnancy and increased risk for preterm birth, focusing mainly on PCBs and OC pesticides [17,18,36]. Two new studies provide little further insight into these relationships, with one finding that maternal levels of chlordecone (a persistent pesticide) are associated with a decreased length of gestation and an increased risk of preterm delivery [37], while another study found no association between a number of OC pesticides in maternal serum and preterm birth [38]. For PFCs, prenatal PFOS [22,39], as well as prenatal PFOA [39], have been reported to be associated with increased odds of preterm delivery in a limited number of studies, though other studies did not report significant effects [25,27].

Much of the research focus lately has turned to the role of nonpersistent chemicals, such as phthalates and BPA, on length of gestation. Higher concentrations of BPA in women in the third trimester of pregnancy were found in women who delivered preterm, compared to women who delivered at term [40,41]; BPA was also associated with an increased odds of preterm delivery in another study [31]. Studies of phthalates similarly report relationships between maternal phthalate levels during pregnancy and decreased gestation length [42,43] or preterm delivery [40]. Some very recent work has begun to take into account the heterogeneous etiologies of preterm birth, as well as the variability of phthalate exposure across pregnancy, thereby improving on previous studies that were unable to account for these factors. These authors also report significant inverse associations between maternal urinary phthalate measurements during pregnancy and the likelihood of a preterm delivery [44,45]. Despite this collection of positive findings, other studies that have reported no association, or even positive associations, between phthalates and gestation length [46,47], highlighting the need for further research in this area.

The current evidence lends some support to the hypothesis that prenatal exposure to EDCs may adversely affect birth outcomes, though caution should be used when interpreting the results of these studies. Due to variation in study designs, assessment of exposures, varying results, and the possibility of publication bias (i.e., negative or nonsignificant findings may be published less frequently than those with positive findings), it is currently difficult to conclude with any certainty whether a relationship exists between EDCs and birth weight, preterm birth, or both.

13.2.2 Male Reproductive Tract Development

Birth anomalies of the male reproductive tract, such as cryptorchidism and hypospadias, appear to be increasing in recent decades [48]. Many believe that EDCs may be playing a role in this increase. A leading hypothesis for a collection of linked conditions in human males exposed to EDCs in utero is termed *testicular dysgenesis syndrome (TDS)*. TDS represents a number of reproductive disorders of varying severity that are associated with disturbed gonadal development, including cryptorchidism, hypospadias, and smaller reproductive organs [49,50]. Later in life, the effects of TDS are hypothesized to manifest as reduced semen quality, infertility, and an increased risk for testicular cancer. The evidence for widespread endocrine disruption among males is thus further fueled by reports of significant secular declines in semen quality [51] and testosterone [52], as well as increased rates of testicular cancer [53], in men over the past 50 years or so. There is also limited evidence of reproductive tract effects in females, but these are generally not thought to manifest until later in life and will not be covered here [54,55].

Several studies have assessed relationships between POPs and male genital birth defects with inconsistent findings [18,48]. This inconsistency is still evident in more recent studies. Studies of persistent pesticides, hexachlorobenzene (HCB) and DDE, a DDT metabolite, have found that maternal serum concentrations during pregnancy are associated with hypospadias [56], and that DDE is also associated with decreased anal position index [57], but not anogenital distance (AGD) or penis size [58]. PBDEs in breast milk have been reported to be associated with risk of cryptorchidism [59], while a different study found that mean mid-maternal pregnancy serum levels of PCB, PBDE, and persistent pesticide concentrations were all higher in mothers of boys born with hypospadias, but these results were not statistically significant [60].

For the nonpersistent EDCs, maternal urinary phthalates during pregnancy have been reported to be inversely associated with AGD [61–63], penis size [62,63], hypospadias [64,65], and incomplete testicular descent in boys [62], though other studies have reported no significant associations [66]. In addition, phthalates in breast milk have been associated with decreases in serum measures of free testosterone and Leydig cell function in young boys [67]. BPA has also been reported to be associated with decreased AGD [32] and hypospadias [65]. For nonpersistent pesticides, maternal atrazine exposure during pregnancy has been shown to be moderately associated with the risk of hypospadias, cryptorchidism, and small penis size [68], while two studies, one of which was a meta-analysis, revealed an increased risk of hypospadias [69,70] and cryptorchidism [69] in boys whose parents were occupationally exposed to pesticides.

While there appears to be some evidence that EDCs may adversely affect the male reproductive tract, these results should be interpreted carefully. Due to varying study designs and exposure assessment methods, especially for nonpersistent EDCs where one measurement of exposure is likely insufficient to adequately represent early-life exposure, and mixed results, definitive conclusions cannot be drawn. Thus, there is evidence that phthalates and possibly other EDCs disrupt early male reproductive development, but additional studies are needed.

13.2.3 Pubertal Development

Recent population trends show shifts in the age of onset and progression of puberty [71,72]. These observed alterations in pubertal timing are a significant public health concern and represent an added risk factor for endocrine-related diseases in adulthood. These changes cannot be fully explained by known predictors, such as living conditions and body mass index (BMI), so exposure to EDCs has been hypothesized to be a significant contributor [73,74].

POPs have been implicated as contributors to the altered timing of pubertal onset. Most frequently, these effects are manifested as earlier menarche in girls or delayed puberty in boys, though results are not always consistent across studies [75,76]. Recently, researchers have reported later gonadarche and pubarche in boys with higher levels of serum HCB, an OC pesticide [77]; later age at puberty in boys with increasing levels of serum PFCs [78]; and earlier age at menarche for girls with higher serum PBDE levels [79]. However, there are also inconsistencies. For example, a recent study found no association between the levels of persistent pesticides in serum and adipose tissues of adolescent girls and precocious puberty [80], while other studies have reported that maternal PCBs are inversely associated with pubertal onset in boys [81], and that higher PFOS, either prenatally or concurrently, is associated with later menarche in girls [78,82].

Until recently, little has been known about the effects of nonpersistent EDCs on pubertal development, but new work has revealed insights into these relationships. Two recent studies reported significant positive associations between high-molecular-weight urinary phthalate metabolites and pubic hair development in girls [83,84]. No such associations were observed for BPA in either study, though other research has found that girls with idiopathic central precocious puberty had significantly higher urinary BPA levels [85]. Among boys, a small study reported that plasma concentrations of high-molecular-weight phthalates were significantly higher in boys with pubertal gynecomastia compared to a control group [86]. In addition, prenatal exposure to phthalates and BPA was associated with greatly reduced odds of adrenarche and slightly reduced odds of puberty in boys, while childhood phthalate exposures were not associated with either adrenarche or puberty [87]. In another recent study, exposure to some phthalates was associated with earlier age at appearance of pubic hair in boys, but no such associations were observed in girls [88].

Recent studies continue to provide some evidence in support of the hypothesis that EDCs may lead to earlier menarche in girls, delayed puberty in boys, or both, though results vary greatly across studies depending on the type of EDC and the timing of EDC exposure. These inconsistent findings across studies point to the need for additional research to elucidate the relationship and mechanisms surrounding the effects of EDC exposure and pubertal development.

13.2.4 Obesity

The prevalence of overweight and obesity is rapidly increasing in the United States and worldwide [89,90]. In addition to diet, physical activity, and genetics, environmental obesogens may play a role in these trends. Obesogens are defined as chemicals that inappropriately alter lipid homeostasis to promote adipogenesis and lipid accumulation. Experimental evidence showing that numerous chemicals may impart these effects is growing [90,91]. Recently, there have been a large number of studies investigating the relationships of EDCs with obesity, BMI, and a number of other related outcomes in young children and adolescents.

Results of studies of POPs have been largely inconsistent [90,92]. Most contemporary studies of persistent pesticides have focused on DDT and its major metabolite, DDE, yielding mixed results. One study found no association between prenatal DDT or DDE and any overweight/obesity-related outcomes in 7-year olds [93], while other studies report that prenatal exposure to DDT, DDE, and PCBs, measured in either maternal serum during pregnancy or umbilical cord serum, are significantly positively associated with BMI, waist circumference, risk of overweight, and risk of obesity (for DDT and DDE) [94] and risk of overweight (for DDT) [95]. In girls, prenatal DDE and PCBs were associated with risk of overweight [95] and increased waist circumference [96], excessive BMI, and increase in BMI over time [96,97]. On the other hand, in a cross-sectional study of adolescents, three serum PCB congeners (138, 153, 180) were actually associated with decreased BMI, but a fourth (118) was positively associated [98]. There is only one study that has looked at the relatively new emerging PFC class of chemicals and obesity, and it found no significant changes in adiposity markers with concurrent levels of PFCs in 8- to 10-year-old children [99].

More recently, the research focus has shifted to the ubiquitous, nonpersistent EDCs and their effects on childhood obesity. The plasticizer BPA has been implicated in a number of studies, with positive associations found between concurrent urinary BPA levels and BMI and risk of obesity or overweight in school-aged girls [100,101], and in both girls and boys [102–104], as well as current growth in 2- to 5-year olds [105]. Studies of prenatal exposure to BPA and obesity-related outcomes in childhood have led to more mixed results. Published studies have found that BPA is associated with increased waist circumference and BMI in 4-year-old children [106]; decreased BMI, percent body fat, and risk of overweight or obese in 9-year-old girls [100]; and no association in 5-year olds [105]. Growing evidence also suggests that childhood exposure to certain phthalates may increase the risk of obesity in children [92,107,108]. Low-molecular-weight phthalates in urine have been found to be associated with BMI and waist circumference in girls [109], obesity in boys [110], obesity in children and adolescents [111,112], and BMI in overweight children [113]. High-molecular-weight phthalates were also associated with obesity in young girls [110]. Research concerning childhood obesity and contemporary-use pesticides is still quite limited. Two studies have looked at adolescent obesity in relation to dichlorophenols, chemicals used in the production of pesticides, and found that concurrent urinary levels were positively associated with BMI, waist circumference, and risk of obesity [114,115]. One additional study assessed prenatal exposure to contemporary-use pesticides by maternal employment in a greenhouse during early pregnancy and performance of specific tasks; it found increased BMI, fat fold, and percentage of body fat in the children of mothers who were the most highly exposed to pesticides during early pregnancy [34].

Further research is still needed to adequately assess whether EDC exposure is associated with childhood obesity and other weight-related outcomes, as well as with related conditions, such as metabolic syndrome, diabetes, and future cardiovascular disease.

13.2.5 Neurodevelopment

Neurodevelopmental disorders are prevalent in the United States and worldwide, with evidence that rates of certain disorders, such as attention-deficit hyperactivity disorder (ADHD) and autism spectrum disorder (ASD), have been increasing in recent years [116–119]. While it is likely that these trends are attributable to numerous factors, including changes in diagnostic practices, there is a growing belief that exposure to EDCs may play a significant role. Human studies have related exposure to EDCs, both in utero and during early childhood, and neurodevelopmental disorders such as decreased IQ, poorer memory, ASD, ADHD, and other behavioral problems [120–123]. Sex steroid hormones are vital to central nervous system development. Thus, developing neuroendocrine systems may be particularly sensitive to EDC exposure [124]. Thyroid hormones also play an essential role in neurodevelopment, in addition to many other functions related to growth and metabolism. There is a growing list of EDCs that have been found capable of disrupting thyroid function (PCBs, PBDEs, pesticides, phthalates, and BPA, in addition to numerous other EDCs) via diverse mechanisms [125–127].

The adverse effects of PCBs and persistent OC pesticides on neurodevelopment and neurological-related outcomes are well documented [128–130], and research on these associations continues to accumulate. Recently, chlordecone, an OC, in cord blood and breast milk was associated with decreased fine motor function in boys [131]; and prenatal DDE was inversely associated with cognitive index, quantitative and verbal skills, and memory in young children [132]. However, another study found no association between prenatal DDT or DDE and tests of mental development at 7 and 8 years of age [133]. Prenatal maternal serum PCBs have been associated with lower psychomotor and mental development (Bayley's scores) [134,135] and reduced scores on the Kauffman Assessment Battery, a test of cognitive development, most significantly in boys [136]. PCBs measured in umbilical cord serum were associated with decreased psychomotor development [134,135], decreased mental development [135], and lower scores on the Conner's continuous performance test of attention and impulse control and the Wechsler Intelligence Scale for Children intelligence test in boys [137]. Prenatal PBDE exposures have been associated with decreased IQ [138,139], increased hyperactivity [138], lower scores on tests of mental development [140], impaired attention, decreased processing speeds, perceptual reasoning, and verbal comprehension [139], and lower scores on tests of psychomotor development [141]. Postnatal exposure to PBDEs has also been reported to be associated with attention deficits, poor social competence [142], and lower scores on tests of psychomotor development [141]. There are a very limited number of studies that have examined the effect of PFCs on neurodevelopment to date. In one, PFOS, but not PFOA, in cord blood was associated with adverse performance on the Comprehensive Developmental Inventory for Infants and Toddlers, particularly the gross-motor domain [143]. Another study found no association between PFC levels early in gestation and behavioral questionnaires at 7 years old [144].

Researchers have also been investigating the effects of nonpersistent EDCs on child neurodevelopment and neurological function. Prenatal BPA exposure has been associated with behavioral problems such as emotional reactivity and aggression [145], externalizing behavior [146], and poorer executive function [147] in young girls, while being associated with anxiety, depression, and aggression in young boys [145,148]. Childhood BPA, on the other hand, is reportedly associated with internalizing, inattention, and hyperactivity in children and externalizing/conduct behaviors in girls alone [148]. Prenatal phthalates have been found to be associated with deficits in mental and motor development in young children [149], lower mental scores in girls [150], and low-molecular-weight phthalate metabolites were associated with aggression, conduct and attention problems, depression, and externalizing problems [151]. Similarly, concurrent levels of high-molecular-weight phthalates have been found to be associated with ADHD in children aged 6–15 years. These associations were stronger in boys than girls [152]. There have also been a large number of studies addressing the adverse neurodevelopmental and neurocognitive effects associated with early-life exposure to nonpersistent pesticides, particularly the OP class of insecticides, and this research has been reviewed in great detail elsewhere [153–155]. A recent study adds to the body of literature finding that prenatal OP exposure is associated with lower scores on newborn behavioral scales [156].

While there is some strong evidence of the negative effects of many EDCs, particularly pesticides, on neurodevelopment, it is not fully understood if these chemicals are inducing neurotoxicity at low levels via an endocrine-related mode of action, their designed neurotoxic mechanism, or some other pathway that is not well understood. More human and toxicological studies of pesticides as possible EDCs are needed to address these underlying questions about the neurodevelopment-related modes of action.

13.3 CONCLUSIONS

While many of the studies reviewed in this chapter add to a growing body of evidence that EDCs may adversely affect child development through altered endocrine function, much more work needs to be carried out before any conclusions can be drawn with certainty. There are some limitations to the current body of work that are likely contributing to the inconsistent results reviewed here. Many studies of the effects of EDCs on children's health have relatively small sample sizes, possibly leaving them without enough statistical power to detect small, but potentially relevant, health effects, and also leading to concerns about multiple comparisons. In addition, many are exploratory, cross-sectional, or both, and have exposure data available for only one point in time. Especially for the nonpersistent EDCs, one point in time is not likely to be reflective of exposure over the long term. Differences in study design, study populations, life stage, data analysis approaches, and strategies for attaining data on exposure, end point, and important covariates all further contribute to the difficulties in comparison across studies and make summarizing the findings difficult.

The adverse health effects following EDC exposures depend on many factors, such as the timing of exposure, level and duration of exposure, type of EDC, and environmental and genetic factors of the individuals. Because of this, there is a great need for well-designed longitudinal studies that measure both exposure and developmental end points at multiple potentially sensitive times. In particular, studies of nonpersistent EDCs must consider intraindividual variability in exposure levels over time. Future research aimed at explaining sexually dimorphic impacts of EDCs on development is also needed, as are studies capable of exploring the health effects resulting from exposure to multiple EDCs simultaneously, designed to more closely reflect the reality of being exposed to chemical mixtures. Research that combines molecular epidemiology and toxicology approaches should be conducted to establish causality and to elucidate specific biological mechanisms of EDCs in humans, individual susceptibility factors, and the stages of development most sensitive to exposure. Finally, more research is needed in the area of exposure science to enable more precise effect estimates in epidemiology studies used for risk assessment, to provide solid data on important exposure sources and pathways for risk management, and to help inform effective regulations. To illustrate the need for this kind of research, consider the example of several phthalates being banned from use in children's toys, as well as BPA from baby bottles, in the United States due to concerns for children's health. The most sensitive exposure period to these chemicals, however, may be the developing fetus, which would likely not be affected by legislation that is geared only toward reducing chemicals in children's toys and baby bottles rather than eliminating them.

Given all of these factors and the large variability across human studies, it is currently impossible to determine individual-level risk and whether there are "safe" levels of exposure to EDCs for children and pregnant women. Although the effect estimates or expected changes in developmental markers reported in individual studies may seem subtle because exposure is ubiquitous, a seemingly small shift in the population distribution for these measures in relation to exposure is of great public health concern. Given the range of potential serious developmental effects, efforts to reduce EDC exposure as a precaution among pregnant women and children are warranted. For persistent EDCs, like PCBs and DDT, which are no longer used in most countries, as well as for more contemporary POPs such as PBDEs, consuming a diet lower in animal fats and adherence to local fishing advisories may reduce exposure. Given that many products in homes, offices, day-care centers, and cars may contain PBDEs or other flame retardants, careful cleaning practices to reduce indoor dust [e.g., cleaning carpets and dusty surfaces regularly using a vacuum cleaner with a high-efficiency particulate air (HEPA) filter] may help to reduce exposure [157]. For nonpersistent EDCs, purchasing consumer goods or personal care products labeled "phthalate-free" or "BPA-free" may help to reduce exposure [158], as well as replacing packaged foods with "fresh" alternatives [159] or conventional produce with organic alternatives [160]. Caution should be taken, however, when new, "safer" products simply replace a high-risk EDC with a new chemical for which we may know even less about its potential toxicity.

While the steps listed here may help reduce exposure to some extent, exposure to most EDCs is multisource, multipathway, and multiroute. Individual exposure scenarios depend on many factors, many of which may not be modifiable through personal choices and activities. Thus, the most effective way to reduce risk is at the regulatory level. However, very few chemicals on the market have been thoroughly tested for endocrine-disrupting potential, and there has been little motivation for chemical producers to do so given the outdated and largely ineffective regulatory framework for controlling chemical risks in the United States [161]. However, the U.S. Environmental Protection Agency (EPA) did enact legislation in 1996 that required special considerations be given to child susceptibility in the agency's risk assessment of pesticides, and that certain chemicals be screened for endocrine activity [162]. This has since resulted in implementation of a more comprehensive Endocrine Disrupting Screening Program, though results of this program are not yet available [163,164].

In conclusion, the current body of work provides evidence that EDCs may adversely affect child development through altered endocrine function (Figure 13.1). Many of the current studies are limited by small sample sizes and cross-sectional study designs that are unable to account for temporal variability in EDC exposure, particularly for nonpersistent chemicals, or identify sensitive windows of susceptibility. Longitudinal studies that measure both exposure and developmental end points at multiple potentially sensitive points in time are needed. Still, given the range of potential serious developmental effects, efforts to reduce EDC exposure as a precaution among pregnant women and children are warranted. To help inform effective regulations, epidemiology should be used in concert with toxicology and exposure science to establish causality and to elucidate specific biological mechanisms of EDCs in humans and identify individual susceptibility factors and sensitive windows of exposure, as well as exposure sources and pathways.

References

[1] Diamanti-Kandarakis E, Bourguignon JP, Giudice LC, Hauser R, Prins GS, Soto AM, et al. Endocrine-disrupting chemicals: an Endocrine Society scientific statement. Endocr Rev 2009;30:293–342.
[2] Schug TT, Janesick A, Blumberg B, Heindel JJ. Endocrine disrupting chemicals and disease susceptibility. J Steroid Biochem Mol Biol 2011;127:204–15.
[3] Titus-Ernstoff L, Troisi R, Hatch EE, Palmer JR, Hyer M, Kaufman R, et al. Birth defects in the sons and daughters of women who were exposed in utero to diethylstilbestrol (DES). Int J Androl 2010;33:377–84.
[4] Landrigan PJ, Miodovnik A. Children's health and the environment: an overview. Mt Sinai J Med 2011; 78:1–10.

[5] Green R, Hauser R, Calafat AM, Weuve J, Schettler T, Ringer S, et al. Use of di(2-ethylhexyl) phthalate-containing medical products and urinary levels of mono(2-ethylhexyl) phthalate in neonatal intensive care unit infants. Environ Health Perspect 2005;113:1222–5.

[6] Calafat AM, Weuve J, Ye X, Jia LT, Hu H, Ringer S, et al. Exposure to bisphenol A and other phenols in neonatal intensive care unit premature infants. Environ Health Perspect 2009;117:639–44.

[7] Caserta D, Mantovani A, Marci R, Fazi A, Ciardo F, La Rocca C, et al. Environment and women's reproductive health. Hum Reprod Update 2011;17:418–33.

[8] Eskenazi B, Chevrier J, Rosas LG, Anderson HA, Bornman MS, Bouwman H, et al. The Pine River statement: human health consequences of DDT use. Environ Health Perspect 2009;117:1359–67.

[9] Meeker JD. Exposure to environmental endocrine disrupting compounds and men's health. Maturitas 2010;66:236–41.

[10] Centers for Disease Control and Prevention. Fourth national report on human exposure to environmental chemicals. Atlanta, GA: Centers for Disease Control & Prevention; 2010.

[11] Foster PM. Disruption of reproductive development in male rat offspring following *in utero* exposure to phthalate esters. Int J Androl 2006;29:140–7. discussion 181–45.

[12] Meeker JD, Sathyanarayana S, Swan SH. Phthalates and other additives in plastics: human exposure and associated health outcomes. Philos Trans R Soc Lond B Biol Sci 2009;364:2097–113.

[13] Meeker JD, Ferguson KK. Phthalates: human exposure and related health effects. In: Schecter A, editor. Dioxins and health (*3rd ed.*). Hoboken, NJ: John Wiley & Sons; 2012.

[14] vom Saal FS, Akingbemi BT, Belcher SM, Birnbaum LS, Crain DA, Eriksen M, et al. Chapel Hill bisphenol A expert panel consensus statement: integration of mechanisms, effects in animals and potential to impact human health at current levels of exposure. Reprod Toxicol 2007;24:131–8.

[15] Braun JM, Hauser R. Bisphenol A. and children's health. Curr Opin Pediatr 2011;23:233–9.

[16] Martin JA, Hamilton BE, Sutton PD, Ventura SJ, Mathews TJ, Osterman MJ. Births: final data for 2008. Natl Vital Stat Rep 2010;59(1):3–71.

[17] Stillerman KP, Mattison DR, Giudice LC, Woodruff TJ. Environmental exposures and adverse pregnancy outcomes: a review of the science. Reprod Sci 2008;15:631–50.

[18] Wigle DT, Arbuckle TE, Turner MC, Berube A, Yang Q, Liu S, et al. Epidemiologic evidence of relationships between reproductive and child health outcomes and environmental chemical contaminants. J Toxicol Environ Health B Crit Rev 2008;11:373–517.

[19] Harley KG, Chevrier J, Schall RA, Sjodin A, Bradman A, Eskenazi B. Association of prenatal exposure to polybrominated diphenyl ethers and infant birth weight. Am J Epidemiol 2011;174:885–92.

[20] Kezios KL, Liu X, Cirillio PM, Kalantzi OI, Wang Y, Petreas MX, et al. Prenatal polychlorinated biphenyl exposure is associated with decreased gestational length but not birth weight: archived samples from the Child Health and Development Studies pregnancy cohort. Environ Health 2012;11:49.

[21] Maisonet M, Terrell ML, McGeehin MA, Christensen KY, Holmes A, Calafat AM, et al. Maternal concentrations of polyfluoroalkyl compounds during pregnancy and fetal and postnatal growth in British girls. Environ Health Perspect 2012;120:1432–7.

[22] Chen MH, Ha EH, Wen TW, Su YN, Lien GW, Chen CY, et al. Perfluorinated compounds in umbilical cord blood and adverse birth outcomes. PLoS One 2012;7:e42474.

[23] Apelberg BJ, Witter FR, Herbstman JB, Calafat AM, Halden RU, Needham LL, et al. Cord serum concentrations of perfluorooctane sulfonate (PFOS) and perfluorooctanoate (PFOA) in relation to weight and size at birth. Environ Health Perspect 2007;115:1670–6.

[24] Washino N, Saijo Y, Sasaki S, Kato S, Ban S, Konishi K, et al. Correlations between prenatal exposure to perfluorinated chemicals and reduced fetal growth. Environ Health Perspect 2009;117:660–7.

[25] Fei C, McLaughlin JK, Tarone RE, Olsen J. Perfluorinated chemicals and fetal growth: a study within the Danish National Birth Cohort. Environ Health Perspect 2007;115:1677–82.

[26] Lignell S, Aune M, Darnerud PO, Hanberg A, Larsson SC, Glynn A. Prenatal exposure to polychlorinated biphenyls (PCBs) and polybrominated diphenyl ethers (PBDEs) may influence birth weight among infants in a Swedish cohort with background exposure: a cross-sectional study. Environ Health 2013;12:44.

[27] Hamm MP, Cherry NM, Chan E, Martin JW, Burstyn I. Maternal exposure to perfluorinated acids and fetal growth. J Expo Sci Environ Epidemiol 2010;20:589–97.

[28] Govarts E, Nieuwenhuijsen M, Schoeters G, Ballester F, Bloemen K, de Boer M, et al. Birth weight and prenatal exposure to polychlorinated biphenyls (PCBs) and dichlorodiphenyldichloroethylene (DDE): a meta-analysis within 12 European Birth Cohorts. Environ Health Perspect 2012;120:162–70.

[29] Johnson PI, Sutton P, Atchley DS, Koustas E, Lam J, Sen S, et al. The navigation guide-evidence-based medicine meets environmental health: systematic review of human evidence for PFOA effects on fetal growth. Environ Health Perspect 2014.

[30] Snijder CA, Heederik D, Pierik FH, Hofman A, Jaddoe VW, Koch HM, et al. Fetal growth and prenatal exposure to bisphenol A: the generation R study. Environ Health Perspect 2013;121:393–8.

[31] Chou WC, Chen JL, Lin CF, Chen YC, Shih FC, Chuang CY. Biomonitoring of bisphenol A concentrations in maternal and umbilical cord blood in regard to birth outcomes and adipokine expression: a birth cohort study in Taiwan. Environ Health 2011;10:94.

[32] Miao M, Yuan W, He Y, Zhou Z, Wang J, Gao E, et al. In utero exposure to bisphenol-A and anogenital distance of male offspring. Birth Defects Res A Clin Mol Teratol 2011;91:867–72.

[33] Zhang Y, Lin L, Cao Y, Chen B, Zheng L, Ge RS. Phthalate levels and low birth weight: a nested case-control study of Chinese newborns. J Pediatr 2009;155:500–4.

[34] Wohlfahrt-Veje C, Main KM, Schmidt IM, Boas M, Jensen TK, Grandjean P, et al. Lower birth weight and increased body fat at school age in children prenatally exposed to modern pesticides: a prospective study. Environ Health 2011;10:79.

[35] Wickerham EL, Lozoff B, Shao J, Kaciroti N, Xia Y, Meeker JD. Reduced birth weight in relation to pesticide mixtures detected in cord blood of full-term infants. Environ Int 2012;47:80–5.

[36] Ferguson KK, O'Neill MS, Meeker JD. Environmental contaminant exposures and preterm birth: a comprehensive review. J Toxicol Environ Health B Crit Rev 2013;16:69–113.

[37] Kadhel P, Monfort C, Costet N, Rouget F, Thome JP, Multigner L, et al. Chlordecone exposure, length of gestation, and risk of preterm birth. Am J Epidemiol 2014;179:536–44.

[38] Basterrechea M, Lertxundi A, Iniguez C, Mendez M, Murcia M, Mozo I, et al. Prenatal exposure to hexachlorobenzene (HCB) and reproductive effects in a multicentre birth cohort in Spain. Sci Total Environ 2014;466-467:770–6.

[39] Whitworth KW, Haug LS, Baird DD, Becher G, Hoppin JA, Skjaerven R, et al. Perfluorinated compounds in relation to birth weight in the Norwegian Mother and Child Cohort Study. Am J Epidemiol 2012;175:1209–16.

[40] Meeker JD, Hu H, Cantonwine DE, Lamadrid-Figueroa H, Calafat AM, Ettinger AS, et al. Urinary phthalate metabolites in relation to preterm birth in Mexico city. Environ Health Perspect 2009;117:1587–92.

[41] Cantonwine D, Meeker JD, Hu H, Sanchez BN, Lamadrid-Figueroa H, Mercado-Garcia A, et al. Bisphenol a exposure in Mexico City and risk of prematurity: a pilot nested case control study. Environ Health 2010;9:62.

[42] Whyatt RM, Adibi JJ, Calafat AM, Camann DE, Rauh V, Bhat HK, et al. Prenatal di(2-ethylhexyl)phthalate exposure and length of gestation among an inner-city cohort. Pediatrics 2009;124:e1213–20.

[43] Latini G, De Felice C, Presta G, Del Vecchio A, Paris I, Ruggieri F, et al. In utero exposure to di-(2-ethylhexyl) phthalate and duration of human pregnancy. Environ Health Perspect 2003;111:1783–5.

[44] Ferguson KK, McElrath TF, Ko YA, Mukherjee B, Meeker JD. Variability in urinary phthalate metabolite levels across pregnancy and sensitive windows of exposure for the risk of preterm birth. Environ Int 2014;70:118–24.

[45] Ferguson KK, McElrath TF, Meeker JD. Environmental phthalate exposure and preterm birth. JAMA Pediatr 2014;168:61–7.

[46] Adibi JJ, Hauser R, Williams PL, Whyatt RM, Calafat AM, Nelson H, et al. Maternal urinary metabolites of di-(2-ethylhexyl) phthalate in relation to the timing of labor in a US multicenter pregnancy cohort study. Am J Epidemiol 2009;169:1015–24.

[47] Wolff MS, Engel SM, Berkowitz GS, Ye X, Silva MJ, Zhu C, et al. Prenatal phenol and phthalate exposures and birth outcomes. Environ Health Perspect 2008;116:1092–7.

[48] Main KM, Skakkebaek NE, Virtanen HE, Toppari J. Genital anomalies in boys and the environment. Best Pract Res Clin Endocrinol Metab 2010;24:279–89.

[49] Skakkebaek NE, Rajpert-De Meyts E, Main KM. Testicular dysgenesis syndrome: an increasingly common developmental disorder with environmental aspects. Hum Reprod 2001;16:972–8.

[50] Kay VR, Bloom MS, Foster WG. Reproductive and developmental effects of phthalate diesters in males. Crit Rev Toxicol 2014;44:467–98.

[51] Swan SH, Elkin EP, Fenster L. The question of declining sperm density revisited: an analysis of 101 studies published 1934–1996. Environ Health Perspect 2000;108:961–6.

[52] Travison TG, Araujo AB, O'Donnell AB, Kupelian V, McKinlay JB. A population-level decline in serum testosterone levels in American men. J Clin Endocrinol Metab 2007;92:196–202.

[53] Huyghe E, Matsuda T, Thonneau P. Increasing incidence of testicular cancer worldwide: a review. J Urol 2003;170:5–11.

[54] Costa EM, Spritzer PM, Hohl A, Bachega TA. Effects of endocrine disruptors in the development of the female reproductive tract. Arq Bras Endocrinol Metabol 2014;58:153–61.

[55] Kay VR, Chambers C, Foster WG. Reproductive and developmental effects of phthalate diesters in females. Crit Rev Toxicol 2013;43:200–19.

[56] Rignell-Hydbom A, Lindh CH, Dillner J, Jonsson BA, Rylander L. A nested case-control study of intrauterine exposure to persistent organochlorine pollutants and the risk of hypospadias. PLoS One 2012;7:e44767.

[57] Torres-Sanchez L, Zepeda M, Cebrian ME, Belkind-Gerson J, Garcia-Hernandez RM, Belkind-Valdovinos U, et al. Dichlorodiphenyldichloroethylene exposure during the first trimester of pregnancy alters the anal position in male infants. Ann N Y Acad Sci 2008;1140:155–62.

[58] Longnecker MP, Gladen BC, Cupul-Uicab LA, Romano-Riquer SP, Weber JP, Chapin RE, et al. *In utero* exposure to the antiandrogen 1,1-dichloro-2,2-bis(*p*-chlorophenyl)ethylene (DDE) in relation to anogenital distance in male newborns from Chiapas, Mexico. Am J Epidemiol 2007;165:1015–22.

[59] Main KM, Kiviranta H, Virtanen HE, Sundqvist E, Tuomisto JT, Tuomisto J, et al. Flame retardants in placenta and breast milk and cryptorchidism in newborn boys. Environ Health Perspect 2007;115:1519–26.

[60] Carmichael SL, Herring AH, Sjodin A, Jones R, Needham L, Ma C, et al. Hypospadias and halogenated organic pollutant levels in maternal mid-pregnancy serum samples. Chemosphere 2010;80:641–6.

[61] Suzuki Y, Yoshinaga J, Mizumoto Y, Serizawa S, Shiraishi H. Foetal exposure to phthalate esters and anogenital distance in male newborns [published online June 22, 2011]. Int J Androl doi:10.1111/j.1365-2605.2011.01190.x.

[62] Swan SH. Environmental phthalate exposure in relation to reproductive outcomes and other health endpoints in humans. Environ Res 2008;108:177–84.

[63] Bustamante-Montes LP, Hernandez-Valero MA, Flores-Pimentel D, Garcia-Fabila M, Amaya-Chavez A, Barr DB, et al. Prenatal exposure to phthalates is associated with decreased anogenital distance and penile size in male newborns. J Dev Orig Health Dis 2013;4:300–6.

[64] Ormond G, Nieuwenhuijsen MJ, Nelson P, Toledano MB, Iszatt N, Geneletti S, et al. Endocrine disruptors in the workplace, hair spray, folate supplementation, and risk of hypospadias: case-control study. Environ Health Perspect 2009;117:303–7.

[65] Choi H, Kim J, Im Y, Lee S, Kim Y. The association between some endocrine disruptors and hypospadias in biological samples. J Environ Sci Health A Tox Hazard Subst Environ Eng 2012;47:2173–9.

[66] Chevrier C, Petit C, Philippat C, Mortamais M, Slama R, Rouget F, et al. Maternal urinary phthalates and phenols and male genital anomalies. Epidemiology 2012;23:353–6.

[67] Main KM, Mortensen GK, Kaleva MM, Boisen KA, Damgaard IN, Chellakooty M, et al. Human breast milk contamination with phthalates and alterations of endogenous reproductive hormones in infants three months of age. Environ Health Perspect 2006;114:270–6.

[68] Agopian AJ, Lupo PJ, Canfield MA, Langlois PH. Case-control study of maternal residential atrazine exposure and male genital malformations. Am J Med Genet A 2013;161A:977–82.

[69] Gaspari L, Paris F, Jandel C, Kalfa N, Orsini M, Daures JP, et al. Prenatal environmental risk factors for genital malformations in a population of 1442 French male newborns: a nested case-control study. Hum Reprod 2011;26:3155–62.

[70] Rocheleau CM, Romitti PA, Dennis LK. Pesticides and hypospadias: a meta-analysis. J Pediatr Urol 2009; 5:17–24.

[71] Euling SY, Herman-Giddens ME, Lee PA, Selevan SG, Juul A, Sorensen TI, et al. Examination of US puberty-timing data from 1940 to 1994 for secular trends: panel findings. Pediatrics 2008;121(Suppl. 3):S172–91.

[72] Aksglaede L, Sorensen K, Petersen JH, Skakkebaek NE, Juul A. Recent decline in age at breast development: the Copenhagen Puberty Study. Pediatrics 2009;123:e932–9.

[73] Mouritsen A, Aksglaede L, Sorensen K, Mogensen SS, Leffers H, Main KM, et al. Hypothesis: exposure to endocrine-disrupting chemicals may interfere with timing of puberty. Int J Androl 2010;33:346–59.

[74] Schoeters G, Den Hond E, Dhooge W, van Larebeke N, Leijs M. Endocrine disruptors and abnormalities of pubertal development. Basic Clin Pharmacol Toxicol 2008;102:168–75.

[75] Buck Louis GM, Gray Jr. LE, Marcus M, Ojeda SR, Pescovitz OH, Witchel SF, et al. Environmental factors and puberty timing: expert panel research needs. Pediatrics 2008;121(Suppl. 3):S192–207.

[76] Ozen S, Goksen D, Darcan S. Agricultural pesticides and precocious puberty. Vitam Horm 2014;94:27–40.

[77] Lam T, Williams PL, Lee MM, Korrick SA, Birnbaum LS, Burns JS, et al. Prepubertal organochlorine pesticide concentrations and age of pubertal onset among Russian boys. Environ Int 2014;73C:135–42.

[78] Lopez-Espinosa MJ, Fletcher T, Armstrong B, Genser B, Dhatariya K, Mondal D, et al. Association of perfluorooctanoic acid (PFOA) and perfluorooctane sulfonate (PFOS) with age of puberty among children living near a chemical plant. Environ Sci Technol 2011;45:8160–6.

[79] Chen A, Chung E, DeFranco EA, Pinney SM, Dietrich KN. Serum PBDEs and age at menarche in adolescent girls: analysis of the National Health and Nutrition Examination Survey 2003–2004. Environ Res 2011;111:831–7.

[80] Ozen S, Darcan S, Bayindir P, Karasulu E, Simsek DG, Gurler T. Effects of pesticides used in agriculture on the development of precocious puberty. Environ Monit Assess 2012;184:4223–32.

[81] Humblet O, Williams PL, Korrick SA, Sergeyev O, Emond C, Birnbaum LS, et al. Dioxin and polychlorinated biphenyl concentrations in mother's serum and the timing of pubertal onset in sons. Epidemiology 2011;22:827–35.

[82] Christensen KY, Maisonet M, Rubin C, Holmes A, Calafat AM, Kato K, et al. Exposure to polyfluoroalkyl chemicals during pregnancy is not associated with offspring age at menarche in a contemporary British cohort. Environ Int 2011;37:129–35.

[83] Wolff MS, Teitelbaum SL, McGovern K, Windham GC, Pinney SM, Galvez M, et al. Phthalate exposure and pubertal development in a longitudinal study of US girls. Hum Reprod 2014.

[84] Watkins DJ, Tellez-Rojo MM, Ferguson KK, Lee JM, Solano-Gonzalez M, Blank-Goldenberg C, et al. In utero and peripubertal exposure to phthalates and BPA in relation to female sexual maturation. Environ Res 2014;134C:233–41.

[85] Durmaz E, Asci A, Erkekoglu P, Akcurin S, Gumusel BK, Bircan I. Urinary bisphenol a levels in girls with idiopathic central precocious puberty. J Clin Res Pediatr Endocrinol 2014;6:16–21.

[86] Durmaz E, Ozmert EN, Erkekoglu P, Giray B, Derman O, Hincal F, et al. Plasma phthalate levels in pubertal gynecomastia. Pediatrics 2010;125:e122–9.

[87] Ferguson KK, Peterson KE, Lee JM, Mercado-Garcia A, Blank-Goldenberg C, Tellez-Rojo MM, et al. Prenatal and peripubertal phthalates and bisphenol A in relation to sex hormones and puberty in boys. Reprod Toxicol 2014;47:70–6.

[88] Mouritsen A, Frederiksen H, Sorensen K, Aksglaede L, Hagen C, Skakkebaek NE, et al. Urinary phthalates from 168 girls and boys measured twice a year during a 5-year period: associations with adrenal androgen levels and puberty. J Clin Endocrinol Metab 2013;98:3755–64.

[89] Wang Y, Lobstein T. Worldwide trends in childhood overweight and obesity. Int J Pediatr Obes 2006; 1:11–25.

[90] La Merrill M, Birnbaum LS. Childhood obesity and environmental chemicals. Mt Sinai J Med 2011;78:22–48.

[91] Grun F, Blumberg B. Minireview: the case for obesogens. Mol Endocrinol 2009;23:1127–34.

[92] Hatch EE, Nelson JW, Stahlhut RW, Webster TF. Association of endocrine disruptors and obesity: perspectives from epidemiological studies. Int J Androl 2010;33:324–32.

[93] Warner M, Aguilar Schall R, Harley KG, Bradman A, Barr D, Eskenazi B. In utero DDT and DDE exposure and obesity status of 7-year-old Mexican-American children in the CHAMACOS cohort. Environ Health Perspect 2013;121:631–6.

[94] Warner M, Wesselink A, Harley KG, Bradman A, Kogut K, Eskenazi B. Prenatal exposure to dichlorodiphenyltrichloroethane and obesity at 9 years of age in the CHAMACOS study cohort. Am J Epidemiol 2014; 179:1312–22.

[95] Valvi D, Mendez MA, Martinez D, Grimalt JO, Torrent M, Sunyer J, et al. Prenatal concentrations of polychlorinated biphenyls, DDE, and DDT and overweight in children: a prospective birth cohort study. Environ Health Perspect 2012;120:451–7.

[96] Tang-Peronard JL, Heitmann BL, Andersen HR, Steuerwald U, Grandjean P, Weihe P, et al. Association between prenatal polychlorinated biphenyl exposure and obesity development at ages 5 and 7 y: a prospective cohort study of 656 children from the Faroe Islands. Am J Clin Nutr 2014;99:5–13.

[97] Verhulst SL, Nelen V, Hond ED, Koppen G, Beunckens C, Vael C, et al. Intrauterine exposure to environmental pollutants and body mass index during the first 3 years of life. Environ Health Perspect 2009;117:122–6.

[98] Dhooge W, Den Hond E, Koppen G, Bruckers L, Nelen V, Van De Mieroop E, et al. Internal exposure to pollutants and body size in Flemish adolescents and adults: associations and dose–response relationships. Environ Int 2010;36:330–7.

[99] Timmermann CA, Rossing LI, Grontved A, Ried-Larsen M, Dalgard C, Andersen LB, et al. Adiposity and glycemic control in children exposed to perfluorinated compounds. J Clin Endocrinol Metab 2014;99:E608–14.

[100] Harley KG, Aguilar Schall R, Chevrier J, Tyler K, Aguirre H, Bradman A, et al. Prenatal and postnatal bisphenol A exposure and body mass index in childhood in the CHAMACOS cohort. Environ Health Perspect 2013;121:514–20. 520e511–6.

[101] Li DK, Miao M, Zhou Z, Wu C, Shi H, Liu X, et al. Urine bisphenol-A level in relation to obesity and overweight in school-age children. PLoS One 2013;8:e65399.

[102] Bhandari R, Xiao J, Shankar A. Urinary bisphenol A and obesity in U.S. children. Am J Epidemiol 2013; 177:1263–70.

[103] Trasande L, Attina TM, Blustein J. Association between urinary bisphenol A concentration and obesity prevalence in children and adolescents. JAMA 2012;308:1113–21.

[104] Wang HX, Zhou Y, Tang CX, Wu JG, Chen Y, Jiang QW. Association between bisphenol A exposure and body mass index in Chinese school children: a cross-sectional study. Environ Health 2012;11:79.

[105] Braun JM, Lanphear BP, Calafat AM, Deria S, Khoury J, Howe CJ, et al. Early life bisphenol a exposure and child body mass index: a prospective cohort study. Environ Health Perspect 2014;122:1239–45.

[106] Valvi D, Casas M, Mendez MA, Ballesteros-Gomez A, Luque N, Rubio S, et al. Prenatal bisphenol a urine concentrations and early rapid growth and overweight risk in the offspring. Epidemiology 2013;24:791–9.

[107] Wolff MS, Teitelbaum SL, Windham G, Pinney SM, Britton JA, Chelimo C, et al. Pilot study of urinary biomarkers of phytoestrogens, phthalates, and phenols in girls. Environ Health Perspect 2007;115:116–21.

[108] Kim SH, Park MJ. Phthalate exposure and childhood obesity. Ann Pediatr Endocrinol Metab 2014;19:69–75.

[109] Hatch EE, Nelson JW, Qureshi MM, Weinberg J, Moore LL, Singer M, et al. Association of urinary phthalate metabolite concentrations with body mass index and waist circumference: a cross-sectional study of NHANES data, 1999–2002. Environ Health 2008;7:27.

[110] Zhang Y, Meng X, Chen L, Li D, Zhao L, Zhao Y, et al. Age and sex-specific relationships between phthalate exposures and obesity in Chinese children at puberty. PLoS One 2014;9:e104852.

[111] Buser MC, Murray HE, Scinicariello F. Age and sex differences in childhood and adulthood obesity association with phthalates: analyses of NHANES 2007–2010. Int J Hyg Environ Health 2014;217:687–94.

[112] Trasande L, Attina TM, Sathyanarayana S, Spanier AJ, Blustein J. Race/ethnicity-specific associations of urinary phthalates with childhood body mass in a nationally representative sample. Environ Health Perspect 2013;121:501–6.

[113] Teitelbaum SL, Mervish N, Moshier EL, Vangeepuram N, Galvez MP, Calafat AM, et al. Associations between phthalate metabolite urinary concentrations and body size measures in New York City children. Environ Res 2012;112:186–93.

[114] Buser MC, Murray HE, Scinicariello F. Association of urinary phenols with increased body weight measures and obesity in children and adolescents. J Pediatr 2014.

[115] Twum C, Wei Y. The association between urinary concentrations of dichlorophenol pesticides and obesity in children. Rev Environ Health 2011;26:215–9.

[116] Boyle CA, Boulet S, Schieve LA, Cohen RA, Blumberg SJ, Yeargin-Allsopp M, et al. Trends in the prevalence of developmental disabilities in US children, 1997–2008. Pediatrics 2011;127:1034–42.

[117] Kim YS, Leventhal BL, Koh YJ, Fombonne E, Laska E, Lim EC, et al. Prevalence of autism spectrum disorders in a total population sample. Am J Psychiatry 2011;168:904–12.

[118] Hertz-Picciotto I, Delwiche L. The rise in autism and the role of age at diagnosis. Epidemiology 2009;20:84–90.

[119] Aguiar A, Eubig PA, Schantz SL. Attention deficit/hyperactivity disorder: a focused overview for children's environmental health researchers. Environ Health Perspect 2010;118:1646–53.

[120] Miodovnik A. Environmental neurotoxicants and developing brain. Mt Sinai J Med 2011;78:58–77.

[121] Weiss B. Endocrine disruptors as a threat to neurological function. J Neurol Sci 2011;305:11–21.

[122] Polanska K, Jurewicz J, Hanke W. Review of current evidence on the impact of pesticides, polychlorinated biphenyls and selected metals on attention deficit/hyperactivity disorder in children. Int J Occup Med Environ Health 2013;26:16–38.

[123] Rossignol DA, Genuis SJ, Frye RE. Environmental toxicants and autism spectrum disorders: a systematic review. Transl Psychiatry 2014;4:e360.

[124] Parent AS, Naveau E, Gerard A, Bourguignon JP, Westbrook GL. Early developmental actions of endocrine disruptors on the hypothalamus, hippocampus, and cerebral cortex. J Toxicol Environ Health B Crit Rev 2011;14:328–45.

[125] Boas M, Feldt-Rasmussen U, Main KM. Thyroid effects of endocrine disrupting chemicals [published online September 10, 2011]. Mol Cell Endocrinol. doi:10.1016/j.mce.2011.09.005.

[126] Miller MD, Crofton KM, Rice DC, Zoeller RT. Thyroid-disrupting chemicals: interpreting upstream biomarkers of adverse outcomes. Environ Health Perspect 2009;117:1033–41.

[127] Preau L, Fini JB, Morvan-Dubois G, Demeneix B. Thyroid hormone signaling during early neurogenesis and its significance as a vulnerable window for endocrine disruption [published online June 27, 2014]. Biochim Biophys Acta doi:10.1016/j.bbagrm.2014.06.015.

[128] Korrick SA, Sagiv SK. Polychlorinated biphenyls, organochlorine pesticides and neurodevelopment. Curr Opin Pediatr 2008;20:198–204.

[129] Rosas LG, Eskenazi B. Pesticides and child neurodevelopment. Curr Opin Pediatr 2008;20:191–7.

[130] Jurewicz J, Hanke W. Prenatal and childhood exposure to pesticides and neurobehavioral development: review of epidemiological studies. Int J Occup Med Environ Health 2008;21:121–32.

[131] Boucher O, Simard MN, Muckle G, Rouget F, Kadhel P, Bataille H, et al. Exposure to an organochlorine pesticide (chlordecone) and development of 18-month-old infants. Neurotoxicology 2013;35:162–8.

[132] Torres-Sanchez L, Schnaas L, Rothenberg SJ, Cebrian ME, Osorio-Valencia E, Hernandez Mdel C, et al. Prenatal *p, p*-DDE exposure and neurodevelopment among children 3.5–5 years of age. Environ Health Perspect 2013;121:263–8.

[133] Jusko TA, Klebanoff MA, Brock JW, Longnecker MP. *In-utero* exposure to dichlorodiphenyltrichloroethane and cognitive development among infants and school-aged children. Epidemiology 2012;23:689–98.

[134] Park HY, Hertz-Picciotto I, Sovcikova E, Kocan A, Drobna B, Trnovec T. Neurodevelopmental toxicity of prenatal polychlorinated biphenyls (PCBs) by chemical structure and activity: a birth cohort study. Environ Health 2010;9:51.

[135] Park HY, Park JS, Sovcikova E, Kocan A, Linderholm L, Bergman A, et al. Exposure to hydroxylated polychlorinated biphenyls (OH-PCBs) in the prenatal period and subsequent neurodevelopment in eastern Slovakia. Environ Health Perspect 2009;117:1600–6.

[136] Tatsuta N, Nakai K, Murata K, Suzuki K, Iwai-Shimada M, Kurokawa N, et al. Impacts of prenatal exposures to polychlorinated biphenyls, methylmercury, and lead on intellectual ability of 42-month-old children in Japan. Environ Res 2014;133:321–6.

[137] Sagiv SK, Thurston SW, Bellinger DC, Altshul LM, Korrick SA. Neuropsychological measures of attention and impulse control among 8-year-old children exposed prenatally to organochlorines. Environ Health Perspect 2012;120:904–9.

[138] Chen A, Yolton K, Rauch SA, Webster GM, Hornung R, Sjodin A, et al. Prenatal polybrominated diphenyl ether exposures and neurodevelopment in U.S. children through 5 years of age: the HOME study. Environ Health Perspect 2014;122:856–62.

[139] Eskenazi B, Chevrier J, Rauch SA, Kogut K, Harley KG, Johnson C, et al. *In utero* and childhood polybrominated diphenyl ether (PBDE) exposures and neurodevelopment in the CHAMACOS study. Environ Health Perspect 2013;121:257–62.

[140] Herbstman JB, Sjodin A, Kurzon M, Lederman SA, Jones RS, Rauh V, et al. Prenatal exposure to PBDEs and neurodevelopment. Environ Health Perspect 2010;118:712–9.

[141] Lynch CD, Jackson LW, Kostyniak PJ, McGuinness BM, Buck Louis GM. The effect of prenatal and postnatal exposure to polychlorinated biphenyls and child neurodevelopment at age twenty four months. Reprod Toxicol 2012;34:451–6.

[142] Gascon M, Vrijheid M, Martinez D, Forns J, Grimalt JO, Torrent M, et al. Effects of pre and postnatal exposure to low levels of polybromodiphenyl ethers on neurodevelopment and thyroid hormone levels at 4 years of age. Environ Int 2011;37:605–11.

[143] Chen MH, Ha EH, Liao HF, Jeng SF, Su YN, Wen TW, et al. Perfluorinated compound levels in cord blood and neurodevelopment at 2 years of age. Epidemiology 2013;24:800–8.

[144] Fei C, Olsen J. Prenatal exposure to perfluorinated chemicals and behavioral or coordination problems at age 7 years. Environ Health Perspect 2011;119:573–8.

[145] Perera F, Vishnevetsky J, Herbstman JB, Calafat AM, Xiong W, Rauh V, et al. Prenatal bisphenol a exposure and child behavior in an inner-city cohort. Environ Health Perspect 2012;120:1190–4.

[146] Braun JM, Yolton K, Dietrich KN, Hornung R, Ye X, Calafat AM, et al. Prenatal bisphenol A exposure and early childhood behavior. Environ Health Perspect 2009;117:1945–52.

[147] Braun JM, Kalkbrenner AE, Calafat AM, Yolton K, Ye X, Dietrich KN, et al. Impact of early-life bisphenol A exposure on behavior and executive function in children. Pediatrics 2011;128:873–82.

[148] Harley KG, Gunier RB, Kogut K, Johnson C, Bradman A, Calafat AM, et al. Prenatal and early childhood bisphenol A concentrations and behavior in school-aged children. Environ Res 2013;126:43–50.

[149] Whyatt RM, Liu X, Rauh VA, Calafat AM, Just AC, Hoepner L, et al. Maternal prenatal urinary phthalate metabolite concentrations and child mental, psychomotor, and behavioral development at 3 years of age. Environ Health Perspect 2012;120:290–5.

[150] Tellez-Rojo MM, Cantoral A, Cantonwine DE, Schnaas L, Peterson K, Hu H, et al. Prenatal urinary phthalate metabolites levels and neurodevelopment in children at two and three years of age. Sci Total Environ 2013;461–462:386–90.

[151] Engel SM, Miodovnik A, Canfield RL, Zhu C, Silva MJ, Calafat AM, et al. Prenatal phthalate exposure is associated with childhood behavior and executive functioning. Environ Health Perspect 2010;118:565–71.

[152] Chopra V, Harley K, Lahiff M, Eskenazi B. Association between phthalates and attention deficit disorder and learning disability in U.S. children, 6–15 years. Environ Res 2014;128:64–9.

[153] Munoz-Quezada MT, Lucero BA, Barr DB, Steenland K, Levy K, Ryan PB, et al. Neurodevelopmental effects in children associated with exposure to organophosphate pesticides: a systematic review. Neurotoxicology 2013;39:158–68.

[154] Saunders M, Magnanti BL, Correia Carreira S, Yang A, Alamo-Hernandez U, Riojas-Rodriguez H, et al. Chlorpyrifos and neurodevelopmental effects: a literature review and expert elicitation on research and policy. Environ Health 2012;11(Suppl. 1):S5.

[155] Burns CJ, McIntosh LJ, Mink PJ, Jurek AM, Li AA. Pesticide exposure and neurodevelopmental outcomes: review of the epidemiologic and animal studies. J Toxicol Environ Health B Crit Rev 2013;16:127–283.

[156] Zhang Y, Han S, Liang D, Shi X, Wang F, Liu W, et al. Prenatal exposure to organophosphate pesticides and neurobehavioral development of neonates: a birth cohort study in Shenyang, China. PLoS One 2014;9:e88491.

[157] Environmental Working Group. Reducing your exposure to PBDEs in your home. <http://www.ewg.org/pbdefree>. [accessed 31.12.11].

[158] Dunagan SC, Dodson RE, Rudel RA, Brody JG. Toxics use reduction in the home: lessons learned from household exposure studies. J Clean Prod 2011;19:438–44.

[159] Rudel RA, Gray JM, Engel CL, Rawsthorne TW, Dodson RE, Ackerman JM, et al. Food packaging and bisphenol A and bis(2-ethyhexyl) phthalate exposure: findings from a dietary intervention. Environ Health Perspect 2011;119:914–20.

[160] Lu C, Toepel K, Irish R, Fenske RA, Barr DB, Bravo R. Organic diets significantly lower children's dietary exposure to organophosphorus pesticides. Environ Health Perspect 2006;114:260–3.

[161] Vogel SA, Roberts JA. Why the toxic substances control act needs an overhaul, and how to strengthen oversight of chemicals in the interim. Health Aff (Millwood) 2011;30:898–905.

[162] Landrigan PJ, Goldman LR. Children's vulnerability to toxic chemicals: a challenge and opportunity to strengthen health and environmental policy. Health Aff (Millwood) 2011;30:842–50.

[163] Harding AK, Daston GP, Boyd GR, Lucier GW, Safe SH, Stewart J, et al. Endocrine disrupting chemicals research program of the U.S. Environmental Protection Agency: summary of a peer-review report. Environ Health Perspect 2006;114:1276–82.

[164] US Environmental Protection Agency. Endocrine Disruptor Screening Program (EDSP). <http://www.epa.gov/endo/>. [accessed 31.12.11].

Effects of Endocrine Disrupters on Immune Function and Inflammation

Rodney R. Dietert

Abstract

Endocrine-disrupting chemicals (EDCs) are among the most hazardous toxicants known. They can affect immune function directly, via action on immune cell surface receptors, or indirectly, through other physiological mediators. Because prolonged immune dysfunction elevates the risk of a myriad of communicable and noncommunicable diseases, EDC-mediated immunotoxicity is a significant human health concern. This chapter describes the immunotoxicity and impact on inflammation associated with priority EDCs (grouped

Endocrine Disruption and Human Health.
DOI: http://dx.doi.org/10.1016/B978-0-12-801139-3.00014-4

together as "the dirty dozen"), as well as for other representative EDCs. Age and sex are significant factors in the susceptibility to EDC-induced immunotoxicity and the likely spectrum of outcomes. Despite the fact that EDCs include many diverse chemicals, there are patterns of immunomodulation that follow EDC exposure. These include targeting of dendritic cell and macrophage function, skewing of T helper mediated functions, and modulation of inflammatory responses in tissues. These combine to affect the risk of disease following EDC exposure.

14.1 INTRODUCTION

Endocrine-disrupting chemicals (EDCs) are represented by approximately 1000 distinct environmental chemicals, drugs, and food components comprising several major categories of known toxicants [e.g., heavy metals, polychlorinated biphenyls (PCBs), dioxins, organotins, flame retardants, polyfluorinated chemicals, herbicides, and pesticides]. EDCs are identified by their capacity to cause biologic disruption of hormone-driven processes in animals, humans, or both, often via their ability to interact with hormone receptors on cells. Because most of them interact with cell-surface or nuclear receptors, they can alter cellular homeostasis at exceedingly low doses. This places them in a special category of toxicants in terms of health risks. In light of the special concern over low-dose adverse effects from EDC exposure, the Endocrine Society of the United States has advocated the use of the precautionary principle in decision making about health risks from potential endocrine disruptors [1].

For those EDCs that have been evaluated for immunotoxicity, the vast majority cause immune disruption. The exact nature of the adverse outcomes for the immune system following an EDC exposure depends upon (1) the exposure dose and the duration of exposure, (2) the developmental life stage of exposure, (3) the sex of the individual, (4) the status of an individual's microbiome, (5) other environmental conditions (e.g., stress, diet, or co-exposure to other toxicants), and (6) the route of exposure.

While the types of immune disruption and health outcomes following EDC exposure are myriad, there are some common patterns that have been observed across different categories of EDCs [2]. For example, Figure 14.1 illustrates that exposure to EDCs is commonly associated with inappropriate inflammatory responses in specific tissues.

In this chapter, certain similarities among EDC-induced immunotoxicity will be emphasized to help provide a framework for considering the types of health risks that have been associated with EDC exposure. While some minimal immune-related exposure information exists for a significant number of the approximately 1000 EDCs, this review will focus on those EDCs that are the greatest environmental concerns, for which we have the most extensive immune-related research and evaluation, or both. For this purpose, we turn to what has been termed by the environmental working group [3] as the "dirty dozen" [i.e., atrazine, bisphenol A (BPA), dioxin, phthalates, perchlorate, polybrominated diphenyl ethers, lead, arsenic, mercury, perfluorinated chemicals, organophosphate pesticides (OPs), and glycol ethers], plus a few additional examples, including the PCBs, additional heavy metals (e.g., cadmium), antibacterial soap products (triclosan), estrogenic food components (e.g., genistein), and drugs (valproate).

**Examples of endocrine disruptor exposure
and reported misregulated tissue inflammation**

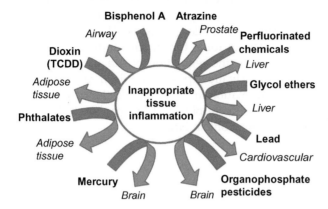

FIGURE 14.1   Examples of EDC exposures that have been reported to result in inappropriate tissue inflammation are illustrated. The EDCs are shown in bold type and are connected to a reported target tissue (indicated in italics) via arrows. (Not all EDCs that have been reported to produce misregulated inflammation are included in this figure.) In addition, many EDCs affect multiple target tissues. Prolonged inappropriate inflammation in tissues often results in tissue pathology, disease, or both.

14.2 IMMUNE AND INFLAMMATORY ALTERATIONS ASSOCIATED WITH THE "DIRTY DOZEN" EDCs

14.2.1 Arsenic

Arsenic is a widespread pollutant, and arsenic exposure has been associated with cardiovascular disease, diabetes, various cancers, neurotoxicity, and immune alterations. Early-life exposure to arsenic has been reported to produce several different immune outcomes, as reviewed by Dangleben et al. [4]. However, two of these stand out: (1) reduced host protection against viral infections, and (2) inappropriate inflammatory responses in the tissues. An increase in childhood infections and the severity of infections has been noted [5], which fits with the observations that arsenic-exposed mice are more susceptible to influenza virus infection and that such exposure predisposes for damaging airway inflammatory responses [6]. These are combined with an exaggerated and often inappropriate inflammatory response. For example, the research of several investigators has shown that prenatal arsenic exposure produces altered pro-inflammatory signaling [7,8], including the overproduction of pro-inflammatory cytokines such as interleukin-6 (IL-6) [9]. Inappropriate immune production of inflammatory mediators facilitates the activation of redox pathways [10], which contributes to tissue pathology and potentially to later-life cancer.

14.2.2 Atrazine

Widespread exposure to the herbicide atrazine occurs through its extensive crop use and the potential for contaminating drinking water. Immunosuppression, including reduced natural killer (NK) cell activity, is one of the presorted outcomes in mice from low-level exposure to atrazine via drinking water [11]. However, prenatal and lactational exposures are reported to produce later-life immune dysregulation in which some immune responses are excessively elevated [12]. This led investigators to suggest that atrazine exposure may contribute to the risk of autoimmune and allergic disease [12]. Alteration in dendritic cell maturation appears to be one potential route for atrazine-induced immune dysregulation [13]. It appears that atrazine may alter the regulation of inflammation in tissues. For example, Rayner et al. [14] reported that early life exposure of Wistar rats to atrazine increased the incidence of specific prostate inflammation in the adult. Similar results with adult male prostate inflammation in Long-Evans rats were obtained by Stanko et al. [15] following late-gestational exposure to an atrazine metabolite mixture.

14.2.3 Bisphenol A

BPA is a chemical found in food and beverage cans, as well as baby bottle and infant food containers with xenoestrogen activity. Because users (including infants) can be exposed to BPA that leaches out of these products, especially in higher temperatures, the long-term outcomes of exposure are a significant concern. Immunologically, exposure to BPA has been associated with increased airway inflammation [16], particularly enhanced allergic inflammation [17]. In animal models, exposure to BPA has been associated with an elevated risk of both eosinophilic airway inflammation [18] and colonic inflammation [19]. O'Brien et al. [20] recently reported that perinatal exposure of mice to BPA via the maternal diet produced long-term mast cell dysregulation that enhances the production of pro-inflammatory mediators in allergic asthma.

14.2.4 Dioxin

Dioxins such as 2,3,7,8-tetrachlorodibenzo-p-dioxin (TCDD) are among the most researched chemicals in the world, with much of the biological activity mediated via interaction with the aryl hydrocarbon (Ah) receptor. Ah hydrocarbon receptor (AhR) signaling has several major effects on different tissues containing immune cells, particularly during development [21]. The impact of AhR signaling on the immune system was recently reviewed by Stockinger et al. [22] and Hanieh [23]. Because there is cross-talk between the pathways for AhR induction and inflammation [24], it is not surprising that AhR agonists such as TCDD exert such a profound effect on immune function and regulation of inflammation. The impact is particularly noticeable during a time of immune challenge, such as with viral infection [25]. There is evidence suggesting that dendritic cells are direct targets of ligands for the AhR, and the skewing of dendritic cell function by exposure to dioxin may play a significant role in altered host responses [26]. Inflammatory pathway genes were found to be significant targets of TCDD-induced alterations in gene expression in adipose tissue, and this is likely to contribute to an elevated risk of inflammation-driven obesity [27].

Exposure to TCDD in early life has been reported to interfere with lymphocyte differentiation, causing an increase in some hematopoietic stem cells but a reduction in B and T lymphocyte differentiation [28]. It also disrupts mucosal immunity, elevating the risk for loss of tolerance and food allergies [29], as well as otitis media [30]. TCDD-induced imbalances in cytokines and increased inflammation appear to play a role in dioxin-elevated risk of liver fibrosis [31], as well as inflammation-driven obesity and diabetes [32,33].

14.2.5 Glycol Ethers

Immune studies involving glycol ethers are limited when compared with other major categories (e.g., heavy metals and dioxins) of EDCs. Among the first studies is that of Exon et al. [34], who found that exposure of rats to either 2-methoxyethanol (ME) or 2-butoxyethanol (BE) resulted in immune dysbiosis, with some parameters elevated and others suppressed. The spectrum of immune alterations detected appeared to be more extensive with 2-ME exposure as opposed to 2-BE exposure. In a study of topical exposure of mice to 2-BE, Singh et al. [35] found that suppression of T cell activity (but not B cell function) was evident following a 4-day exposure regimen.

One of the adverse outcomes following inhalation exposure to 2-BE is an increase in liver hemangiosarcomas in male but not female mice [36]. A current model of 2-BE effects seen in mice suggests that 2-BE induces macrophage activation and inflammation in the liver involving Kupffer cells (liver macrophages). Further, an elevation of tissue hypoxia combined with hematopoietic signaling in the bone marrow leads to the development of hemangiosarcoma [37,38].

14.2.6 Lead

The heavy metal lead has gained notoriety as a neurotoxicant with blood lead levels associated with adverse outcomes having fallen repeatedly during the past few decades. However, the developing immune system appears to be approximately as sensitive to lead exposure as is the neurological system. Several key immune and inflammatory alterations have been attributed to lead exposure. These include a skewing of Th helper function in favor of Th2- over Th1-driven responses [39] and a concomitant elevation in immunoglobulin E (IgE) production [40]. The sensitivity of Th alteration to lead appears to emerge developmentally near the midpoint of gestational development [41]. The immune Th skewing caused by lead has host response ramifications. Th1-driven responses to virus infections and tumors can be blunted. In contrast, the propensity for Th2-based responses has been associated with an elevated risk for certain allergic diseases, such as asthma, in some populations of children [42]. Lead has also been reported to exacerbate autoimmunity in an animal model of lupus [43].

One of the serious outcomes following exposure to lead is the dysregulation of inflammation. Several factors change, starting with innate immune cells and ending with inappropriately directed and/or unresolving inflammation in tissues [44]. Lead exposure can produce elevated arachidonate on cell surfaces, which contributes to elevated prostaglandin production [45] and elevated reactive oxygen species production by innate immune cells [46]. The increased propensity for exaggerated inflammation is thought to contribute to the association of elevated blood lead levels with increased risk of both hypertension and cardiovascular disease [47].

14.2.7 Mercury

Mercury has overlapping effects on the immune system with the other heavy metals (i.e., arsenic, cadmium, and lead). However, among these metals, exposure to mercury is most closely associated with elevated risk of multiple autoimmune conditions as an outcome of immunotoxicity [48]. It also promotes inflammatory disease via induction of both the ecyclooxygenase-2 and inducible nitric oxide synthase genes [49].

Pollard and Kono [50] argue that mercury induces autoimmunity in individuals with a genetic predisposition and that the process involves alterations among innate immune cells that utilize nucleic acid-binding and toll-like receptors and need increased pro-inflammatory cytokine production. In contrast, type I interferon production does not appear to be involved [50]. The role of altered innate immune cell responses was also noted by Nyland et al. [51], who found that prior mercury exposure caused a problematic, macrophage-driven response to viral infection in mice, leading to cardiac inflammation and an increased likelihood of autoimmunity. Mercury exposure affects the function of many organs; among these are the brain and neurological system, which are vulnerable to oxidative-induced damage [52].

Methylmercury acts to disrupt mitochondrial function, which begins a cascade that reduces adenosine triphosphate (ATP) synthesis and increases lipid, protein, and DNA peroxidation. It concomitantly decreases glutathione levels, increasing the risk for inflammatory-driven oxidative damage in tissues [53].

14.2.8 Organophosphate Pesticides

As a group, the organophosphate pesticides (OPs) have received less priority for immunotoxicity evaluation when compared with some other categories of EDCs (e.g., dioxins, plasticizers, and the heavy metals). Certainly, one reason for this involves the extreme sensitivity of the neurological system to OPs. As a result, much more attention has been given to neurotoxicologic evaluation of OPs than to immune-driven adverse outcomes. However, immune studies do exist and may not be unrelated to neurotoxicity as an end point of OP exposure.

Immunotoxicity studies tend to show that OPs disrupt the balance of immune function, particularly following early life exposures. There is evidence suggesting that these immune observations are relevant to several species, including humans [54,55]. Sensitive immune targets appear to be the dendritic cells [56] and macrophages [57]. Oxidative imbalances in tissues during immune responses are among the apparent outcomes of OP exposure [58].

Immunotoxicity from OP exposure may be part of the process, resulting in OP-induced neurotoxicity. Sunkaria et al. [59] have hypothesized that OP activation of resident microglia (brain macrophages) and their subsequent apoptosis following inflammatory mediator release contribute significantly to OP-induced neurotoxicity. This hypothesis has additional research support [60].

14.2.9 Perchlorate

Perchlorate, usually encountered in the form of ammonium perchlorate, is an oxidant used in rocket fuel and in some fertilizers. It is one of the contaminants found in drinking water. Most of the toxic and endocrine-disrupting action of perchlorate appears to be through its targeting of the thyroid, leading to hypothyroidism [61]. Immune studies of perchlorate are limited. In a recent draft review of perchlorate toxicity and safety limits, the U.S. Environmental Protection Agency (EPA) identified three immune observations of perchlorate immunotoxicity: (1) a reduction of in vitro phagocytic activity by peritoneal macrophages, (2) the enhancement of the plaque-forming cell (PFC) assay response to sheep erythrocytes as an antigen, and (3) enhancement of the local lymph node assay response with 2,4-dinitrochlorobenzene used as the eliciting agent [62]. The enhanced PFC result is difficult to interpret since the assay was originally designed to detect immunosuppression as the primary outcome. Because the effect on the thyroid is the primary low-dose adverse outcome and the previous immune studies included a limited spectrum of parameters (some in vitro), it may be useful to consider this EDC as incompletely characterized for immune and inflammatory effects.

14.2.10 Perfluorinated Chemicals

Fluorochemicals have been used in a variety of industrial and consumer products based on their ability to repel water as well as oil. Their endocrine-disrupting activity centers around sex hormone disruption that affects male reproductive health following early life exposure [63]. Among the perfluorinated chemicals most examined for immunotoxicity is perfluorooctanoic acid (PFOA). Several recent investigations suggest that this is a particularly hazardous disruptor of immune homeostasis, producing numerous disease-promoting outcomes [64]. PFOA can activate the alpha isotype of peroxisome proliferator-activated receptors (PPARs). Evidence suggests that some (but not all) of its immunotoxicity may involve PPAR-mediated events [65], since PPARα-null mice still show evidence of PFOA-induced alterations in inflammatory gene transcription [66].

Exposure to PFOA is associated with altered lymphoid population and cytokine levels, as well as reduced adaptive immune responses in mice [65,67,68]. In two different investigations with humans, low-level PFOA serum concentration has been associated with significantly reduced antibody responses to routine childhood vaccines [69,70]. These results suggest that in utero exposure to PFOA can contribute to childhood immunosuppression and elevated risk of infections.

Not all immune-related functions are suppressed by PFOA exposure. It has been suggested that PFOA increases inappropriate tissue inflammation, resulting in pathologies and disease in neurological and other systems [71]. In particular, exposure to PFOA appears to deplete glutathione reserves and epigenetically alters glutathione transferase expression [72], increasing the risk of oxidative damage focused on tissues like the liver [73]. Among the elevated inflammatory mediators contributing to hepatic damage are IL-6, cyclooxygenase-2, and C-reactive protein [74]. Adding to the risk, the hepatic inflammatory damage induced by PFOA is exacerbated by a high-fat diet intake [73]. Among the targets of PFOA are mast cells. After exposure, mast cells increase the production and release of tumor necrosis factor (TNF)-α, IL-1β, IL-6, IL-8, and histamine, thereby increasing the inflammatory component of allergic responses [75].

14.2.11 Phthalates

Phthalates are in a category known as *plasticizers*, in that they help to increase the flexibility of plastics. They can be found in many other industrial and consumer products, including food containers, medical devices, personal care products, paint coatings, and the enteric coating on some pill forms of pharmaceuticals. There is evidence to suggest that they are endocrine disruptors [76,77]. Among numerous phthalates, observations have been made regarding phthalate exposure and immune alterations. To date, the most extensively examined phthalate for effects on the immune system is di-(2-ethylhexyl) phthalate (DEHP).

Several different studies have been conducted across different species, age groups, and sexes. The most prevalent finding suggests that phthalates and their metabolites have the capacity to skew immune function and enhance some forms of tissue inflammation, heightening the risk of and severity of certain immune-based diseases (e.g., allergy). For example, in a prospective birth cohort study, Wang et al. [78] reported that the urine phthalate metabolite level in the serum of 2-year-olds was positively correlated with IgE levels. Also, the metabolite level when stratified by quartiles was positively correlated with atopic dermatitis. In the National Health and Nutrition Examination Survey (NHANES) for 2005–2006, Hoppin et al. [79] reported a positive association of phthalate metabolites with allergic symptoms and sensitization in adults, but not in children (6–17 years of age). In mice, exposure to dibutyl phthalate was shown to alter the activity of macrophages, which affected their antigen presentation capacity [80]. Palleschi et al. [81] found that human granulocytes were inappropriately activated following exposure to DEHP.

In a more comprehensive study in rats, Tonk et al. [82] reported increased age-based immune sensitivity to DEHP in the juvenile rat compared with that of the adult. Among the parameters affected were the T-dependent antibody response, NK activity, and macrophage production of TNF-α.

Two studies suggest that exposure to DEHP is associated with increased inflammatory oxidation. Campioli et al. [83] found that in utero exposure of Sprague Dawley rats to DEHP resulted in increased adipose tissue inflammatory markers (e.g., TNF-α) across several doses, and this association was also reflected in the serum of offspring at the highest exposure dose. In addition, gene expression analysis showed alteration in both immune response and inflammatory-associated genes.

14.2.12 Polybrominated Compounds (Flame Retardants)

Chemicals such as polybrominated biphenyls (PBBs), polybrominated diphenyl ethers (PBDEs), and other polybrominated chemicals (e.g., tetrabromobisphenol A, hexabromocyclododecane) have been used in a variety of industrial and home-use products as burn-inhibiting flame retardants. The first category used, the PBBs, were employed to replace the highly toxic PCBs. But as toxicity concern arose with PBBs, they gave way to a myriad of at least 200 PBDEs (then thought to be less toxic than PBBs). However, the potential toxicity and endocrine-disrupting capacities of even the more recently employed brominated flame retardants have become a significant concern [84].

Immune assessment of both human and animal exposure to flame retardants dates back at least 35 years [85,86]. Following continuous exposure of mice to PBDE into adulthood, Zeng et al. [87] found that Th1-driven acquired immune function was suppressed, which was reflected in reduced IFN-γ production, as well as antigen-specific CD8 T cell numbers, proliferation, and function. PBDE-reduced Th1 function is consistent with the finding that exposure of mice to this EDC (producing increased tissue levels of this pollutant) is associated with increased titers of virus (human coxsackievirus B3) in the liver [88] and impaired production of cytokines that are important in antiviral defense in the host [89]. Exposure of mice to some flame retardants has been reported to disrupt cytokine production during the course of viral infection, resulting in inappropriate host tissue immune responses [90].

The effects of PBDE exposure also extend to innate immune cells. Hennigar et al. [91] found that direct exposure of porcine macrophages to PBDE reduced production of pro-inflammatory cytokines (e.g., TNF-α and IL-6). Fair et al. [92] reported that in vivo exposure of adult mice by oral gavage resulted in reduced NK activity and numbers of both peripheral blood monocytes and certain T cell subpopulations. Early life exposure to PBDE was found to reduce the size of both primary and secondary lymphoid organs in the young offspring [93].

14.3 INFORMATION ON OTHER EDCs

Beyond the "dirty dozen" EDCs, several others have been examined for their immunotoxicity and impact on inflammatory processes. Cadmium overlaps in adverse immune effects with several of the other heavy metals. A naturally occurring metal, it is a byproduct of mining and is used in a variety of products from batteries, stabilizers, coatings, and pigments to newer products such as solar panels. It has no identified physiological benefit and has been shown to be an endocrine disruptor [94]. One of the major effects of exposure to cadmium is a shift to a pro-oxidative state through the overproduction of pro-inflammatory cytokines (TNF-α and IL-6) [95]. Cyclooxygenase activity can increase via COX-2 activation [96], and this combination increases the risk of oxidative tissue damage [97]. Immune cell alterations are also driven by cadmium. For example, Chakraborty et al. [98] found that cadmium exposure of mice alter the phenotype and function of dendritic cells. With early life exposure of mice, Holásková et al. [99] reported an alteration in thymic and spleen lymphoid populations by cadmium. The immune cell population differences were associated with altered acquired immune responses, but these outcomes differed between males and females. This is a frequently observed aspect of developmental exposures to EDCs. Sex-specific differences in later life immune outcomes are common following early life exposures to EDCs.

Another persistent pollutant with significant endocrine-disrupting and immunotoxic capacities are the PCBs. These preceded the brominated compounds as flame retardants until their toxicities became fully evident. They are still problematic as environmental contaminants. As with many other EDCs, PCBs appear to skew Th-driven immune function and exacerbate tissue-inflammatory responses. With early life exposures, PCBs appear to elevate the risk of allergic sensitization [100] and childhood asthma [101] while simultaneously suppressing the responses to common childhood vaccines [102,103]. PCBs have also been implicated in vascular inflammatory disease [104]. Finally, exposure to some PCB congeners appears to affect the risk of non-Hodgkin lymphoma [105].

Table 14.1 includes additional examples of EDCs that have been reported to exhibit immunomodulatory or immunotoxic effects [106–116]. The categories include products from antimicrobial soap (triclosan), naturally occurring phytoestrogens in food (genistein), antimollusk (tributyltin) and antifungal (vinclozolin) compounds, drugs (valproate), mycotoxins (zearalenone), and industrial organics (acetaldehyde and nonylphenol). Information

TABLE 14.1   Examples of Other Endocrine Disruptors and Reported Immune Effects

Chemical/Drug	Category	Species	Effect	Reference(s)
Acetaldehyde	Volatile organic compound	Mouse	Exacerbation of airway allergic inflammation in an asthma model	[106]
Genistein	Food component	Rat (perinatal)/ human (adult)	Sex-specific alterations in NK cell activity following early life exposure; anti-inflammatory action with exposures in older adults	[107,108]
Nonylphenol	Alkylphenol	Human (cells)/ mouse	Increased proinflammatory cytokine production by plasmacytoid dendritic cells in human cells; increased allergic lung inflammation in mice	[109]
Tributylin	Organotin biocide	Mouse	Increased thymocyte apoptosis and suppression of both humoral and cell-mediated immune responses	[110]
Triclosan	Anti-microbial in soap	Human	Increased risk of allergic sensitization; anti-inflammatory actions	[111,112]
Valproate	Anti-convulsive drug	Mouse/human (cells)	Prenatal exposure elevates postnatal intestinal inflammation; altered human dendritic cell differentiation via histone deacetylase-inhibiting activity	[113,114]
Vinclozolin	Fungicide	Mouse	Increased risk of macrophage and lymphocyte-driven inflammation in nonlymphoid tissues following embryonic exposure	[115]
Zearalenone	Mycotoxin	Rat	Thymic atrophy	[116]

in this table reveals the importance of both the age of exposure and sex. This can be seen with genistein. For example, perinatal exposure to genistein is generally viewed as problematic for the developing immune system, whereas postmenopausal genistein intake by adult women may produce quite different outcomes and be useful for dampening some inappropriate forms of tissue inflammation. Given the large numbers of EDCs in the environment and the increasing recognition that immune disruption is a major part of risk for both communicable and noncommunicable diseases, this information base is likely to increase in the near future.

14.4 CONCLUSIONS

Purported EDCs, numbering at approximately 1000, are among the most problematic risk factors for human and animal health. By definition, these chemicals and drugs affect hormone systems, and often at low doses of exposure. The immune system, including those immune cells residing in nonlymphoid tissues, is a significant target of EDCs. Perinatal exposure of the immune system can produce long-lasting effects and contribute to an elevated risk of both childhood and adult disease. Significant sex-based differences in immune outcome have been noted for EDCs. Most EDCs examined to date produce the suppression of some immune capacities and inappropriate enhancement of others via disrupted regulation of the immune system. In addition, most alter tissue regulation and the course of tissue inflammation by acting on innate immune cells. Observed changes in EDC-affected tissue inflammation depend upon (1) the specific EDC, (2) the age of exposure, (3) the sex of the exposed, (4) the age at assessment, and (5) the types of inflammatory pathways examined (e.g., neutrophil-, macrophage-, or eosinophil-driven inflammation).

Acknowledgments

The author declares there is no conflict of interest in the preparation of this chapter. He also thanks Janice Dietert, Performance Plus Consulting, for her editorial assistance.

References

[1] Diamanti-Kandarakis E, Bourguignon JP, Giudice LC, Hauser R, Prins GS, et al. Endocrine-disrupting chemicals: an Endocrine Society scientific statement. Endocr Rev 2009;30:293–342.
[2] Dietert RR. Misregulated inflammation as an outcome of early-life exposure to endocrine-disrupting chemicals. Rev Environ Health 2012;27(2–3):117–31.
[3] Environmental Working Group. Dirty dozen list of endocrine disruptors. Online article. <http://www.ewg.org/research/dirty-dozen-list-endocrine-disruptors>; October 28, 2013 [accessed 19.06.14].
[4] Dangleben NL, Skibola CF, Smith MT. Arsenic immunotoxicity: a review. Environ Health 2013;12(1):73.
[5] Farzan SF, Korrick S, Li Z, Enelow R, Gandolfi AJ, Madan J, et al. In utero arsenic exposure and infant infection in a United States cohort: a prospective study. Environ Res 2013;126:24–30.
[6] Ramsey KA, Foong RE, Sly PD, Larcombe AN, Zosky GR. Early life arsenic exposure and acute and long-term responses to influenza A infection in mice. Environ Health Perspect 2013;121(10):1187–93.
[7] Fry RC, Navasumrit P, Valiathan C, Svensson JP, Hogan BJ, et al. Activation of inflammation/NF-kappaB signaling in infants born to arsenic-exposed mothers. PLoS Genet 2007;3:e207.
[8] Bailey KA, Laine J, Rager JE, Sebastian E, Olshan A, Smeester L, et al. Prenatal arsenic exposure and shifts in the newborn proteome: interindividual differences in tumor necrosis factor (TNF)-responsive signaling. Toxicol Sci 2014;139(2):328–37.
[9] Qi Y, Zhang M, Li H, Frank JA, Dai L, Liu H, et al. Autophagy inhibition by sustained over-production of IL-6 contributes to arsenic-induced carcinogenesis. Cancer Res 2014;74(14):3740–52. May 15. pii: canres.3182.2013.
[10] Bourdonnay E, Morzadec C, Fardel O, Vernhet L. Arsenic increases lipopolysaccharide-dependent expression of interleukin-8 gene by stimulating a redox-sensitive pathway that strengthens p38-kinase activation. Mol Immunol 2011;48(15–16):2069–78.
[11] Zhao S, Liu J, Zhao F, Liu W, Li N, Suo Q, et al. Sub-acute exposure to the herbicide atrazine suppresses cell immune functions in adolescent mice. Biosci Trends 2013;7(4):193–201.
[12] Rowe AM, Brundage KM, Schafer R, Barnett JB. Immunomodulatory effects of maternal atrazine exposure on male Balb/c mice. Toxicol Appl Pharmacol 2006;214(1):69–77.
[13] Filipov NM, Pinchuk LM, Boyd BL, Crittenden PL. Immunotoxic effects of short-term atrazine exposure in young male C57BL/6 mice. Toxicol Sci 2005;86(2):324–32.
[14] Rayner JL, Enoch RR, Wolf DC, Fenton SE. Atrazine-induced reproductive tract alterations after transplacental and/or lactational exposure in male Long-Evans rats. Toxicol Appl Pharmacol 2007;218(3):238–48.
[15] Stanko JP, Enoch RR, Rayner JL, Davis CC, Wolf DC, et al. Effects of prenatal exposure to a low dose atrazine metabolite mixture on pubertal timing and prostate development of male Long-Evans rats. Reprod Toxicol 2010;30:540–9.
[16] Spanier AJ, Kahn RS, Kunselman AR, Hornung R, Xu Y, et al. Prenatal exposure to bisphenol A and child wheeze from birth to 3 years of age. Environ Health Perspect 2012;120:916–20.

[17] Bauer SM, Roy A, Emo J, Chapman TJ, Georas SN, Lawrence BP. The effects of maternal exposure to bisphenol A on allergic lung inflammation into adulthood. Toxicol Sci 2012;130(1):82–93.

[18] Midoro-Horiuti T, Tiwari R, Watson CS, Goldblum RM. Maternal bisphenol a exposure promotes the development of experimental asthma in mouse pups. Environ Health Perspect 2010;118:273–7.

[19] Braniste V, Jouault A, Gaultier E, Polizzi A, Buisson-Brenac C, et al. Impact of oral bisphenol A at reference doses on intestinal barrier function and sex differences after perinatal exposure in rats. Proc Natl Acad Sci USA 2010;107:448–53.

[20] O'Brien E, Dolinoy DC, Mancuso P. Perinatal bisphenol A exposures increase production of pro-inflammatory mediators in bone marrow-derived mast cells of adult mice. J Immunotoxicol 2014;11(1):84–9.

[21] Hogaboam JP, Moore AJ, Lawrence BP. The aryl hydrocarbon receptor affects distinct tissue compartments during ontogeny of the immune system. Toxicol Sci 2008;102:160–70.

[22] Stockinger B, Di Meglio P, Gialitakis M, Duarte JH. The aryl hydrocarbon receptor: multitasking in the immune system. Annu Rev Immunol 2014;32:403–32.

[23] Hanieh H. Toward understanding the role of aryl hydrocarbon receptor in the immune system: current progress and future trends. Biomed Res Int 2014;2014:520763.

[24] Vogel CF, Khan EM, Leung PS, Gershwin ME, Chang WL, Wu D, et al. Cross-talk between aryl hydrocarbon receptor and the inflammatory response: a role for nuclear factor-κB. J Biol Chem 2014;289(3):1866–75.

[25] Jin GB, Moore AJ, Head JL, Neumiller JJ, Lawrence BP. Aryl hydrocarbon receptor activation reduces dendritic cell function during influenza virus infection. Toxicol Sci 2010;116:514–22.

[26] Jin GB, Winans B, Martin KC, Lawrence BP. New insights into the role of the aryl hydrocarbon receptor in the function of CD11c(+) cells during respiratory viral infection. Eur J Immunol 2014;44(6):1685–98.

[27] Kim MJ, Pelloux V, Guyot E, Tordjman J, Bui LC, et al. Inflammatory pathway genes belong to major targets of persistent organic pollutants in adipose cells. Environ Health Perspect 2012;120:508–14.

[28] Ahrenhoerster LS, Tate ER, Lakatos PA, Wang X, Laiosa MD. Developmental exposure to 2,3,7,8 tetrachlorodibenzo-*p*-dioxin attenuates capacity of hematopoietic stem cells to undergo lymphocyte differentiation. Toxicol Appl Pharmacol 2014;277(2):172–82.

[29] Ishikawa S. Children's immunology, what can we learn from animal studies: impaired mucosal immunity in the gut by 2,3,7,8-tetrachlorodibenzo-*p*-dioxin (TCDD): a possible role for allergic sensitization. J Toxicol Sci 2009;34(Suppl. 2):SP349–SP361.

[30] Miyashita C, Sasaki S, Saijo Y, Washino N, Okada E, et al. Effects of prenatal exposure to dioxin-like compounds on allergies and infections during infancy. Environ Res 2011;111:551–8.

[31] Pierre S, Chevallier A, Teixeira-Clerc F, Ambolet-Camoit A, Bui LC, Bats AS, et al. Aryl hydrocarbon receptor-dependent induction of liver fibrosis by dioxin. Toxicol Sci 2014;137(1):114–24.

[32] Sugai E, Yoshioka W, Kakeyama M, Ohsako S, Tohyama C. *In utero* and lactational exposure to 2,3,7,8-tetrachlorodibenzo-*p*-dioxin modulates dysregulation of the lipid metabolism in mouse offspring fed a high-calorie diet. J Appl Toxicol 2014;34(3):296–306.

[33] Warner M, Mocarelli P, Brambilla P, Wesselink A, Samuels S, Signorini S, et al. Diabetes, metabolic syndrome, and obesity in relation to serum dioxin concentrations: the Seveso women's health study. Environ Health Perspect 2013;121(8):906–11.

[34] Exon JH, Mather GG, Bussiere JL, Olson DP, Talcott PA. Effects of subchronic exposure of rats to 2-methoxyethanol or 2-butoxyethanol: thymic atrophy and immunotoxicity. Fundam Appl Toxicol 1991;16(4):830–40.

[35] Singh P, Zhao S, Blaylock BL. Topical exposure to 2-butoxyethanol alters immune responses in female BALB/c mice. Int J Toxicol 2001;20(6):383–90.

[36] Klaunig JE, Kamendulis LM. Mode of action of butoxyethanol-induced mouse liver hemangiosarcomas and hepatocellular carcinomas. Toxicol Lett 2005;156(1):107–15. 28.

[37] Kamendulis LM, Corthals SM, Klaunig JE. Kupffer cells participate in 2-butoxyethanol-induced liver hemangiosarcomas. Toxicology 2010;270(2–3):131–6.

[38] Laifenfeld D, Gilchrist A, Drubin D, Jorge M, Eddy SF, Frushour BP, et al. The role of hypoxia in 2-butoxyethanol-induced hemangiosarcoma. Toxicol Sci 2010;113(1):254–66.

[39] Gao D, Mondal TK, Lawrence DA. Lead effects on development and function of bone marrow-derived dendritic cells promote Th2 immune responses. Toxicol Appl Pharmacol 2007;222(1):69–79.

[40] Heo Y, Lee BK, Ahn KD, Lawrence DA. Serum IgE elevation correlates with blood lead levels in battery manufacturing workers. Hum Exp Toxicol 2004;23(5):209–13.

3. CONCERNS FOR HUMAN HEALTH

[41] Bunn TL, Parsons PJ, Kao E, Dietert RR. Exposure to lead during critical windows of embryonic development: differential immunotoxic outcome based on stage of exposure and gender. Toxicol Sci 2001;64(1):57–66.

[42] Pugh Smith P, Nriagu JO. Lead poisoning and asthma among low-income and African American children in Saginaw, Michigan. Environ Res 2011;111(1):81–6.

[43] Hudson CA, Cao L, Kasten-Jolly J, Kirkwood JN, Lawrence DA. Susceptibility of lupus-prone NZM mouse strains to lead exacerbation of systemic lupus erythematosus symptoms. J Toxicol Environ Health A 2003;66(10):895–918.

[44] Leifer CA, Dietert RR. Early life environment and developmental immunotoxicity in inflammatory dysfunction and disease. Toxicol Environ Chem 2011;93(7):1463–85.

[45] Knowles SO, Donaldson WE. Dietary modification of lead toxicity: effects on fatty acid and eicosanoid metabolism in chicks. Comp Biochem Physiol C 1990;95:99–104.

[46] Pineda-Zavaleta AP, García-Vargas G, Borja-Aburto VH, Acosta-Saavedra LC, Vera Aguilar E, et al. Nitric oxide and superoxide anion production in monocytes from children exposed to arsenic and lead in region Lagunera, Mexico. Toxicol Appl Pharmacol 2004;198:283–90.

[47] Vaziri ND. Mechanisms of lead-induced hypertension and cardiovascular disease. Am J Physiol Heart Circ Physiol 2008;295:H454–65.

[48] Motts JA, Shirley DL, Silbergeld EK, Nyland JF. Novel biomarkers of mercury-induced autoimmune dysfunction: a cross-sectional study in Amazonian Brazil. Environ Res 2014;132C:12–18.

[49] Park HJ, Youn HS. Mercury induces the expression of cyclooxygenase-2 and inducible nitric oxide synthase. Toxicol Ind Health 2013;29(2):169–74.

[50] Pollard KM, Kono DH. Requirements for innate immune pathways in environmentally induced autoimmunity. BMC Med 2013;11:100. http://dx.doi.org/10.1186/1741-7015-11-100.

[51] Nyland JF, Fairweather D, Shirley DL, Davis SE, Rose NR, Silbergeld EK. Low-dose inorganic mercury increases severity and frequency of chronic coxsackievirus-induced autoimmune myocarditis in mice. Toxicol Sci 2012;125(1):134–43.

[52] Fujimura M, Cheng J, Zhao W. Perinatal exposure to low-dose methylmercury induces dysfunction of motor coordination with decreases in synaptophysin expression in the cerebellar granule cells of rats. Brain Res 2012;1464:1–7.

[53] Carocci A, Rovito N, Sinicropi MS, Genchi G. Mercury toxicity and neurodegenerative effects. Rev Environ Contam Toxicol 2014;229:1–18.

[54] Thrasher JD, Heuser G, Broughton A. Immunological abnormalities in humans chronically exposed to chlorpyrifos. Arch Environ Health 2002;57(3):181–7.

[55] Galloway T, Handy R. Immunotoxicity of organophosphorous pesticides. Ecotoxicology 2003;12(1–4):345–63.

[56] Schäfer M, Koppe F, Stenger B, Brochhausen C, Schmidt A, Steinritz D, et al. Influence of organophosphate poisoning on human dendritic cells. Chem Biol Interact 2013;206(3):472–8.

[57] Proskocil BJ, Bruun DA, Jacoby DB, van Rooijen N, Lein PJ, Fryer AD. Macrophage TNF-α mediates parathion-induced airway hyperreactivity in guinea pigs. Am J Physiol Lung Cell Mol Physiol 2013;304(8):L519–29.

[58] Astiz M, Diz-Chaves Y, Garcia-Segura LM. Sub-chronic exposure to the insecticide dimethoate induces a proinflammatory status and enhances the neuroinflammatory response to bacterial lypopolysaccharide in the hippocampus and striatum of male mice. Toxicol Appl Pharmacol 2013;272(2):263–71.

[59] Sunkaria A, Wani WY, Sharma DR, Gill KD. Dichlorvos exposure results in activation induced apoptotic cell death in primary rat microglia. Chem Res Toxicol 2012;25(8):1762–70.

[60] Binukumar BK, Bal A, Gill KD. Chronic dichlorvos exposure: microglial activation, proinflammatory cytokines and damage to nigrostriatal dopaminergic system. Neuromolecular Med 2011;13(4):251–65.

[61] Yu KO, Narayanan L, Mattie DR, Godfrey RJ, Todd PN, Sterner TR, et al. The pharmacokinetics of perchlorate and its effect on the hypothalamus–pituitary–thyroid axis in the male rat. Toxicol Appl Pharmacol 2002;182:148–59.

[62] United States Environmental Protection Agency, DRAFT Public Health Goal for PERCHLORATE in Drinking Water, Prepared by Pesticide and Environmental Toxicology, Branch Office of Environmental Health Hazard Assessment California Environmental Protection Agency, <http://www.oehha.ca.gov/water/phg/pdf/120612Perchloratedraft.pdf?utm_source=120712Perchlorate&utm_campaign=Perchlorate+2012&utm_medium=email>; 2012 [accessed 19.06.14].

3. CONCERNS FOR HUMAN HEALTH

[63] Vested A, Ramlau-Hansen CH, Olsen SF, Bonde JP, Kristensen SL, Halldorsson TI, et al. Associations of *in utero* exposure to perfluorinated alkyl acids with human semen quality and reproductive hormones in adult men. Environ Health Perspect 2013;121(4):453–8. 458e1-5.

[64] DeWitt JC, Peden-Adams MM, Keller JM, Germolec DR. Immunotoxicity of perfluorinated compounds: recent developments. Toxicol Pathol 2012;40(2):300–11.

[65] DeWitt JC, Shnyra A, Badr MZ, Loveless SE, Hoban D, Frame SR, et al. Immunotoxicity of perfluorooctanoic acid and perfluorooctane sulfonate and the role of peroxisome proliferator-activated receptor alpha. Crit Rev Toxicol 2009;39(1):76–94.

[66] Rosen MB, Abbott BD, Wolf DC, Corton JC, Wood CR, Schmid JE, et al. Gene profiling in the livers of wild-type and PPARalpha-null mice exposed to perfluorooctanoic acid. Toxicol Pathol 2008;36(4):592–607.

[67] Yang Q, Abedi-Valugerdi M, Xie Y, Zhao XY, Möller G, Nelson BD, et al. Potent suppression of the adaptive immune response in mice upon dietary exposure to the potent peroxisome proliferator, perfluorooctanoic acid. Int Immunopharmacol 2002;2(2–3):389–97.

[68] Son HY, Lee S, Tak EN, Cho HS, Shin HI, Kim SH, et al. Perfluorooctanoic acid alters T lymphocyte phenotypes and cytokine expression in mice. Environ Toxicol 2009;24(6):580–8.

[69] Grandjean P, Andersen EW, Budtz-Jørgensen E, Nielsen F, Mølbak K, Weihe P, et al. Serum vaccine antibody concentrations in children exposed to perfluorinated compounds. JAMA 2012;307(4):391–7.

[70] Granum B, Haug LS, Namork E, Stølevik SB, Thomsen C, Aaberge IS, et al. Pre-natal exposure to perfluoroalkyl substances may be associated with altered vaccine antibody levels and immune-related health outcomes in early childhood. J Immunotoxicol 2013;10(4):373–9.

[71] Hu Q, Franklin JN, Bryan I, Morris E, Wood A, DeWitt JC. Does developmental exposure to perflurooc-tanoic acid (PFOA) induce immunopathologies commonly observed in neurodevelopmental disorders? Neurotoxicology 2012;33(6):1491–8.

[72] Tian M, Peng S, Martin FL, Zhang J, Liu L, Wang Z, et al. Perfluorooctanoic acid induces gene promoter hypermethylation of glutathione-S-transferase Pi in human liver L02 cells. Toxicology 2012;296(1–3):48–55.

[73] Tan X, Xie G, Sun X, Li Q, Zhong W, Qiao P, et al. High fat diet feeding exaggerates perfluorooctanoic acid-induced liver injury in mice via modulating multiple metabolic pathways. PLoS One 2013;8(4):e61409.

[74] Yang B, Zou W, Hu Z, Liu F, Zhou L, Yang S, et al. Involvement of oxidative stress and inflammation in liver injury caused by perfluorooctanoic acid exposure in mice. Biomed Res Int 2014;2014:409837.

[75] Singh TS, Lee S, Kim HH, Choi JK, Kim SH. Perfluorooctanoic acid induces mast cell-mediated allergic inflammation by the release of histamine and inflammatory mediators. Toxicol Lett 2012;210(1):64–70.

[76] Martino-Andrade AJ, Morais RN, Botelho GG, Muller G, Grande SW, Carpentieri GB, et al. Coad-ministration of active phthalates results in disruption of foetal testicular function in rats. Int J Androl 2009;32(6):704–12.

[77] Schug TT, Janesick A, Blumberg B, Heindel JJ. Endocrine disrupting chemicals and disease susceptibility. J Steroid Biochem Mol Biol 2011;127(3–5):204–15.

[78] Wang IJ, Lin CC, Lin YJ, Hsieh WS, Chen PC. Early life phthalate exposure and atopic disorders in children: a prospective birth cohort study. Environ Int 2014;62:48–54.

[79] Hoppin JA, Jaramillo R, London SJ, Bertelsen RJ, Salo PM, Sandler DP, et al. Phthalate exposure and allergy in the U.S. population: results from NHANES 2005–2006. Environ Health Perspect 2013;121(10):1129–34.

[80] Li L, Li HS, Song NN, Chen HM. The immunotoxicity of dibutyl phthalate on the macrophages in mice. Immunopharmacol Immunotoxicol 2013;35(2):272–81.

[81] Palleschi S, Rossi B, Diana L, Silvestroni L. Di(2-ethylhexyl)phthalate stimulates Ca(2+) entry, chemotaxis and ROS production in human granulocytes. Toxicol Lett 2009;187(1):52–7.

[82] Tonk EC, Verhoef A, Gremmer ER, van Loveren H, Piersma AH. Relative sensitivity of developmental and immune parameters in juvenile versus adult male rats after exposure to di(2-ethylhexyl) phthalate. Toxicol Appl Pharmacol 2012;260(1):48–57.

[83] Campioli E, Martinez-Arguelles DB, Papadopoulos V. *In utero* exposure to the endocrine disruptor di-(2-ethylhexyl) phthalate promotes local adipose and systemic inflammation in adult male offspring. Nutr Diabetes 2014;4:e115.

[84] Hood E. Endocrine disruption and flame-retardant chemicals. Environ Health Perspect 2006;114(2):A112.

[85] Bekesi JG, Roboz J, Anderson HA, Roboz JP, Fischbein AS, Selikoff IJ, et al. Impaired immune function and identification of polybrominated biphenyls (PBB) in blood compartments of exposed Michigan dairy farmers and chemical workers. Drug Chem Toxicol 1979;2(1–2):179–91.

3. CONCERNS FOR HUMAN HEALTH

[86] Fowles JR, Fairbrother A, Baecher-Steppan L, Kerkvliet NI. Immunologic and endocrine effects of the flame-retardant pentabromodiphenyl ether (DE-71) in C57BL/6J mice. Toxicology 1994;86(1–2):49–61.

[87] Zeng W, Wang Y, Liu Z, Khanniche A, Hu Q, Feng Y, et al. Long-term exposure to decabrominated diphenyl ether impairs CD8 T-cell function in adult mice. Cell Mol Immunol 2014;11(4):367–76. April 7. http://dx.doi.org/10.1038/cmi.2014.16.

[88] Lundgren M, Darnerud PO, Ilbäck NG. The flame-retardant BDE-99 dose-dependently affects viral replication in CVB3-infected mice. Chemosphere 2013;91(10):1434–8.

[89] Lundgren M, Darnerud PO, Blomberg J, Friman G, Ilbäck NG. Polybrominated diphenyl ether exposure suppresses cytokines important in the defence to coxsackievirus B3 infection in mice. Toxicol Lett 2009;184(2):107–13.

[90] Watanabe W, Shimizu T, Sawamura R, Hino A, Konno K, Hirose A, et al. Effects of tetrabromobisphenol A, a brominated flame retardant, on the immune response to respiratory syncytial virus infection in mice. Int Immunopharmacol 2010;10(4):393–7.

[91] Hennigar SR, Myers JL, Tagliaferro AR. Exposure of alveolar macrophages to polybrominated diphenyl ethers suppresses the release of pro-inflammatory products *in vitro*. Exp Biol Med (Maywood) 2012;237(4):429–34.

[92] Fair PA, Stavros HC, Mollenhauer MA, DeWitt JC, Henry N, Kannan K, et al. Immune function in female B(6) C(3)F(1) mice is modulated by DE-71, a commercial polybrominated diphenyl ether mixture. J Immunotoxicol 2012;9(1):96–107.

[93] Hong SK, Sohn KH, Kim IY, Lee JK, Ju JH, Kim JH, et al. Polybrominated diphenyl ethers orally administration to mice were transferred to offspring during gestation and lactation with disruptions on the immune system. Immune Netw 2010;10(2):64–74.

[94] Henson MC, Chedrese PJ. Endocrine disruption by cadmium, a common environmental toxicant with paradoxical effects on reproduction. Exp Biol Med (Maywood) 2004;229(5):383–92.

[95] Alghasham A, Salem TA, Meki AR. Effect of cadmium-polluted water on plasma levels of tumor necrosis factor-α, interleukin-6 and oxidative status biomarkers in rats: protective effect of curcumin. Food Chem Toxicol 2013;59:160–4.

[96] Huang YY, Xia MZ, Wang H, Liu XJ, Hu YF, Chen YH, et al. Cadmium selectively induces MIP-2 and COX-2 through PTEN-mediated Akt activation in RAW264.7 cells. Toxicol Sci 2014;138(2):310–21.

[97] Almenara CC, Broseghini-Filho GB, Vescovi MV, Angeli JK, Faria Tde O, Stefanon I, et al. Chronic cadmium treatment promotes oxidative stress and endothelial damage in isolated rat aorta. PLoS One 2013;8(7):e68418.

[98] Chakraborty K, Chatterjee S, Bhattacharyya A. Modulation of phenotypic and functional maturation of murine bone-marrow-derived dendritic cells (BMDCs) induced by cadmium chloride. Int Immunopharmacol 2014;20(1):131–40.

[99] Holásková I, Elliott M, Hanson ML, Schafer R, Barnett JB. Prenatal cadmium exposure produces persistent changes to thymus and spleen cell phenotypic repertoire as well as the acquired immune response. Toxicol Appl Pharmacol 2012;265(2):181–9.

[100] Grandjean P, Poulsen LK, Heilmann C, Steuerwald U, Weihe P. Allergy and sensitization during childhood associated with prenatal and lactational exposure to marine pollutants. Environ Health Perspect 2010;118(10):1429–33.

[101] Hansen S, Strøm M, Olsen SF, Maslova E, Rantakokko P, Kiviranta H, et al. Maternal concentrations of persistent organochlorine pollutants and the risk of asthma in offspring: results from a prospective cohort with 20 years of follow-up. Environ Health Perspect 2014;122(1):93–9.

[102] Heilmann C, Budtz-Jørgensen E, Nielsen F, Heinzow B, Weihe P, Grandjean P. Serum concentrations of antibodies against vaccine toxoids in children exposed perinatally to immunotoxicants. Environ Health Perspect 2010;118(10):1434–8.

[103] Stølevik SB, Nygaard UC, Namork E, Haugen M, Meltzer HM, Alexander J, et al. Prenatal exposure to polychlorinated biphenyls and dioxins from the maternal diet may be associated with immunosuppressive effects that persist into early childhood. Food Chem Toxicol 2013;51:165–72.

[104] Petriello MC, Newsome B, Hennig B. Influence of nutrition in PCB-induced vascular inflammation. Environ Sci Pollut Res Int 2014;21(10):6410–8.

[105] Freeman MD, Kohles SS. Plasma levels of polychlorinated biphenyls, non-Hodgkin lymphoma, and causation. J Environ Public Health 2012;2012:258981.

[106] Kawano T, Matsuse H, Fukahori S, Tsuchida T, Nishino T, Fukushima C, et al. Acetaldehyde at a low concentration synergistically exacerbates allergic airway inflammation as an endocrine-disrupting chemical and as a volatile organic compound. Respiration 2012;84(2):135–41.

[107] Guo TL, White Jr KL, Brown RD, Delclos KB, Newbold RR, Weis C, et al. Genistein modulates splenic natural killer cell activity, antibody-forming cell response, and phenotypic marker expression in F(0) and F(1) generations of Sprague-Dawley rats. Toxicol Appl Pharmacol 2002;181(3):219–27.

[108] Bime C, Wei CY, Holbrook J, Smith LJ, Wise RA. Association of dietary soy genistein intake with lung function and asthma control: a post-hoc analysis of patients enrolled in a prospective multicentre clinical trial. Prim Care Respir J 2012;21(4):398–404.

[109] Hung CH, Yang SN, Wang YF, Liao WT, Kuo PL, Tsai EM, et al. Environmental alkylphenols modulate cytokine expression in plasmacytoid dendritic cells. PLoS One 2013;8(9):e73534.

[110] Chen Q, Zhang Z, Zhang R, Niu Y, Bian X, Zhang Q. Tributyltin chloride-induced immunotoxicity and thymocyte apoptosis are related to abnormal Fas expression. Int J Hyg Environ Health 2011;214(2):145–50.

[111] Savage JH, Matsui EC, Wood RA, Keet CA. Urinary levels of triclosan and parabens are associated with aeroallergen and food sensitization. J Allergy Clin Immunol 2012;130(2):453–60. e7.

[112] Barros SP, Wirojchanasak S, Barrow DA, Panagakos FS, Devizio W, Offenbacher S. Triclosan inhibition of acute and chronic inflammatory gene pathways. J Clin Periodontol 2010;37(5):412–8.

[113] de Theije CG, Koelink PJ, Korte-Bouws GA, Lopes da Silva S, Korte SM, Olivier B, et al. Intestinal inflammation in a murine model of autism spectrum disorders. Brain Behav Immun 2014;37:240–7.

[114] Arbez J, Lamarthée B, Gaugler B, Saas P. Histone deacetylase inhibitor valproic acid affects plasmacytoid dendritic cells phenotype and function. Immunobiology 2014;219(8):637–43. Mar 29. pii: S0171-2985(14)00061-8.

[115] Anway MD, Leathers C, Skinner MK. Endocrine disruptor vinclozolin induced epigenetic transgenerational adult-onset disease. Endocrinology 2006;147(12):5515–23.

[116] Hueza IM, Raspantini PC, Raspantini LE, Latorre AO, Górniak SL. Zearalenone, an estrogenic mycotoxin, is an immunotoxic compound. Toxins (Basel) 2014;6(3):1080–95.

3. CONCERNS FOR HUMAN HEALTH

Endocrine Disruption and Disorders of Energy Metabolism

Philippa D. Darbre

Abstract

This chapter discusses emerging evidence that exposure to endocrine-disrupting chemicals (EDCs) can interfere in endocrine regulation of energy metabolism, and in so doing, lead to the development of obesity, metabolic syndrome, type 2 diabetes, and cardiovascular disease. The prevalence of obesity has increased markedly in recent decades, and although genetic predisposition, excessive food intake, and lack of exercise all contribute to the trend, evidence is accumulating that some EDCs, termed *obesogens*, can disrupt lipid homeostasis, promoting adipogenesis and lipid accumulation and leading to weight gain and obesity. Worldwide incidence of type 2 diabetes is also rising, having already doubled over the past three decades, and some EDCs have been shown capable of disrupting glucose homeostasis and giving rise to hyperglycemia and insulin resistance. Emerging evidence that EDCs may affect cardiovascular disease is discussed, as are the wider implications of the obesogenic activity of EDCs being able to increase body burdens of lipophilic environmental pollutant chemicals.

15.1 INTRODUCTION

In the human body, the endocrine system plays a central role in regulating the utilization of fuels, including carbohydrate, fats, and protein. Hormones are responsible for the storage of excess fuel in times of plenty and mobilization of stored fuel in times of need. Alteration to any of these hormonally controlled processes can be expected to lead to imbalances in metabolism. Diseases resulting from disordered metabolism, such as obesity, metabolic syndrome, type 2 diabetes, and cardiovascular disease (CVD), are continuing to rise in human populations. Established risk factors are genetic predisposition, excessive food intake, and lack of exercise, but these alone cannot account for the disease trends. This chapter discusses the emerging evidence that exposure to endocrine-disrupting chemicals (EDCs) may also be involved.

15.2 EDCs AND OBESITY

In Western countries, a body mass index (BMI) of 25–30 kg/m^2 is considered overweight and of greater than 30 kg/m^2 as obese. (BMI is obtained by dividing a person's weight in kilograms by the square of their height in meters.) The incidence of obesity has risen sharply over recent decades in many parts of the world, as shown by statistics collated by the Organisation for Economic Cooperation and Development (OECD) and given in Figure 15.1 [1]. In the United Kingdom, over 20% of adults are now obese, and in the United States, over 30% of adults are obese (Figure 15.1) [1]. Furthermore, obesity in children is

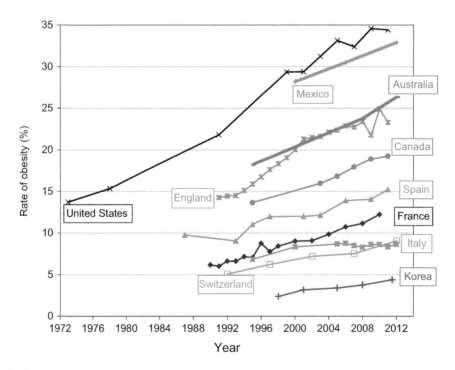

FIGURE 15.1 Trends to increasing obesity in 10 OECD countries. Age- and gender-adjusted rates of obesity and overweight in 2005 OECD standard populations. Measured height and weight in Australia, England, Korea, Mexico, and the United States; self-reported in other countries. No projections were produced in 2010 for Australia, Mexico, and Switzerland. *Source: Reproduced with permission from the 2014 OECD Obesity update [1]; OECD analysis of health survey data.*

also increasing in Westernized countries; in the United States, around 20% of children aged 3–17 years are obese (Figure 15.2) [1]. Although genetic predisposition and excessive food intake coupled with lack of exercise all contribute to these trends, evidence has been accumulating that exposure to some EDCs can interfere in regulation of energy metabolism, causing an altered balance toward weight gain and obesity in spite of normal diet and exercise patterns. This was first proposed in a review in 2002 [2], and such EDCs have now been termed *obesogens* [3,4]. An especially sensitive time frame for exposure has been found to be either prior to birth in utero or in the neonatal period [4], and this has been discussed in Chapter 13.

Animal models have shown that exposure of pregnant mice to tributyltin results in offspring that are heavier than those not exposed [5]. Neonatal mice exposed to the synthetic estrogen diethylstilbestrol (DES) have also been reported to have increased body weight [6]. Figure 15.3 shows a representative photomicrograph at 4–6 months of age of control and neonatal DES-treated female mice: the mice were treated on days 1–5 of age with 1 μg DES/kg body weight/day, and obesity was evident by 4–6 months of age [6]. Other animal models have shown that exposure to some polychlorinated biphenyls (PCBs) [7] and bisphenol A (BPA) [8] can also predispose animals to weight gain and obesity.

There are some epidemiological studies supporting the concept that exposure to EDCs may cause weight gain in children [9–11]. The strongest evidence comes from studies showing that babies born to mothers who smoked tobacco had a low birth weight but were at

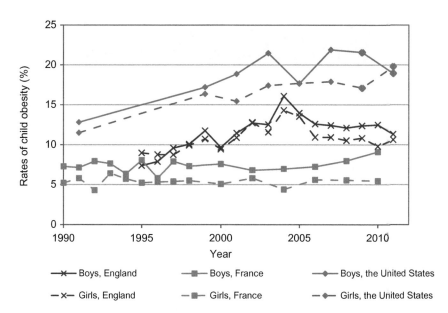

FIGURE 15.2   Trends in child obesity for children aged 3–17 years for the United States, England, and France. Note: Age-standardized rates, 2005 OECD standard population. Measured height and weight in England and the United States, self-reported in France. Rates are based on World Health Organization (WHO) child obesity threshold. *Source: Reproduced with permission from the 2014 OECD Obesity update [1]; OECD estimates based on national health surveys.*

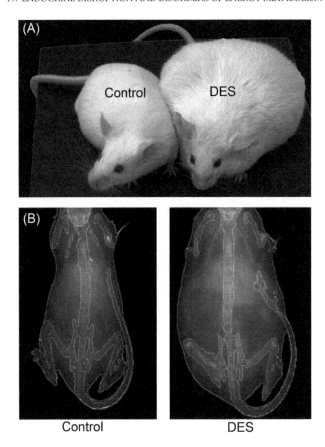

FIGURE 15.3   Effects of exposure to DES in the neonatal period on obesity of mice at 4–6 months of age. (A) Photographs and (B) Piximus densitometry images for control and DES-treated mice show a difference in body size. *Source: Reproduced with permission from Newbold et al. [3].*

increased risk of obesity, metabolic syndrome, and CVD later in life [12]; and meta-analysis of multiple studies confirms that early life exposure to some components of tobacco smoke can lead to later obesity [13]. Other studies have shown that exposures to dichlorodiphe-nyldichloroethylene (DDE), some PCBs, hexachlorobenzene, polybrominated biphenyls, beta-hexachlorocyclohexane, oxychlordane, some dioxins, some furans [14], and phthalates [15,16] are associated with increased body weight.

15.2.1 Mechanisms of Action

Obesogens cause weight gain by altering lipid homeostasis to promote adipogenesis and lipid accumulation, and this may occur by multiple mechanisms, including the following:

- Increasing the number of fat cells (adipocytes)
- Increasing the size of fat cells (adipocytes), storage of fat per cell, or both
- Altering endocrine pathways responsible for control of adipose tissue development

- Altering hormones that regulate appetite, satiety, and food preferences
- Altering basal metabolic rate
- Altering energy balance to favor storage of calories
- Altering insulin sensitivity and lipid metabolism in endocrine tissues such as pancreas, adipose tissue, liver, gastrointestinal tract, brain, and muscle

Obesogens can act to increase adipocyte number and volume by interfering with transcriptional regulators that control lipid flux, adipocyte proliferation, and adipocyte differentiation, particularly through the peroxisome proliferator-activated receptors (namely, PPARα, -δ, and −γ; see Chapter 6). Activation of the retinoid X receptor (RXR)–PPARα heterodimer stimulates β-oxidation breakdown of fatty acids [17]. In contrast, activation of RXR-PPARγ favors the differentiation of adipocyte progenitors and preadipocytes in adipose tissue and regulates lipid biosynthesis and storage [18]. Both tributyltin and tiphenyltin have been shown to stimulate adipogenesis in vitro and in vivo. They are nanomolar affinity ligands for the RXR-PPARγ heterodimer [5,19] and stimulate 3T3-L1 preadipocytes to differentiate into adipocytes [5,19,20] in a PPARγ-dependent manner [21,22]. Cell culture studies using the 3T3L1 model have also shown that both BPA [23] and nonylphenol [24] can promote adipogenesis. The phthalate metabolite mono(2-ethyl-hexyl)phthalate (MEHP) is a known potent and selective activator of PPARγ [25] that promotes differentiation of 3T3-L1 cells into adipocytes [26]. Although many phthalates are more active on PPARα than on PPARγ [27], it may be the metabolites that act by PPARγ to cause weight gain. Urinary phthalate metabolites are present in more than 75% of the U.S. population in excess of several micrograms per liter (see Chapter 2) [28], and an epidemiological study has noted an association between phthalate metabolites and increased waist circumference [15]. More recently, the alkyl esters of p-hydroxybenzoic acid (parabens) have also been shown to promote adipocyte differentiation in 3T3-L1 cells [29]. Adipogenic potency increased with the linear length of the alkyl chain [29] and was associated with PPARγ activation [30]. It seems increasingly likely that any ligand for PPARγ will be able to influence adipogenesis and obesity [30]. This poses the question as to whether mixtures of such ligands may also be able to stimulate adipogenesis at lower concentrations than each alone, as already has been shown for the estrogenic effects of EDCs on breast cancer cell growth (see Chapter 10).

Mature adipocytes are generated from multipotent stromal cells (MSCs) of fetal and adult tissues [31]. These MSCs can differentiate into several different cell types in vitro, including not only adipose tissue but also bone, cartilage, and muscle; and exposure of pregnant mice to tributyltin produced MSCs that differentiated preferentially into adipocytes rather than bone and that showed epigenetic alterations in the methylation status of some adipogenic genes [21]. This demonstrates that at least tributyltin can act by altering both recruitment and differentiation of fat cells. A sensitive time for such alterations would be during development of adipose tissue in early life, which may explain the windows of sensitivity during fetal or early postnatal life for the development of obesity (see Chapter 13).

In addition to PPARs, other nuclear receptors also affect adipose tissue development [32]. Steroid hormones can influence lipid storage and fat deposition. Estrogenic hormone replacement therapy can protect against many age- and menopause-related changes in adipose depot remodeling [33]. Dietary soy phytoestrogens, such as genistein and daidzein, modulate estrogen receptor signaling and reverse truncal fat accumulation in postmenopausal women and in ovariectomized rodent models [34,35]. However, fetal or neonatal estrogen exposure can lead to obesity later in life. Offspring of rodents treated with phytoestrogens during pregnancy or lactation developed obesity at puberty [36], especially the males [37]. Neonatal exposure to DES initially led to depressed body weight but was followed by long-term weight gain in adulthood in female mice [38,39], although not in male mice [40]. It therefore follows that any EDCs with estrogenic activity may act to mimic estrogen action on adipogenesis. While some EDCs may act directly through cellular receptors, other EDCs may act less directly, by stimulating estrogen synthesis. Adipose tissue is known to be a site of estrogen synthesis, and the cytoplasm of adipocytes contains the cytochrome P450 enzyme aromatase, which converts testosterone to estrogen (see Chapter 3). Several EDCs are now known to be able to influence intracellular aromatase activity [41] and could therefore act indirectly to raise intracellular levels of estrogen in adipocytes, with consequent increase in obesity not only in women, but also in men [42].

Another mechanism of EDC action may be through altering the energy balance between energy intake and energy expenditure. This can occur by altering appetite, satiety, and food preferences. It can also occur through altering physical activity, resting metabolic rate, adaptive thermogenesis, and growth rates. Although BPA has been shown to induce obesity in experimental studies [8] and is present in more than 90% of urine samples in the United States [43], any association between human serum BPA levels and fat mass remains inconsistent [44]. However, more recently, BPA levels have been found to correlate with circulating levels of adiponectin, leptin, and ghrelin in humans, suggesting that BPA may also act by interfering with hormonal control of hunger and satiety [45].

15.3 EDCs AND METABOLIC SYNDROME

Metabolic syndrome is a disorder of energy metabolism, which has become very common in the United States, with a prevalence of 24% of the adult population and rising to 43.5% for those aged 60–69 years [46]. It is characterized by the presence of at least three of the following five symptoms [47]:

1. Central obesity, with waist circumference greater than or equal to 102 cm in men or 88 cm in women.
2. Impaired fasting blood glucose level greater than or equal to 6.1 mM.
3. Elevated blood pressure greater than or equal to 130/85 mmHg.
4. Decreased serum high-density lipoprotein levels less than 40 mg/dL (men) or 50 mg/dL (women).
5. Increased serum triglycerides greater than or equal to 1.7 mM.

In addition to being a risk factor, metabolic syndrome has been considered a precursor to type 2 diabetes [48]. Several studies have now been published linking metabolic syndrome with exposure to persistent organic pollutants (POPs) [49].

15.4 EDCs AND TYPE 2 DIABETES

Diabetes mellitus is a metabolic condition characterized by elevated blood glucose levels. Under normal homeostasis, hormones maintain a constant blood glucose level by

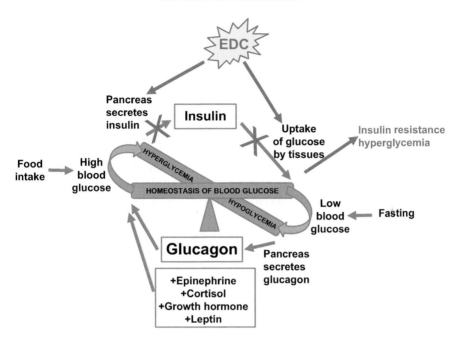

FIGURE 15.4 EDC interference in the homeostatic control of blood glucose. Increased levels of blood glucose stimulate the pancreas to secrete insulin into the blood, which stimulates the uptake of glucose into tissues to restore homeostasis. Decreased levels of blood glucose stimulate the pancreas to secrete glucagon which, together with other hormones, acts to release glucose from tissues and restore homeostasis. EDCs may interfere to cause insulin resistance and maintenance of hyperglycemia.

the combined actions of insulin, glucagon, epinephrine (adrenalin), and cortisol. Fasting blood glucose levels are kept within a narrow range of 4–6 mM, with levels rising only temporarily after a meal to around 8 mM. When glucose levels rise in the blood (hyperglycemia), insulin is secreted into the blood by the beta cells of the pancreas, and it signals to the tissues to take up excess glucose, which is then converted into the storage compounds glycogen (in liver and muscle) and triacylglycerols (in adipose tissue) (Figure 15.4). When glucose levels fall in the blood (hypoglycemia), glucagon is secreted by the alpha cells of the pancreas and causes responsive tissues such as liver to break down glycogen and increase gluconeogenesis to release glucose into the blood (Figure 15.4). Epinephrine (adrenalin), cortisol, and growth hormone act with glucagon to oppose the action of insulin and protect the body from hypoglycemia. Failure of glucose homeostasis in diabetes leads to damaging consequences, especially for nerves and blood vessels. There are two main types of diabetes caused by different mechanisms of failure. Type 1 diabetes (insulin-dependent diabetes mellitus or juvenile diabetes) is an autoimmune condition in which the cells of the pancreas that produce insulin are destroyed. Type 2 diabetes (noninsulin-dependent diabetes mellitus or adult onset diabetes) accounts for at least 90% of all cases of diabetes and results from either inadequate insulin production or resistance to insulin activity.

Type 2 diabetes is one of the fastest-growing worldwide health problems, and in 2010, worldwide prevalence was reported to have risen to 6.4% of the world population for adults aged 20–79 years [50], with estimates of a doubling over the past three decades (from 153 million people affected in 1980 to 347 million in 2008 [51]). Although once considered an adult condition usually occurring in later life (therefore termed *adult onset diabetes*), there has been a dramatic rise over the past three decades in cases in childhood. In 1980, pediatric cases of type 2 diabetes were rare, but by 2012, the rise was such that it now affects 1 in 500 children and adolescents in the United States [52]. The speed of increase in the diabetes epidemic cannot be explained solely by established risk factors such as genetic background, poor diet, and lack of exercise, and EDCs have been implicated [53,54]. Epidemiological studies and animal models demonstrate an association between exposure to a range of POPs and type 2 diabetes [49]. Animal models have shown that BPA can disrupt glucose homeostasis, giving rise to hyperglycemia and glucose intolerance following in utero exposure [55], perinatal exposure [56,57], and long-term exposure in adults [58]. Epidemiological studies also report an association between urinary concentrations of BPA and phthalate metabolites with development of type 2 diabetes [59].

The role of estrogen signaling in regulating glucose homeostasis through ERα- and ERβ-mediated mechanisms has been recognized for some time [60], including modulation of insulin sensitivity and pancreatic insulin secretion [61]. Furthermore, estrogen may also act via a G-protein coupled membrane estrogen receptor to alter insulin secretion [62]. Therefore, it should not be surprising that EDCs with estrogenic activity can also influence insulin sensitivity and glucose homeostasis. However, there does appear to be a difference with length of time of exposure. For BPA, doses of 10 and $100\,\mu g/kg$ have been reported in mice to reduce blood glucose and increase blood insulin over a two-day period, but by longer times of four days, the mice became hyperinsulinemic and insulin-resistant [63]. In addition to affecting insulin, estradiol, DES, and BPA have been reported to suppress calcium spikes that regulate glucagon secretion following low blood glucose levels [64], and so effects may be mediated through modulating not only insulin, but also glucagon.

15.5 EDCs AND CVD

CVD includes all the diseases of the heart and circulation, including coronary heart disease (angina), heart failure, congenital heart disease, and stroke. All these diseases may be caused by narrowing of the arteries from gradual buildup of fatty material on the walls. Obesity [65], metabolic syndrome [66], and diabetes [67] are risk factors for CVD; therefore, it has been suggested that EDCs may also play a role in CVD [68].

The global population is repeatedly exposed to BPA from its use in plastics, and there are detectable levels of metabolites in human urine worldwide [43,69]. Epidemiological studies have shown an association between higher BPA concentrations in urine and cardiovascular diagnoses using studies in the National Health and Nutrition Examination Survey (NHANES) program in the United States for both 2003–2004 and 2005–2006 cohorts [70–72] and using independent European data [73]. Associations between higher BPA exposure (reflected in higher urinary concentrations) and incident coronary artery disease over 10 years of follow-up in the European study showed similar trends to previously reported cross-sectional findings in the more highly exposed NHANES respondents [73]. Peripheral arterial disease (PAD) is a subclinical measure of atherosclerotic vascular disease and an independent risk factor for CVD, and NHANES data from 2003–2004 showed a positive association between increased levels of BPA and PAD [74].

15.6 FINAL COMMENTS ON OBESOGENS AND DISEASE

It is clear that obesity is an underlying risk factor for many chronic diseases, not only diabetes and CVD, but also many cancers [75]. Whether it is the laying down of the fat per se, that obesity is a marker of more general metabolic disorder, or other related mechanisms remains unclear. However, many environmental pollutant chemicals (including EDCs) are lipophilic, and POPs in particular are known to bioaccumulate in body fat over the years (see Chapter 2). It therefore follows that increasing fat deposition through obesity will be associated with a greater body burden of EDCs. Since EDCs are obesogenic as well as lipophilic, their ability to increase fat deposition, which will then enable more EDCs to be retained in the body, could create a continuous spiral of increasing fat deposition and increasing EDC body burden (Figure 15.5). Furthermore, the obesogenic nature of EDCs

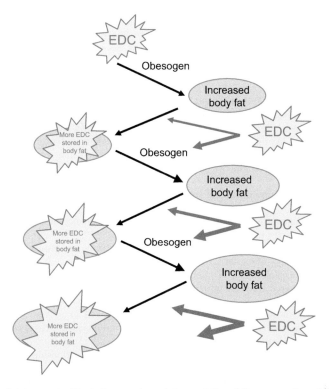

FIGURE 15.5   The "vicious spiral" of obesogenic activity and lipophilic properties of EDCs. The obesogenic activity of EDCs can result in increased body fat: since EDCs are lipophilic, more of them will be stored as the amount of body fat increases. This may occur with an upward trend to more body fat and more stored EDCs, increasing the body burden of EDCs.

3. CONCERNS FOR HUMAN HEALTH

will enable other environmental chemicals with lipophilic properties to also be retained in the increasing fat stores of the body, and such chemicals may be able to act in complementary mechanisms to exacerbate disease processes. For example, in considering the hallmarks of cancer [76], although EDCs may be able to enable sustained proliferation in endocrine-responsive tissues, their obesogenic activity may then cause further accumulation of other environmental chemicals with other properties capable of driving other hallmarks necessary for cancer development. In this way, the obesogenic activity of EDCs may have an even wider impact on disease processes than previously predicted.

References

[1] OECD. Obesity Update, <www.oecd.org/health/obesity-update.htm>; June 2014.
[2] Baillie-Hamilton PF. Chemical toxins: a hypothesis to explain the global obesity epidemic. J Altern Complement Med 2002;8:185–92.
[3] Newbold RR, Padilla-Banks E, Jefferson WN. Environmental estrogens and obesity. Mol Cell Endocrinol 2009;304:84–9.
[4] Janesick A, Blumberg B. Endocrine disrupting chemicals and the developmental programming of adipogenesis and obesity. Birth Defects Res C Embryo Today 2011;93:34–50.
[5] Grün F, Watanabe H, Zamanian Z, Maeda L, Arima K, Cubacha R, et al. Endocrine-disrupting organotin compounds are potent inducers of adipogenesis in vertebrates. Mol Endocrinol 2006;20:2141–55.
[6] Newbold RR, Padilla-Banks E, Snyder RJ, Jefferson WN. Developmental exposure to estrogenic compounds and obesity. Birth Defects Res Part A Clin Mol Teratol 2005;73:478–80.
[7] Arsenescu V, Arsenscu RI, King V, Swanson H, Cassis LA. Polychlorinated biphenyl-77 induces adipocyte differentiation and proinflammatory adipokines and promotes obesity and atherosclerosis. Environ Health Perspect 2008;116:761–8.
[8] vom Saal FS, Nagel SC, Coe BL, Angle BM, Taylor JA. The estrogenic endocrine disrupting chemical bisphenol A (BPA) and obesity. Mol Cell Endocrinol 2012;354:74–84.
[9] Verhulst SL, Nelen V, Hond ED, Koppen G, Beunckens C, Vael C, et al. Intrauterine exposure to environmental pollutants and body mass index during the first 3 years of life. Environ Health Perspect 2009;117:122–6.
[10] Heindel JJ. The obesogen hypothesis of obesity: overview and human evidence. In: Lustig RH, editor. *Obesity before birth*, Endocrine updates, 30. New York, NY: Springer; 2011.
[11] LaMerrill M, Birnbaum LS. Childhood obesity and environmental chemicals. Mt Sinai J Med 2011;78: 22–48.
[12] Power C, Jefferis BJ. Fetal environment and subsequent obesity: a study of maternal smoking. Int J Epidemiol 2002;31:413–9.
[13] Oken E, Levitan EB, Gillman MW. Maternal smoking during pregnancy and child overweight: systematic review and meta-analysis. Int J Obes 2008;32:201–10.
[14] Tang-Peronard JL, Andersen HR, Jensen TK, Heitmann BL. Endocrine-disrupting chemicals and obesity development in humans: a review. Obes Rev 2011;12:622–36.
[15] Stahlhut RW, van Wijngaarden E, Dye TD, Cook S, Swan SH. Concentrations of urinary phthalate metabolites are associated with increased waist circumference and insulin resistance in adult U.S. males. Environ Health Perspect 2007;115:876–82.
[16] Hatch EE, Nelson JW, Qureshi MM, Weinberg J, Moore LL, Singer M, et al. Association of urinary phthalate metabolite concentrations with body mass index and waist circumference: a cross-sectional study of NHANES data, 1999–2002. Environ Health 2008;7:27.
[17] Ferre P. The biology of peroxisome proliferator-activated receptors: relationship with lipid metabolism and insulin sensitivity. Diabetes 2004;53(Suppl. 1):S43–50.
[18] Rosen ED, Sarraf P, Troy AE, Bradwin G, Moore K, Milstone DS, et al. PPAR γ is required for the differentiation of adipose tissue *in vivo* and *in vitro*. Mol Cell 1999;4:611–7.
[19] Kanayama T, Kobayashi N, Mamiya S, Nakanishi T, Nishikawa J. Organotin compounds promote adipocyte differentiation as agonists of the peroxisome proliferator-activated receptor gamma/retinoid X receptor pathway. Mol Pharmacol 2005;67:766–74.

[20] Inadera H, Shimomura A. Environmental chemical tributyltin augments adipocyte differentiation. Toxicol Lett 2005;159:226–34.

[21] Kirchner S, Kieu T, Chow C, Casey S, Blumberg B. Prenatal exposure to the environmental obesogen tributyltin predisposes multipotent stem cells to become adipocytes. Mol Endocrinol 2010;24:526–39.

[22] Li X, Ycaza J, Blumberg B. The environmental obesogen tributyltin chloride acts via peroxisome proliferator activated receptor gamma to induce adipogenesis in murine 3T3-L1 preadipocytes. J Steroid Biochem Mol Biol 2011;127:9–15.

[23] Masuno H, Kidani T, Sekiya K, Sakayama K, Shiosaka T, Yamamoto H, et al. Bisphenol A in combination with insulin can accelerate the conversion of 3T3-L1 fibroblasts to adipocytes. J Lipid Res 2002;43:676–84.

[24] Masuno H, Okamoto S, Iwanami J, Honda K, Shiosaka T, Kidani T, et al. Effect of 4-nonylphenol on cell proliferation and adipocyte formation in cultures of fully differentiated 3T3-L1 cells. Toxicol Sci 2003;75:314–20.

[25] Maloney EK, Waxman DJ. Trans-activation of PPARα and PPARγ by structurally diverse environmental chemicals. Toxicol Appl Pharmacol 1999;161:209–18.

[26] Feige JN, Gelman L, Rossi D, Zoete V, Métivier R, Tudor C, et al. The endocrine disruptor monoethyl-hexyl-phthalate is a selective peroxisome proliferator-activated receptor γ modulator that promotes adipogenesis. J Biol Chem 2007;282:19152–66.

[27] Hurst CH, Waxman DJ. Activation of PPARα and PPARγ by environmental phthalate monoesters. Toxicol Sci 2003;74:297–308.

[28] Silva MJ, Barr DB, Reidy JA, Malek NA, Hodge CC, Caudill SP, et al. Urinary levels of seven phthalate metabolites in the U.S. population from the National Health and Nutrition Examination Survey (NHANES) 1999–2000. Environ Health Perspect 2004;112:331–8.

[29] Hu P, Chen X, Whitener RJ, Boder ET, Jones JO, Porollo A, et al. Effects of parabens on adipocyte differentiation. Toxicol Sci 2013;131:56–70.

[30] Pereira-Fernandes A, Demaegdt H, Vandermeiren K, Hectors TL, Jorens PG, Blust R, et al. Evaluation of a screening system for obesogenic compounds: screening of endocrine disrupting compounds and evaluation of the PPAR dependency of the effect. PLoS One 2013;8:e77481.

[31] da Silva Meirelles L, Caplan AI, Nardi NB. In search of the *in vivo* identity of mesenchymal stem cells. Stem Cells 2008;26:2287–99.

[32] Law J, Bloor I, Budge H, Symonds ME. The influence of sex steroids on adipose tissue growth and function. Horm Mol Biol Clin Invest 2014;19:13–24.

[33] Haarbo J, Marslew U, Gotfredsen A, Christiansen C. Postmenopausal hormone replacement therapy prevents central distribution of body fat after menopause. Metabolism 1991;40:1323–6.

[34] Kim HK, Nelson-Dooley C, Della-Fera MA, Yang JY, Zhang W, Duan J, et al. Genistein decreases food intake, body weight, and fat pad weight and causes adipose tissue apoptosis in ovariectomized female mice. J Nutr 2006;136:409–14.

[35] Wu J, Oka J, Tabata I, Higuchi M, Toda T, Fuku N, et al. Effects of isoflavone and exercise on BMD and fat mass in postmenopausal Japanese women: a 1-year randomized placebo-controlled trial. J Bone Miner Res 2006;21:780–9.

[36] Ruhlen RL, Howdeshell KL, Mao J, Taylor JA, Bronson FH, Newbold RR, et al. Low phytoestrogen levels in feed increase fetal serum estradiol resulting in the "fetal estrogenization syndrome" and obesity in CD-1 mice. Environ Health Perspect 2008;116:322–8.

[37] Penza M, Montani C, Romani A, Vignolini P, Pampaloni B, Tanini A, et al. Genistein affects adipose tissue deposition in a dose-dependent and gender-specific manner. Endocrinology 2006;147:5740–51.

[38] Newbold RR, Padilla-Banks E, Jefferson WN. Adverse effects of the model environmental estrogen diethylstilbestrol are transmitted to subsequent generations. Endocrinology 2006;147(Suppl. 6):S11–7.

[39] Newbold RR, Padilla-Banks E, Snyder RJ, Jefferson WN. Perinatal exposure to environmental estrogens and the development of obesity. Mol Nutr Food Res 2007;51:912–7.

[40] Newbold RR, Padilla-Banks E, Jefferson WN, Heindel JJ. Effects of endocrine disruptors on obesity. Int J Androl 2008;31:201–8.

[41] Whitehead SA, Rice S. Endocrine-disrupting chemicals as modulators of sex steroid synthesis. Best Pract Res Clin Endocrinol Metab 2006;20:45–61.

[42] Williams G. Aromatase up-regulation, insulin and raised intracellular oestrogens in men, induce adiposity, metabolic syndrome and prostate disease, via aberrant ER-α and GPER signalling. Mol Cell Endocrinol 2012;351:269–78.

[43] Calafat AM, Ye X, Wong LY, Reidy JA, Needham LL. Exposure of the U.S. population to bisphenol A and 4-tertiary-octylphenol: 2003–2004. Environ Health Perspect 2008;116:39–44.

[44] Oppeneer SJ, Robien K. Bisphenol A exposure and associations with obesity among adults: a critical review. Public Health Nutr 2014;14:1–17.

[45] Rönn M, Lind L, Örberg J, Kullberg J, Söderberg S, Larsson A, et al. Bisphenol A is related to circulating levels of adiponectin, leptin and ghrelin, but not to fat mass or fat distribution in humans. Chemosphere 2014;112:42–8.

[46] Ford ES, Giles WH, Dietz WH. Prevalence of metabolic syndrome among US adults: findings from the third National Health and Nutrition Examination Survey. JAMA 2002;287:356–9.

[47] NCEP ATP-III Third report of the National Cholesterol Education Program (NCEP) Expert Panel on Detection, Evaluation, and Treatment of High Blood Cholesterol in Adults (Adult Treatment Panel III) final report. Circulation 2002;106:3143–421.

[48] Lorenzo C, Okoloise M, Williams K, Stern MP, Haffner SM. The metabolic syndrome as predictor of type 2 diabetes: the San Antonio Heart Study. Diabetes Care 2003;26:3153–9.

[49] Crinion WJ. The role of persistent organic pollutants in the worldwide epidemic of type 2 diabetes mellitus and the possible connection to farmed Atlantic salmon (*Salmo salar*). Altern Med Rev 2011;16:301–13.

[50] Shaw JE, Sicree RA, Zimmet PZ. Global estimates of the prevalence of diabetes for 2010 and 2030. Diabetes Res Clin Pract 2010;87:4–14.

[51] Danaei G, Finucane MM, Lu Y, Singh GM, Cowan MJ, Paciorek CJ, et al. National, regional, and global trends in fasting plasma glucose and diabetes prevalence since 1980: systematic analysis of health examination surveys and epidemiological studies with 370 country-years and 2.7 million participants. Lancet 2011;378:31–40.

[52] Cizza G, Brown RJ, Rothe KI. Rising incidence and challenges of childhood diabetes. A mini review. J Endocrinol Invest 2012;35:541–6.

[53] Alonso-Magdalena P, Quesada I, Nadal A. Endocrine disruptors in the etiology of type 2 diabetes mellitus. Nat Rev Endocrinol 2011;7:346–53.

[54] Thayer KA, Heindel JJ, Bucher JR, Gallo MA. Role of environmental chemicals in diabetes and obesity: a National Toxicology Program workshop review. Environ Health Perspect 2012;120:779–89.

[55] Alonso-Magdalena P, Vieira E, Soriano S, Menes L, Burks D, Quesada I, et al. Bisphenol A exposure during pregnancy disrupts glucose homeostasis in mothers and adult male offspring. Environ Health Perspect 2010;118:1243–50.

[56] Wei J, Lin Y, Li Y, Ying C, Chen J, Song L, et al. Perinatal exposure to bisphenol A at reference dose predisposes offspring to metabolic syndrome in adult rats on a high-fat diet. Endocrinology 2011;152:3049–61.

[57] Liu J, Yu P, Qian W, Li Y, Zhao J, Huan F, et al. Perinatal bisphenol A exposure and adult glucose homeostasis: identifying critical windows of exposure. PLoS One 2013;8:e64143.

[58] Marmugi A, Lasserre F, Beuzelin D, Ducheix S, Huc L, Polizzi A, et al. Adverse effects of long-term exposure to bisphenol A during childhood leading to hyperglycaemia and hypercholesterolemia in mice. Toxicology 2014;325:133–43.

[59] Sun Q, Cornelis MC, Townsend MK, Tobias DK, Eliassen AH, Franke AA, et al. Association of urinary concentrations of bisphenol A and phthalate metabolites with risk of type 2 diabetes: a prospective investigation in the Nurses' Health Study (NHS) and NHSII cohorts. Environ Health Perspect 2014;122:616–23.

[60] Ropero AB, Alonso-Magdalena P, Quesada I, Nadal A. The role of estrogen receptors in the control of energy and glucose homeostasis. Steroids 2008;73:874–9.

[61] Alonso-Magdalena P, Ropero AB, Carrera MP, Carrera MP, Cederroth CR, Baquié M, et al. Pancreatic insulin content regulation by the estrogen receptor ER alpha. PLoS One 2008;3:e2069.

[62] Nadal A, Rovira JM, Laribi O, Leon-quinto T, Andreu E, Ripoll C, et al. Rapid insulotropic effect of 17beta-estradiol via a plasma membrane receptor. FASEB J 1998;12:1341–8.

[63] Alonso-Magdalena P, Morimoto S, Ripoli C, Fuentes E, Nadal A. The estrogenic effect of bisphenol A disrupts pancreatic beta-cell function *in vivo* and induces insulin resistance. Environ Health Perspect 2006;114:106–12.

[64] Alonso-Magdalena P, Laribi O, Ropero AB, Fuentes E, Ripoli C, Soria B, et al. Low doses of bisphenol A and diethylstilbestrol impair Ca^{2+} signals in pancreatic alpha-cells through a nonclassical membrane estrogen receptor within intact islets of Langerhans. Environ Health Perspect 2005;113:969–77.

[65] Bastien M, Poirier P, Lemieux I, Després JP. Overview of epidemiology and contribution of obesity to cardiovascular disease. Prog Cardiovasc Dis 2014;56:369–81.

[66] Papakonstantinou E, Lambadiari V, Dimitriadis G, Zampelas A. Metabolic syndrome and cardiometabolic risk factors. Curr Vasc Pharmacol 2013;11:858–79.

[67] Sarwar N, Gao P, Seshasai SR, Gobin R, Kaptoge S, Di Angelantonio E, et al. Diabetes mellitus, fasting blood glucose concentration, and risk of vascular disease: a collaborative meta-analysis of 102 prospective studies. Lancet 2010;375:2215–22.

[68] Kirkley AG, Sargis RM. Environmental endocrine disruption of energy metabolism and cardiovascular risk. Curr Diab Rep 2014;14:494.

[69] Ye XB, Pierik FH, Hauser R, Duty S, Angerer J, Park MM, et al. Urinary metabolite concentrations of organophosphorous pesticides, bisphenol A, and phthalates among pregnant women in Rotterdam, the Netherlands: the Generation R study. Environ Res 2008;108:260–7.

[70] Lang IA, Galloway TS, Scarlett A, Henley WE, Depledge M, Wallace RB, et al. Association of urinary bisphenol A concentration with medical disorders and laboratory abnormalities in adults. JAMA 2008;300:1303.

[71] vom Saal FS, Myers JP. Bisphenol A and risk of metabolic disorders. JAMA 2008;300:1353–5.

[72] Melzer D, Rice NE, Lewis C, Henley WE, Galloway TS. Association of urinary bisphenol a concentration with heart disease: evidence from NHANES 2003/06. PLoS One 2010;5:e8673.

[73] Melzer D, Osborne NJ, Henley WE, Cipelli R, Young A, Money C, et al. Urinary bisphenol A: a concentration and risk of future coronary artery disease in apparently healthy men and women. Circulation 2012;125:1482–90.

[74] Shankar A, Teppala S, Sabanayagam C. Bisphenol A and peripheral arterial disease: results from the NHANES. Environ Health Perspect 2012;120:1297–300.

[75] Berger NA. Obesity and cancer pathogenesis. Ann NY Acad Sci 2014;1311:57–76.

[76] Hanahan D, Weinberg RA. Hallmarks of cancer: the next generation. Cell 2011;144:646–74.

PUBLIC POLICY
AND REGULATORY
CONSIDERATIONS

An Introduction to the Challenges for Risk Assessment of Endocrine Disrupting Chemicals

Philippa D. Darbre

Endocrine Disruption and Human Health.
DOI: http://dx.doi.org/10.1016/B978-0-12-801139-3.00016-8

Abstract

This chapter outlines some of the principles on which regulation of endocrine disrupting chemicals (EDCs) depends, and provides an introduction to the concepts of hazard, weight of evidence and risk. Challenges for the regulation of chemicals which act through endocrine mechanisms are discussed. The value and limitations of different types of evidence for the assessment process and the approach of constructing adverse outcome pathways to identify key events and representative endpoints are described. Contributions to the regulatory processes by government, regulatory bodies (national and international), non-government organisations, the media, citizen responsibility and the precautionary principle are outlined.

16.1 INTRODUCTION

A body of evidence, accumulated over recent decades and presented in the first three sections of this book, points to serious long-term consequences if nothing is done to stem the tide of increasing exposure of the human population to endocrine-disrupting chemicals (EDCs). The controversy is now not what the science demonstrates, but the interpretation placed on the science by those with differing points of view and the willpower to act on the science. Realization of the magnitude of the implications of endocrine disruption [1–3] has caused considerable controversy and conflict. At one extreme are those who would like to turn the clock back to live in a world where artificial chemicals are no longer present, and at the other extreme are those for whom economics overrides concern for the environment or human health. The majority of the population live on the continuum in between, acknowledging that some artificial chemicals have brought benefits, but then getting caught up in the whirlwind of modern life, consuming more and more chemicals without further consideration. It is said that "the road to hell is paved with good intentions," and many environmental chemicals have been brought into existence for valid reasons. The problem is how to respond when chemicals brought in for a good initial purpose are then found to have endocrine-disrupting properties. Drugs are extensively tested before release, and even then they are acknowledged to have side effects, but they are taken on the understanding that the benefits will outweigh the adverse consequences. Most environmental chemicals have never even been tested before release, and adverse consequences may fall heavily on those who never had any benefits to counter them. Furthermore, those who have benefited, be it for financial (producer) or lifestyle (consumer) gain, have shown inadequate moral willpower to participate in resolving the consequences, preferring rather to defend the status quo. There is undoubtedly a need for governments to regulate the use of EDCs at the national and international levels. However, there is also a need for producers to be willing to make adjustments for the public good, and for every consumer to start to understand the implications of endocrine disruption and to act responsibly. This chapter outlines some of the principles on which regulatory action depends, and the final three chapters of this book will discuss regulatory needs in the context of EDCs in food (Chapter 17), in water supplies (Chapter 18), and in personal care products (Chapter 19).

16.2 RISK ASSESSMENT FOR EDCs

Risk assessment is a prerequisite for any regulatory action by government. It requires identification of the hazard, assessment of the likely exposure, and consideration of the susceptibility of a person or population (Figure 16.1).

16.2.1 What Is Hazard?

A *hazard* is anything that has the potential to cause harm or, in the context of this book, an adverse health effect in a person, persons, or population of people. Identification of hazards requires knowledge of the types of adverse health effects that could be caused by exposure to one or more EDCs, and hazard characterization requires assessment of the extent and quality of evidence supporting this identification. The scientific evidence may be based on human epidemiology, clinical experience, animal models, or cell culture/in vitro laboratory studies, and involves consideration of both toxicokinetics and toxicodynamics. *Toxicokinetics* considers how the body absorbs, distributes, metabolizes, and eliminates EDCs. *Toxicodynamics* focuses on the mechanisms of EDC actions, including receptor binding, receptor-mediated actions on gene expression or cell functions, and physiological effects in the whole body (animal or human). All approaches have their pros and cons, and consensus is best based on multiple approaches in what is termed *weight of evidence.* Given that extensive controlled testing of EDCs on humans is not possible, weight of evidence is defined as "consideration made in a situation where there is uncertainty, and which is used to ascertain whether the evidence or information surrounding one side of a cause or argument is greater than that supporting the other side" [4].

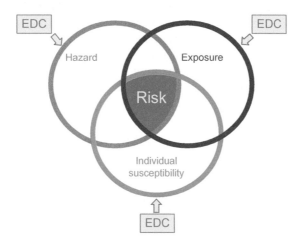

FIGURE 16.1   Components of a risk assessment for EDCs. *Hazard* involves identifying the potency and action of the EDC; *exposure* requires measurement of the amount external to the body and the amount taken into the body; and *individual susceptibility* requires an understanding of how well a person or population may cope with the exposure, especially related to the ease and speed of clearance of the EDC from the body.

16.2.2 What Is Risk?

A *risk* arises when it is possible that a hazard will actually cause harm. The risk has to be assessed, therefore, both for the likelihood of harm being done and for the extent of harm that would be inflicted. For an EDC, this evaluation will depend on the potency and action of the chemical itself (the hazard), the exposure level (the amount external to the body and the amount taken into the body), and individual susceptibility (how well that person or population may cope with the exposure, and especially related to the ease and speed of clearance of the EDC from the body) (Figure 16.1).

Potency and action require consideration of the relation between dose of EDC and likely response. For EDCs, responses may be nonlinear, nonmonotonic, or both (see Chapter 7), which runs counter to classical toxicology, where a higher dose of chemical is expected to give a greater toxicity. Dose-response assessment is broadly a two-step process: first, considering all data available for different assay systems; and second, using this data to extrapolate back to the lowest dose where no effect is observed, often called the *threshold value*. With a margin of error, a no observed adverse effect level (NOAEL) can then be estimated. As with some genotoxic carcinogens [5–8], EDCs may not always have a threshold value for adverse effects [9].

Exposure assessment involves measuring or estimating the magnitude, frequency, and duration of human exposure to an EDC, both in the present and projected into the future. It requires also consideration of the size, nature, and types of human populations exposed to the EDC. Exposure can be measured directly, but more often it is estimated indirectly through measured concentrations in the sources of exposure, and estimates of human intake over time by the relevant route of entry [inhalation, oral, or dermal (see Chapter 2)].

The susceptibility of individuals to EDCs may be influenced by age, gender, genetic background, or presence of other co-risk factors. Genetic background may have many facets resulting from genetic polymorphisms or epigenetic variations, with a range of outcomes. However, one important outcome would be variations in absorption, metabolism, and elimination of an EDC [10]. The presence of multiple EDCs acting by the same or complementary mechanisms may also influence susceptibility [11]. An emerging major influence is the stage of life at which exposure occurs, and many studies now point to early life exposures in utero or the perinatal stage increasing susceptibility to adverse effects in adult life (see Chapter 13) [12].

16.2.3 Importance of Assessing Chemical Mixtures

A main challenge for EDCs is the identification of hazard and risk based not on one EDC, but on multiple EDCs. It is an environmental reality that the human body is exposed to thousands of EDCs from a range of different sources, and both hazard and risk are most likely to result from complex mixtures of EDCs, not to just one EDC. At the current time, most assessments are based on the relation between a single chemical and an adverse health effect, but the reality is that each single EDC may play differing proportional roles in a causative mixture effect. The research need for the future will be to incorporate mixture effects into all studies so that a greater portfolio of mixtures can be generated. The "something-from-nothing" effect demonstrates clearly that cell culture end points [13–15] and biomarkers in animal models [16] can be reached by mixtures of chemicals at concentrations at which each chemical individually would have given no measureable response. Using the case of paraben esters as an example of assessing potential adverse effects on the human breast from comparing measurements of their concentrations in human breast tissue [17] and their concentrations needed for in vitro assays of growth of human breast cancer cells [18], experimental studies showed that some breast tissue samples contain sufficient concentration of one paraben to enable breast cancer cell growth in vitro, but other tissues have sufficient concentration only when all five parabens are mixed [18]. Assessing the effects of parabens on human breast tissue, therefore, must be carried out considering concentrations not of just one, but all five paraben esters [19]. This begs the further question of how much of other EDCs were in those same breast tissue samples and what would have happened if the entire EDC content had been mixed together. At the current time, there are insufficient measurements of EDCs in a single human tissue sample to make such assessments possible. Most measurements have been made on only one chemical, or at most one group of chemicals, and given the very nonparametric distribution of EDCs in human tissues [17,20], this creates uncertainty until full profiles of EDCs can be measured.

16.2.4 Importance of Assessing in Accordance with Mechanisms of Endocrine Action

EDCs challenge current principles of hazard and risk assessment for chemicals because their actions are not nonspecific; rather, they are targeted through biological receptors. Certain principles of endocrinology, therefore, need to be taken into account in assessments of EDCs, and these have been extensively reviewed recently [21]. In brief, the principles are illustrated diagrammatically in Figure 16.2 and detailed as follows:

- Each hormone may act on more than one tissue and may act on different tissues in different ways. An effect on one tissue, therefore, may not predict an effect on another.
- Hormones act throughout life from conception to death, but their effects may differ at different life stages. Exposures during early embryonic and fetal life will influence tissue development, and therefore, effects of disruption would become permanent. Exposures in adult life may be more dependent on continued exposure, and some may be reversible upon cessation of exposure.
- Hormone actions are receptor-mediated. The response of a tissue is, therefore, dependent on the presence of receptors, the concentration of receptors and presence of co-factors that may enhance or repress the hormone effects. The response will also depend on the affinity of the hormone for the receptor.
- Hormones act at low doses, as they have high affinity for their receptors.
- In general, receptor occupancy is low and small changes in hormone concentration can produce large effects. This means that within their effective concentration range, dose responses are nonlinear.
- Dose responses may also be nonmonotonic. Many hormones are known to have different effects at lower than at higher concentrations. Higher levels of EDC exposure/tissue concentration, therefore, may not reflect higher incidence of an adverse effect, but may even signal a separate problem. This fact is discussed in detail in Chapter 7.

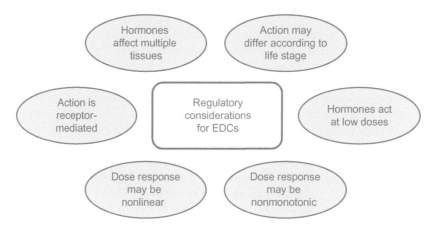

FIGURE 16.2   Endocrine principles that need to guide risk assessment for EDCs, as reviewed by Vandenberg et al. [21].

16.3 VALUE AND LIMITATIONS OF DIFFERENT TYPES OF EVIDENCE

Scientific evidence of EDC actions may be from human epidemiology, clinical studies, animal models, cell culture assays, or cell-free systems, and a range of assays have been described in detail in Chapters 3–6. The challenges for assessment of hazard and risk are how to weight the different approaches, and this requires the use of standardized procedures. The U.S. Environmental Protection Agency (EPA) is developing an Endocrine Disrupter Screening Program (EDSP) [22] and test guidelines are also being assembled by the Organisation for Economic Cooperation and Development (OECD) [23] and the European Union (EU) [24,25]. The precautionary approach of the European Union in weighting the evidence is not without controversy [26,27]. Under the EDSP, the EPA has separated the assessment into a two-tier screening and testing process [22], and this approach has influenced development of testing guidelines in other countries, although ranking within each tier remains under debate [28]:

- Tier 1 screening identifies chemicals that have the potential to interact with the endocrine system.
- Tier 2 testing determines the endocrine-related effects caused by each chemical and obtains information about effects at different doses and different life stages.

The challenge for EDCs is designing tests that cover the entire range of potential endocrine actions. Most test guidelines now incorporate testing for estrogen, androgen, and thyroid hormone disruption, but given the extent of actions of the endocrine system, there are many other endocrine-disrupting actions that remain inadequately covered, and probably also some that remain still to be characterized.

16.3.1 Adverse Outcome Pathways and Representative End Points

Construction of adverse outcome pathways (AOPs) [29] provides an approach to enabling assessment of the complexity by which EDCs may influence endocrine health. An AOP provides a conceptual framework that aims to causally link exposure to an EDC with a sequential and/or branching chain of events at different levels of biological organization, leading to an adverse health outcome. Events along the pathway may include molecular actions, cellular effects, whole organ responses, whole body responses, consequences for a whole population, or any combination thereof [29] (Figure 16.3). This provides a model to support risk assessment based on mechanistic reasoning, but identification of the representative end points for predicting adverse outcomes is of central importance, especially if measurements cannot be made at every step of the AOP, if any one EDC does not act at every step in an AOP, or if multiple EDCs act by complementary mechanisms, requiring combined actions to create the adverse outcome. The extent to which molecular actions can predict later disease outcomes, or the extent to which early reproductive disturbance can be used as an indicator of later reproductive disorders, remain crucial questions for developing reliable risk assessments.

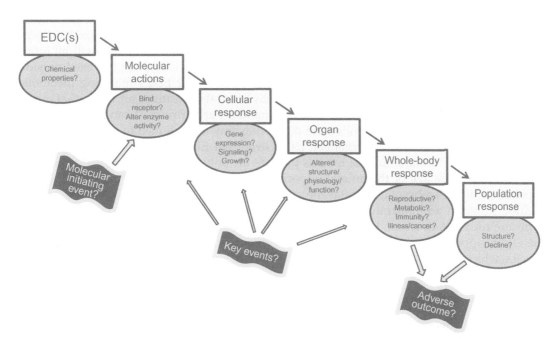

FIGURE 16.3   An AOP may link exposure to EDCs with a series of events at different levels of biological organization (i.e., molecular, cellular, organ, whole body, and population), leading to an adverse health outcome [29]. There may be a molecular initiating event, such as binding of the EDC to a hormone receptor or to an enzyme responsible for endogenous hormone synthesis. This may lead through a series of key events to adverse health outcomes such as impaired reproduction, impaired development, reduced immunity, altered metabolism, cancer, and other ill health.

16.3.2 Values and Limitations of Cell-Free Versus Whole-Cell Assays

Cell-free assays give a very high level of reproducibility, specificity, and sensitivity for detection of a specific event. Receptor-binding assays, especially using recombinant receptors, give very reliable and reproducible dose-response curves, and therefore accurate relative binding affinities of a ligand for a receptor. Such assays can also be amenable to a high degree of automation, and therefore high throughput screening. However, they lack the whole-cell context, which may influence how the event may be modified in the context of a whole cell. For example, binding of a ligand to a receptor may be altered by the presence of other cellular proteins and is no indication as to whether that ligand would act as an agonist or an antagonist within a whole cell. Furthermore, if it is the metabolite of the ligand that has endocrine-disrupting activity, this would not be observed in a cell-free system. The use of cell culture systems can overcome these limitations while still allowing reproducibility. Using a range of cell lines from different tissues can offer the option of investigating differing cell contexts and there are also options to allow for testing in primary cell cultures, in co-cultures of mixed cells (e.g., epithelial and stromal cells mixed), and in organ explants.

16.3.3 Values and Limitations of Animal Models Versus In Vitro Assays

In vitro assays may offer many advantages for screening, but they lack the ability to predict overriding biological effects resulting from indirect as well as direct actions. Absorption, distribution, biological availability, metabolism, and elimination will all influence the ultimate effect on a target organ, and these processes cannot be modeled outside the whole animal. In vitro assays may give false negatives for EDCs requiring metabolic activation not present in the assay system, but may give false positives for EDCs that might undergo rapid metabolic inactivation and elimination. Furthermore, it can be argued that by definition, a chemical can be endocrine-disrupting only if it is linked to a specific adverse endocrine outcome in a whole organism [30]. Given that EDCs cannot be tested in a controlled manner in humans, animal models provide the only option. Animal models have to take account of the age of the animal, especially when assessing effects in adult life from exposure in early embryonic or fetal life, and also need to incorporate multigenerational studies. Route of administration is another important factor and needs to mirror human exposure routes. Animal models also have to take account of species/strain variability, and the effects appearing in one type of animal may not predict for effects in another strain or species, which always leaves open the uncertainty of relevance to the human body.

16.3.4 How to Relate In Vitro to In Vivo Effects in Humans?

Cell culture offers the only option for controlled testing of EDCs directly on human cells, but the difficulty remains as to how to relate effects observed with cultured human cells in vitro with what might happen in vivo in the human body. Widespread administration of diethylstilbestrol (DES) to prevent miscarriage in early pregnancy was a unique event, where effects of exposure to an EDC could be investigated both on the fetus in utero and on the adult mother across a wide population of people, and results could be compared with effects observed in vitro in human cells and in animal models [31]. Future research for other

EDCs will rely on integrating cell culture models with measurements of tissue concentrations of EDCs and the use of epidemiological approaches. A major limitation at the current time concerns having adequate numbers of measurements of EDC concentrations in relevant human tissues and measurements of multiple EDCs in single-tissue samples.

16.4 HOW IS REGULATION BROUGHT ABOUT IN DIFFERENT COUNTRIES?

Regulation is brought about through government action and therefore differs in different countries. In the United States, EDCs are regulated by the EPA. In Canada, EDCs fall within the remit of the government Chemicals Management Plan, launched in 2006 and led jointly by Environment Canada and Health Canada. In the European Union, EDCs are now managed under the Registration, Evaluation, Authorisation, and restriction of CHemicals (REACH) legislation, which was passed in 2006 and came into force in 2007 with implementation phased in over the next decade. REACH applies to chemicals imported or produced in the European Union, and is managed by the European Chemicals Agency (ECHA), which has its headquarters in Helsinki, Finland. Several countries outside the European Union are also moving towards adopting REACH regulations, including China, Croatia, Serbia, Switzerland, and Turkey. Under the REACH legislation, member states can nominate Substances of Very High Concern to a candidate list for restriction or authorization [32].

Although traditionally, chemical regulation has been primarily the domain of national governments, regulation of hazardous chemicals (including EDCs) has stimulated some international initiatives. International cooperation, trade, and travel have created a global economy/community that enables chemicals to cross international boundaries, and this development has served to turn the issue of chemical exposure from a national issue to one of international global proportions. This has been of particular concern in terms of high-production-volume chemicals (see Chapter 1), chemicals that can bioaccumulate, and chemicals with endocrine-disrupting properties. Therefore, it has stimulated the establishment of the following international agreements on regulation:

- The Rotterdam Convention of the United Nations Environment Programme (UNEP; www.pic.int) was established to promote shared responsibility and cooperative efforts in the international trade of certain hazardous chemicals in order to protect human health and the environment from potential harm. The text of the Convention was adopted in 1998 at a conference in Rotterdam, the Netherlands, and it entered into force in 2004.
- The Stockholm Convention (www.pops.int) is a global treaty to protect human health and the environment from persistent organic pollutants (POPs). Initially it concerned 12 classes of POP (see Chapter 1), entered into force in 2004 and was signed by over 150 countries. Since then, further compounds have continued to be added on a rolling basis.

16.5 ROLE OF NONGOVERNMENTAL ORGANIZATIONS

Nongovernmental organization (NGO) is a term used for a group that is not part of a government, is nonprofit, and is set up on a voluntary basis by ordinary citizens. An NGO may be established on a local, national, or international level to address issues in support of the public good. NGOs are task-oriented and driven by people with a common interest to perform a variety of service and humanitarian functions, to bring citizen concerns to governments, to advocate and monitor policies, and to encourage political participation through the provision of information. Several NGOs have championed the issue of endocrine disruption from an early stage and have played a significant role in disseminating information, establishing international awareness, and campaigning for regulatory action on EDCs [33].

16.6 ROLE OF THE MASS MEDIA AND CITIZEN RESPONSIBILITY

The mass media have also contributed significantly to the arena of endocrine disruption through broadcast media (e.g., radio, television, and film), print media (e.g., newspapers, magazines, and books) and the Web. The widespread dissemination of information has had both positive and negative effects, probably roughly equally. On the one hand, mass advertising has served to encourage increasing consumption of a range of consumer goods containing EDCs and has fueled the widespread use of chemicals by portraying them as essential for daily life. On the other hand, reports and documentaries have served to bring awareness of the underlying problems to the general public and to bring education concerning issues of EDCs on a worldwide basis. Many initiatives to remove EDCs from consumer products are now finding their origins in media coverage and resulting generation of public concern, as well as more traditional routes of scientific output and risk assessment. There is little doubt that the general public would wish to contribute to resolving the issues of EDCs, but the problem remains of how to supply accurate educational information in which the public can have confidence. The magnitude of often-conflicting information supplied through the media can cause confusion, and the social pressure to use all the "latest" consumer products provides strong cultural opposition to the simple precautionary measure of not using so many chemicals in daily life.

16.7 PRECAUTIONARY PRINCIPLE

The Precautionary Principle basically reiterates the old sayings "Better safe than sorry" and "Look before you leap" and states that "If an action or policy has a suspected risk of causing harm to the public or to the environment, in the absence of scientific consensus that the action or policy is not harmful, the burden of proof that it is not harmful falls on those taking an action." Concerns for the environment led to the Precautionary Principle being endorsed at an international level initially in the World Charter for Nature by the UN General Assembly in 1982 and was endorsed for EDCs in the Wingspread Statement of 1998 [34]. The European Commission issued a communication on the Precautionary Principle in February 2000 [35], adopted the principle in Article 191 of the Treaty of Lisbon in 2007, and since then, the principle has come to inform much EU policy, including decisions on EDCs under REACH. Use of the Precautionary Principle will inevitably always evoke strong responses from those with differing perspectives, but there is a growing awareness within governments and within national and international regulatory bodies that the issue of EDCs must be tackled. However, with such a complex science and with the challenge that EDCs pose to existing regulatory frameworks, the question is how to strike the appropriate balance between sufficient protection and excessive caution.

References

[1] Diamanti-Kandarakis E, Bourgignon JP, Giudice LC, Hauser R, Prins GS, Soto AM, et al. Endocrine-disrupting chemicals: an Endocrine Society scientific statement. Endocr Rev 2009;30:293–342.

[2] Bergman A, Heindel JJ, Jobling S, Kidd KA, Zoeller RT, editors. The state of the science of endocrine disrupting chemicals—2012. United Nations Environment Programme (UNEP) and World Health Organisation (WHO). Geneva, Switzerland: World Health Organisation Press; 2013. <http://unep.org/pdf/9789241505031_eng.pdf>.

[3] European Environment Agency (EEA). The impacts of endocrine disrupters on wildlife, people and their environments. The Weybridge + 15 (1996–2011) report. Luxemburg: Publications Office of the European Union; 2012. ISBN 978-92-9213-307-B.

[4] Balls M, Amcoff P, Bremer S, Casati S, Coecke S, Clothier R, et al. The principles of weight of evidence validation of test methods and testing strategies. The report and recommendations of ECVAM workshop 58. Altern Lab Anim 2006;34:603–20.

[5] Neumann HG. Risk assessment of chemical carcinogens and thresholds. Crit Rev Toxicol 2009;39:449–61.

[6] Gillespie Z, Pulido O, Vavasour E. Risk assessment approaches for carcinogenic food contaminants. Int Food Risk Analysis J 2011;1:1–18. <http://cdn.intechopen.com/pdfs-wm/20835.pdf>.

[7] SCHER, SCCP, SCENIHR. Risk assessment methodologies and approaches for genotoxic and carcinogenic substances. Brussels: European Commission; 2009. <http://ec.europa.eu/health/ph_risk/committees/04_scher/docs/scher_o_113.pdf>.

[8] Committee on Carcinogenicity of Chemicals in Food, Consumer Products and the Environment. Risk characterisation methods. COC/G 06—version 1.0, <https://www.gov.uk/government/uploads/system/uploads/attachment_data/file/315883/Risk_characterisation_methods.pdf>; 2012.

[9] Vandenberg LN, Colborn T, Hayes TB, Heindel JJ, Jacobs Jr. DR, Lee DH, et al. Hormones and endocrine-disrupting chemicals: low-dose effects and nonmonotonic dose responses. Endocr Rev 2012;33:378–455.

[10] Edwards TM, Myers JP. Environmental exposures and gene regulation in disease etiology. Environ Health Perspect 2007;115:1264–70.

[11] Darbre PD, Fernandez MF. Environmental oestrogens and breast cancer: long-term low-dose effects of mixtures of various chemical combinations. J Epidemiol Community Health 2013;67:203–5.

[12] Schug TT, Janesick A, Blumberg B, Heindel JJ. Endocrine disrupting chemicals and disease susceptibility. J Steroid Biochem Mol Biol 2011;127:204–15.

[13] Rajapakse N, Silva E, Kortenkamp A. Combining xenoestrogens at levels below individual no-observed-effect concentrations dramatically enhances steroid hormone action. Environ Health Perspect 2002;110:917–21.

[14] Silva E, Rajapakse N, Kortenkamp A. Something from "nothing"—eight weak estrogenic chemicals combined at concentrations below NOECs produce significant mixture effects. Environ Sci Technol 2002;36:1751–6.

[15] Kortenkamp A. Ten years of mixing cocktails: a review of combination effects of endocrine-disrupting chemicals. Environ Health Perspect 2007;115(Suppl. 1):98–105.

[16] Brian JV, Harris CA, Scholze M, Backhaus T, Booy P, Lamoree M, et al. Accurate prediction of the response of freshwater fish to a mixture of estrogenic chemicals. Environ Health Perspect 2005;113:721–8.

[17] Barr L, Metaxas G, Harbach CAJ, Savoy LA, Darbre PD. Measurement of paraben concentrations in human breast tissue at serial locations across the breast from axilla to sternum. J Appl Toxicol 2012;32:219–32.

[18] Charles AK, Darbre PD. Combinations of parabens at concentrations measured in human breast tissue can increase proliferation of MCF-7 human breast cancer cells. J Appl Toxicol 2013;33:390–8.

[19] Darbre PD, Harvey PW. Parabens can enable hallmarks and characteristics of cancer in human breast epithelial cells: a review of the literature with reference to new exposure data and regulatory status. J Appl Toxicol 2014;34:925–38.

[20] Porta M, Pumarega J, Gasull M. Number of persistent organic pollutants detected at high concentrations in a general population. Environ Int 2012;44:106–11.

[21] Vandenberg LN, Colborn T, Hayes TB, Heindel JJ, Jacobs Jr. DR, Lee DH, et al. Regulatory decisions on endocrine disrupting chemicals should be based on the principles of endocrinology. Reprod Toxicol 2013;38:1–15.

[22] The U.S. Environmental Protection Agency Endocrine Disruptor Screening Program. <http://www.epa.gov/endo/>.

[23] OECD (Organisation for Economic Cooperation and Development). Draft guidance document on standardised test guidelines for evaluating chemicals for endocrine disruption, <http://www.oecd.org/chemicalsafety/testing/50459967.pdf>; 2012.

[24] European Food Safety Authority (EFSA) Scientific Committee. Scientific opinion on the hazard assessment of endocrine disruptors: scientific criteria for identification of endocrine disruptors and appropriateness of existing test methods for assessing effects mediated by these substances on human health and the environment. EFSA J 2013;11:3132.

[25] Munn S, Goumenou M. Report of the endocrine disrupters—Expert Advisory Group (ED EAG): key scientific issues relevant to the identification and characterisation of endocrine disrupting substances, <http://ec.europa.eu/dgs/jrc/index.cfm?id=1410&dt_code=NWS&obj_id=16530&ori=RSS>; 2013.

[26] Dietrich DR, et al. Scientifically unfounded precaution drives European Commission's recommendations on EDC regulation, while defying common sense, well-established science and risk assessment principles. Chem Biol Interact 2013;205:A1–A5.

[27] Bergman Å, Andersson AM, Becher G, van den Berg M, Blumberg B, Bjerregaard P, et al. Science and policy on endocrine disrupters must not be mixed: a reply to a "common sense" intervention by toxicology journal editors. Environ Health 2013;12:69.

[28] Borgert CJ, Stuchal LD, Mihaich EM, Becker RA, Bentley KS, Brausch JM, et al. Relevance weighting of tier 1 endocrine screening endpoints by rank order. Birth Defects Res B Dev Reprod Toxicol 2014;101:90–113.

[29] Ankley GT, Bennett RS, Erickson RJ, Hoff DJ, Hornung MW, Johnson RD, et al. Adverse outcome pathways: a conceptual framework to support ecotoxicology research and risk assessment. Environ Toxicol Chem 2010;29:730–41.

[30] Testai E, Galli CL, Dekant W, Marinovich M, Piersma AH, Sharpe RM. A plea for risk assessment of endocrine disrupting chemicals. Toxicology 2013;314:51–9.

[31] Harris RM, Waring RH. Diethylstilboestrol—a long-term legacy. Maturitas 2012;72:108–12.

[32] European Chemicals Agency (ECHA). <http://echa.europa.eu>.

[33] CHEMTrust. CHEMTrust overview of key scientific statements on endocrine disrupting chemicals (EDCs) 1991–2013, <http://www.chemtrust.org.uk/wp-content/uploads/Scientific-Statements-on-EDCs-V2-Dec20132.pdf>; January 2014.

[34] The Wingspread Consensus Statement on the Precautionary Principle. <http://www.sehn.org/wing.html>; 1998.

[35] Commission of the European Communities. Communication from the commission on the precautionary principle. Brussels, <http://ec.europa.eu/dgs/health_consumer/library/pub/pub07_en.pd>; 2000.

17

Regulatory Considerations for Endocrine Disrupters in Food

Gerard M. Cooke and Rekha Mehta

Abstract

Endocrine disrupters, chemicals that interfere with normal hormone activity, may get into foods by several different routes, including food-packaging materials, environmental pollutants, and natural plant components. Regulatory decisions regarding food additives and pesticides are based on files that are comparatively data-rich. However, food processing and cooking-induced chemicals, herbal remedies, and supplements can be data-poor, and one can see the complexity surrounding regulatory efforts when it comes to those chemicals in food. Assessments of chemical effects on reproduction require research data on gamete production,

Endocrine Disruption and Human Health.
DOI: http://dx.doi.org/10.1016/B978-0-12-801139-3.00017-X

fertilization, fetal development, and postnatal sexual development. Several validated assays exist to test for possible endocrine disruptive effects at these different stages. However, strategies are needed to assess health or epigenetic effects emerging during later life stages by endocrine disrupter exposure during fetal or pubertal development.

17.1 INTRODUCTION

Endocrine disrupters are chemicals that interfere with normal hormone activity. In a broad sense, chemicals detected in foods that can cause endocrine disruption may be considered either contaminants or are natural constituents of the foodstuffs that have hormonal activity. They can arrive in the food from several different and food-specific routes. Some examples include pesticides that are sprayed onto food while it is growing on the farm; industrial chemicals that through runoff into waterways can contaminate the ground where crops are growing and are absorbed by the plants; food-packaging materials from which chemicals can migrate into the food; feed given to meat-producing animals and fish bred in fish farms that may be contaminated with endocrine-disrupting chemicals (EDCs); seafood caught in waterways that may be contaminated with chemicals; chemicals that are natural to the ground where crops are grown; and natural food components that have endocrine properties (such as isoflavones in soy). These are all sources for possible human exposure to chemicals, some of which may have endocrine-disrupting properties. Add to these situations chemicals that are produced during food processing and cooking that may also have endocrine effects, and the issue of humans taking food supplements and herbal remedies for which there are extremely limited research data available, and one can see the complexity surrounding regulatory efforts when it comes to chemicals in food. Food additives, pesticides, and veterinary drugs are tested extensively for general and reproductive toxicity, and any effects on mammalian reproduction in these tests are required to be indicated during premarket submissions, leading to more confidence in regulatory decision making. For chemicals that may have endocrine effects, the situation becomes even more complex due to the nature of the reproductive process and the need to assess gamete production, fertilization, fetal development, and sexual development to adulthood. There are, therefore, several assays that have been developed and validated to test for possible endocrine-disruptive effects of chemicals in these different stages.

The aim of this chapter is to raise awareness of food-implicated endocrine-disrupting substances and to describe the recommended testing strategies that will provide the relevant data for making regulatory decisions.

17.2 MANUFACTURED FOOD CONTAMINANTS

17.2.1 Pesticides

Pesticides that have been investigated for endocrine-disruptive activities are too numerous to list here. However, some examples that have been documented include the herbicide atrazine, which induces hermaphroditism in frogs and has effects on steroidogenesis in several in vitro systems; organotins used as antifouling agents, including tributyltin, which causes imposex (i.e., females developing male sex organs) in aquatic mollusks and is an inhibitor of aromatase activity; and organophosphates (OPs), which have neurotoxic effects in insects, but some epidemiological studies indicate that prenatal exposure to some OP pesticides may affect the learning development and motor skills of young children [1–4].

When pesticides are submitted to regulatory agencies for approval, sufficient data are supplied by the manufacturer. In contrast to other food contaminants that are possible endocrine disrupters, pesticides are considered data-rich. This is due to the data requirements from several different toxicity tests for chemical safety assessment. Governments in North America, Europe, and Australasia all have their own specific offices that deal with submissions. In Canada, the Pest Management Regulatory Agency (PMRA) of Health Canada receives submissions and is responsible for ensuring the safety of use and the approval process [5]. The occurrence of pesticide residue in foodstuffs where the chemical is used is also important information supplied by the manufacturer. Persistence in the environment has to be a consideration in the approval process, as once the pesticide migrates from the site of intended use through runoff and enters the waterways, there can be absorption into other foodstuffs, such as fish and seafood.

17.2.2 Food Packaging and the Migration of Chemicals into Food

Food packaging and storage materials that come into contact with food consist mostly of plastics and cardboard. The migration of chemicals from the packaging material is a complex but measurable process and depends on the type of material, the properties of the foodstuff (liquid or solid, pH, fat content, etc.), and whether environmental conditions such as heating are involved [6]. Examples of chemicals that are known components of plastics and are considered candidates for causing endocrine disruption are benzophenone, nonylphenol, bisphenol A (BPA), phthalates, and tributyltin. Benzophenone is a component of printing ink used in packaging and has the ability to migrate from the outside of a printed paperboard to the inside, where it can come into contact with the food. Further, the use of recycled paper in the manufacture of paperboard can lead to increased quantities of benzophenone in the packaging material. A comprehensive review of the migration of chemicals from many different polymers used in food packaging has been published [6]. The measurement of the chemicals that leach or migrate out of plastics involves immersion of the plastic in a container with a food "simulant" such as water or a 10% ethanol solution, and after a certain amount of time, the liquid simulant is analyzed for chemicals that have migrated into it. The effect of heating (conventional and microwave) is also measured, as heating tends to increase the rate of migration of chemicals out of the plastic. As an example, Nam et al. [7] showed an elevated migration of BPA from baby bottles with higher temperatures and an increased number of uses (Table 17.1). While the major components that migrate are known for most plastics, the final packaging material may also contain unidentified chemicals termed *nonintentionally added substances* chemically produced by the plastic or the source materials used in the packaging material manufacturing process [8]. Clearly, the food would be exposed to these nonintentional chemicals, but there are no data concerning their toxicity. For the most part, toxicity testing has only considered single components, such as BPA or an individual phthalate; therefore, the toxicity of the entire leachate is unknown. Interestingly, the few studies that have tested

TABLE 17.1   Migration of BPA from Baby Bottles Under Different Conditions

(a) Effect of Temperature

	Temperature (°C)				
	40	50	60	80	95
New baby bottles: BPA (ppb)	0.03	0.04	0.06	0.12	0.13
Baby bottles used for 6 months: BPA (ppb)	0.2	0.4	0.88	1.4	18.5

(b) Effect of Repeated Use

	Number of uses			
	1–10	11–45	60–100	6 Months
BPA (ppb)	0 to 1	~1	1 to 3	18.5

Values approximated from data presented in Ref. [7].

whole leachates have shown that the effects cannot be solely attributed to the major component or putative mixture components, and a more comprehensive approach may be necessary [9,10]. Furthermore, the endocrine-disruptive possibilities of food-packaging materials have not been given the same attention as genotoxic and mutagenic effects [11,12]. However, individual chemical toxicity testing has shown that some components can act as steroid hormone mimics that interact with steroid receptors in in vitro and in vivo rodent models, where they have effects on the reproductive process. For the feto-maternal unit, there are few studies that have examined the absorption, distribution, metabolism, and excretion characteristics of food-packaging materials for estimations of fetal exposure, especially during early pregnancy when the organ systems are being established [13,14]. Infants are consumers of baby foods and formula that are packaged and heat-treated, and later in life, children are large consumers of packaged snack foods (e.g., juice boxes) where the portions are small but have a large surface area–to-volume ratio that would lead to higher levels of migrated chemicals in their food. In addition, their small size per unit weight means that in general, the food consumption of children is higher than adults, and consequently, their chemical exposure estimates will be higher than for adults. Thus, for the purposes of regulating putative endocrine disrupters migrating from packaging into food for fetuses, infants, and children, direct extrapolation from adult exposure levels would be inaccurate; hence, risk assessment for infants takes into consideration these additional parameters.

17.2.3 Chemicals Formed During Cooking and in Heat Treatment Processes

Some chemicals are formed during the process of cooking food or in canning and jarring processes. Furan is a volatile etherlike chemical formed by heating food. The source material for furan formation is debatable, with fats, carbohydrates, and ascorbic acid all having been postulated as precursors for furan formation. The major food source for human furan exposure is coffee. Furan is considered to be a carcinogen due to its ability to cause liver tumors in rodents [15–17]. However, recent studies have shown that furan may affect male reproductive function [18], and thus further research is necessary to determine if furan is an endocrine disrupter. This may be relevant because the heating of jarred foods such as baby food means that the furan does not escape, and as a result, the infant may be exposed to levels that could have deleterious effects. Acrylamide is a chemical that can form in some foods during high-temperature cooking processes such as frying, roasting, and baking. It is formed from sugars and the amino acid asparagine. It does not come from the environment or food-packaging materials. Acrylamide was shown to cause cancer when animals were exposed to very high doses. It is not known if acrylamide is an endocrine disruptor, but some effects on rat thyroid gland morphology [19] and on the hypothalamus-pituitary-thyroid (HPT) axis [20] have been reported. Nitrosamines are formed by the reaction between amines and a nitrosating agent. Foods such as cured meats contain nitrite, and thus such foods will contain nitrosamines and nitrosamides [21]. These food constituents can cause cancer, and a relationship between maternal ingestion and childhood brain tumor incidence has been reported [22]. Thus, there is the possibility that nitrosamines or nitrosamides may be endocrine disrupters, but at present, studies confirming this likelihood are few.

17.2.4 Food Contaminants Resulting from Veterinary Practices

There are other aspects of food-contaminant regulation that deserve passing mention. Veterinary health practices often result in human food containing residues from treatment of animals with antibiotics and hormones, and animal feed that may be contaminated with pesticides and heavy metals presents possibilities for endocrine disruption in human pregnancy [23]. The hormonal compounds are synthetically produced xenobiotics and have estrogenic (i.e., oestradiol-17β and its esters; zeranol), androgenic (i.e., testosterone and esters; trenbolone acetate) or progestogenic (i.e., progesterone; melengestrol acetate) activity [24]. In the developed world, most countries have regulations that abide by set standards or maximum residue limits (MRLs) and inspection agencies that analyze food products for such residues to determine the safety of the foods for human consumption. In Canada, the responsibility to set standards rests with Health Canada's Veterinary Drugs Directorate [25], and the enforcement of these standards is conducted by the Canadian Food Inspection Agency [26]. However, regarding foods being imported or exported, food inspection systems at the sender and receiver countries will be involved. In Canada, other government departments that play a role in food importation include the Department of Foreign Affairs, Trade, and Development and the Canada Border Services Agency; Environment Canada will become involved if the products come under the Convention of International Trade in Endangered Species of Wild Flora and Fauna, also known as the Washington Convention, to which Canada is a signatory [26].

17.3 NATURALLY OCCURRING FOOD CONTAMINANTS

17.3.1 Heavy Metals

Heavy metals that contaminate food and are putative endocrine disrupters include mercury, arsenic, and cadmium. Such metals can enter the food chain from natural earth deposits where crops are grown, but also industrial effluents from mining or manufacturing processes. Exposure in utero to mercury in the form of methylmercury has been shown to have deleterious effects on cognitive development in fetuses and infants [27,28]. Inorganic arsenic is toxic and is ingested by humans through drinking water and food. Arsenic in fish and mollusks that are used as human food primarily takes the form of arsenobetaine (and to a lesser extent arsenocholine). These organic forms of arsenic are formed in vivo through detoxification of ingested inorganic arsenic. Arsenobetaine is minimally absorbed through the human gut and is not considered to be toxic [29]. The results of a recent investigation into the possible endocrine-disruptive properties of arsenobetaine support the conclusion that arsenobetaine consumption during pregnancy would not have deleterious effects for the fetus [30]. Cadmium is known to be toxic to the reproductive system affecting the hypo-thalamic-pituitary-gonadal (HPG) axis at all levels with damage caused to both ovarian and testicular function [31,32]. It is found naturally in the earth and also enters the environment through industrial processes that have cadmium as a waste product. Crops grown in soils with high cadmium content have to be monitored, and other foods that contain cadmium include aquatic species, especially shellfish, which absorb cadmium from the water. The Food Directorate in Health Canada and the Canadian Food Inspection Agency have the responsibility of testing foods for contaminant levels, including heavy metals. Some years ago, it was discovered that durum wheat grown in western Canada had higher cadmium levels because of the cadmium content of the soil in that part of the country. Although the levels were always lower than the internationally recognized limits, this problem was rectified through the discovery that cadmium absorption is regulated by a single dominant gene, and therefore it was possible to select wheat with low levels of this allele, with a resultant decrease in the cadmium content of the wheat. Consequently, the cadmium levels in the wheat grown in Canada are no longer an issue [33].

17.4 NATURAL FOOD CONSTITUENTS

17.4.1 Phytoestrogens

Some foodstuffs naturally contain chemicals that have hormonal activity. The estrogenic activity of some plant phytoestrogens is well known to farmers because of their effects on reproduction in ruminants, causing subfertility and in some cases permanent infertility [34,35]. With regard to human consumption, isoflavones in soy, coumestrol in alfalfa, and lignans in flax are well-known examples of dietary phytoestrogens. Of these, the soy phytoestrogens genistein and daidzein have received the most attention since these interact with the estrogen receptor (ER) almost as well as estradiol itself [36,37]. Soy consumption is thought to be beneficial for cardiovascular health, menopause, and osteoporosis and for reducing the incidence of certain cancers, such as breast and prostate cancer. This is largely based on epidemiological evidence showing that Asians living in Asia have lower incidences of cardiovascular disease and hormone-dependent cancers, but when they immigrate to North America or Europe, they begin to have the same risks for these diseases and complaints as the local residents. Since a major lifestyle difference is the amount of soy in the diet, it has been concluded that soy components are beneficial to human health. On the

TABLE 17.2   Serum Phytoestrogen Levels in Some Male Populations

	Serum phytoestrogens (nmol/L)		
	Equol	Daidzein	Genistein
Infants[a]	17	1160	1640
Japanese men	99	283	493
UK men	<1.0	18	33

Values quoted in Refs. [41,42].
[a]Four-month-old boys fed exclusively soy based infant formula.

other hand, because of their estrogenic activity, the possibility that soy phytoestrogens may act as endocrine disrupters has been raised [38–40]. This may be of particular significance for babies for whom soy-based infant formula may be their only source of nutrition; and this would mean that they are exposed to considerable quantities of genistein and daidzein, as is clear from the studies of Morton et al. [41] and Setchell et al. [42] and shown in Table 17.2. Animal models have shown that exposure to genistein in utero, neonatally, or both can lead to alterations in reproductive development [43]. Manufacturers of infant formula argue that babies have been fed soy-based formula for many decades and their subsequent fertility does not appear to be impaired. To determine the degree of endocrine disruption that soy isoflavones may be causing to humans, large-scale comprehensive prospective studies are needed where the sexual development and fertility of infants that were fed soy formula are followed.

Genistein has also been demonstrated to function as an estrogen agonist, antagonist, or selective ER modulator in animal models of hormone-dependent cancers [44]. Thus, depending on the dose and the stage at which exposure occurs during infant development, genistein alone or dietary isoflavones suppress or stimulate estrogen-dependent mammary gland tumors in rodents [45–48]. Prenatal and postnatal exposure to dietary soy isoflavones also suppresses the growth of colon tumors in male rats, with ER-β as a suggested critical mediator in mitigating cancer-preventive effects of soy isoflavones [49]. These are some examples of endocrine disrupters that have challenged traditional concepts in toxicology and risk assessment. Hence, an extensive discussion is currently occurring in the scientific literature on two major characteristics of endocrine disrupters: low-dose effects and nonmonotonic dose–response curves. This has resulted in a recommendation for a suspect endocrine-disruptor testing strategy to include the use of a wider range of doses, extending well into the low-dose range to facilitate accurate risk analysis [50,51].

17.4.2 Natural Health Products

In Canada, the Food Directorate of Health Canada is responsible for the regulation of foods marketed as natural health products [52]. The Natural and Non-prescription Health Products Directorate of Health Canada regulates the safety of herbal remedies and homeopathic treatments [53]. Thus, for example, if folate is added to foods as a fortification, then the regulation is the responsibility of the Food Directorate, but if folate is sold as a supplement, then

TABLE 17.3   Folate Levels in Women

Percentile	Age (Years)		
	14–18	19–30	31–50
75th	710	1149	1592
95th	812	1642	2275
99th	954	1577	2489

Data extrapolated from Ref. [54].
Women in the 1st to 50th percentiles all consumed folate below
the recommended upper limit of 1000 dietary folate equivalents.

the regulation is the responsibility of the Natural and Non-prescription Health Products Directorate. In general, herbal remedies and homeopathic treatments are considered to have good safety profiles when used according to traditional practices. These practices are often historically rooted in hundreds of years of human experience and are often accompanied by documented safety considerations, which are routinely applied to products on the market. Regardless, the active constituents in these preparations have often not been identified by conventional scientific study. From the perspective of endocrine disruption, some natural health products (e.g., indole-3-carbinol/diindolylmethane present in broccoli and other crucifers; and tongkat ali, a popular Malaysian herbal plant) are known to increase or decrease endocrine activity. However, when used as directed, they have not demonstrated modulation above or below normal human physiological ranges. Some supplements have been added to foods (e.g., fortification of milk with vitamin D, and bread, cereals, and other grain products with folate). Folate is an interesting case because insufficient folate in the diet of a pregnant woman may lead to the fetus developing neural tube defects such as spina bifida or anencephaly. Furthermore, the development of these diseases occurs within the first month of pregnancy, often before the woman realizes she is pregnant. Consequently, in an effort to ensure that women take in enough folate, fortification of food was implemented, and women are urged to take multivitamins as well. However, in North America at least, it now appears that the problem is not one of folate deficiency, but that folate intake is actually *exceeding* the recommended levels. Bailey et al. [54] have shown that in women older than 19 years, folate intake by the 75th percentile and higher was above the recommended upper limit of 1000 dietary folate equivalents (Table 17.3) and also that the excess was due to supplement usage, as dietary folate intake alone was below the upper limit. Excessive folate intake has not been studied extensively, but a study with pregnant mice given a high-folate diet showed that some changes in gene methylation were evident in the livers of the fetuses [55]. Thus, while folate has not been described as an endocrine disrupter, clearly, more research is needed here, as epigenetic changes that occur as a consequence of maternal nutrition at the time of conception could be an important modulator of normal fetal development. As might be expected, folate intake by men in North America reflects the same levels as by women, but the physiological significance of this is not known [55]. Ginseng is a popular herbal remedy purported

TABLE 17.4   Serum Testosterone in Male Rats Treated with Extracts from Some Natural Health Products

	Serum testosterone in	
	Control (%)	Treated (%)
Tribulus alatus	100	2600
Garcinia kola	100	138
Camellia sinensis	100	409

Data extrapolated from Refs. [57–59].

to be antidiabetic, antihypertensive, anticancer, and beneficial in memory enhancement. Some active components of ginseng have been shown to be embryotoxic in vitro, suggesting the possibility of a teratogenic effect in vivo. However, recent studies have shown that these fears are probably unfounded, as female mice orally administered an extract of Korean red ginseng exhibited no adverse effects on fertility or fetal survival and no fetal abnormalities or developmental problems were identified [56]. Some herbal remedies that need attention with respect to endocrine disruption are those that may have aphrodisiac properties. Some of these have been reported to increase serum testosterone levels in male rats, which in some cases elevated the serum testosterone 5-fold and in one case 18-fold [57–59] (Table 17.4)! Quite apart from the hyperandrogenizing effect of these treatments on male reproductive physiology, the possibility exists that exposure of pregnant females to such treatments may have deleterious effects on fetal sexual development.

17.5 ASSAY MODELS FOR ENDOCRINE DISRUPTIVE ACTIVITY

The regulatory process requires the assessment of all the data available for the toxicity of a chemical, and part of this process is to assign weight to the studies where the data provide the greatest confidence for making the decision [60]. Mechanistic aspects of toxicity are often produced from in vitro assays such as hormone receptor interaction, and while these studies help considerably, the need for toxicity data from living systems remains essential. The need for animal studies to determine the endocrine-disruptive capacity of food contaminants and constituents persists and will continue to do so until tests that do not need live animals are developed and validated. The search for the best criteria on which to base regulatory decisions is an ongoing process; determining which tests are the most appropriate and which data should be given the most weight is part of the process (for a recent approach, see Ref. [60]). To meet such challenges, the chemical Test Guidelines (TGs) program of the Organisation of Economic Development (OECD), for example, provides access to a collection of internationally agreed testing methods used by governments, industry, and independent laboratories to assess the safety of chemical products. These guidelines are primarily used in regulatory safety testing and are updated regularly in consultation with global expert scientists in government, academia, and industry to keep pace with progress in science and regulatory needs [61]. The 2011 OECD Revised Conceptual Framework for Testing and Assessment of Endocrine Disrupters lists the OECD TGs and standardized mammalian and nonmammalian test methods available that can be used to evaluate chemicals for endocrine disruption (OECD GD 150, 2012) [62]. This framework is intended to provide a guide to the tests available rather than a testing strategy [62].

There are tests available for general toxicity of chemicals that include reproductive aspects [61]. The repeated-dose 28-day (OECD 407) and 90-day Oral Toxicity (OECD 408) studies use weanling rats and in-life observations of general health, followed by clinical biochemistry and histopathology of many physiological systems, including reproductive tissues. Clearly, these can be extended to include serum estimations of reproductive end points such as steroids, thyroid hormones, and gonadotropins. However, endocrine disruption requires assessments that are more specific to reproduction.

In the United States, a tiered approach to the testing of chemicals for endocrine disruption was developed and adopted [63]. Tier 1 tests include in vitro assessments of androgen and ER interaction using cells in culture, steroidogenic enzyme activities, amphibian metamorphosis, fish short-term reproduction assays, and the Herschberger and Uterotrophic and male and female pubertal bioassays for androgenic and estrogenic properties of chemicals. Figure 17.1 lists some in vivo and in vitro mammalian assay tests available for endocrine-disruptive activity.

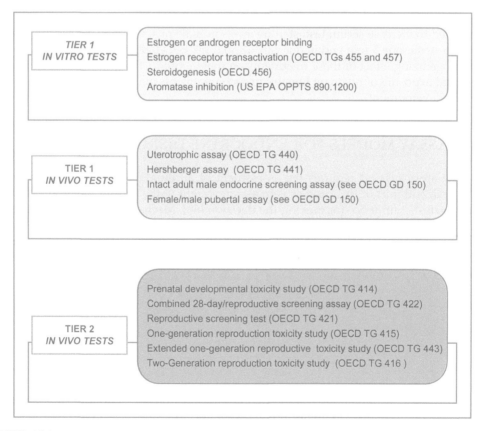

FIGURE 17.1   Some mammalian assay models for endocrine-disruptive activity. OECD TGs are found in Ref. [61]. OECD Guidance Document 150 is in Ref. [62].

17.5.1 Tier 1 In Vitro Tests

Tests for ER binding of chemicals can use rat uterine cytosol as a source of the ER for competitive binding assays, but now cell lines are available that can measure if a chemical causes transcriptional activation of the ER (OECD 455 and 457) [61]. Similarly, for interactions with the androgen receptor (AR), rat prostate cytosol is used as a source of AR for competitive binding assays. However, to date, no cell-based transactivation assay is validated for assessment of the interaction of chemicals with the AR.

The effects of chemicals on steroidogenesis in vitro can be assessed using the human cell line H295R (OECD 456) for androgen biosynthesis and human recombinant microsomes can be purchased and used to determine effects on aromatase activity [61].

17.5.2 Tier 1 In Vivo Tests

Nonmammalian in vivo tier 1 tests for toxic effects on the thyroid and HPG axis are the Amphibian Metamorphosis Assay (AMA), where frog tadpoles are exposed to the chemical and tadpole metamorphosis and thyroid histology are examined; and for the HPG axis, the Fish Short-Term Reproduction Assay, where fathead minnows are exposed and reproductive success is determined. Neither of these assays is considered definitive for endocrine disruption, but along with other tests, they would indicate whether further tests are warranted.

Two short-term tests for screening chemicals for estrogenic/antiestrogenic or androgenic/antiandrogenic effects in a mammalian system (rats) are the Uterotrophic Bioassay (OECD 440) and the Hershberger Bioassay (OECD 441) [61]. The Uterotrophic Bioassay, illustrated in Figure 17.2, can be done in two ways, with the preferred method being as follows: Post Natal Day (PND) 18 female pups are dosed for three consecutive days, and 24 h after the last dose, the pups are sacrificed and their uteruses weighed. Estrogenic chemicals will cause an increase in uterine weight compared to vehicle-dosed controls. The second method is less preferable because it requires the additional intervention of ovariectomy in 6- to 8-week-old female rats, followed by a 14-day period to allow the uterus to regress and then dosing with the chemical for 3 (or even up to 7) consecutive days. At sacrifice, the uterine weight is recorded. In these studies, ethinyl-estradiol serves as a positive control. The Uterotrophic Bioassay is considered effective for estrogenic compounds but is less reliable for antiestrogenic chemicals.

The Hershberger Bioassay involves castrating PND 42 male rats and allowing 7 days for the accessory sex organs to regress. Dosing with chemicals is done for 10 consecutive days and then at sacrifice, the ventral prostate, seminal vesicles, levator ani-bulbocavernosus muscle, paired Cowper's glands, and the glans penis are weighed. Androgenic chemicals will increase the weights of these tissues compared with vehicle-dosed controls. Testosterone propionate is a suitable positive control, and in the case of detecting anti-androgenic chemicals, rats dosed with both testosterone propionate and the chemical of interest will exhibit reductions in the weights of the same tissues compared with rats dosed only with testosterone propionate. Careful adjustment of the testosterone propionate dose will allow effective detection of anti-androgenic chemicals.

The Pubertal Rat Female and Male Assays are also short term tests to examine for chemical effects on vaginal opening in females and preputial separation in males, these being

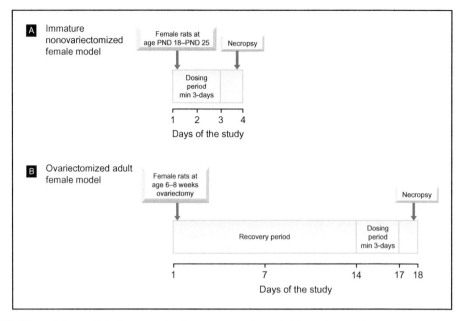

FIGURE 17.2   Scheme of the Uterotrophic Bioassay in Rodents (OECD TG 440). The test substance is administered daily by oral gavage or subcutaneous injection to at least two treatment groups of experimental animals for
an administration period of three consecutive days for the immature nonovariectomized model and a minimum
administration period of three consecutive days for the ovariectomized adult model. The animals are necropsied
approximately 24 h after the last dose. For estrogen agonists, a statistically significant increase in the mean uterine
weight of a test group indicates a positive response in this bioassay. *Source: Adapted from OECD TG 440 [61].*

estrogen and androgen driven events, respectively. PND 22 female rats are dosed with the
chemical daily until PND 42 and observed for the day when vaginal opening occurs and
subsequently, vaginal swabs are taken to assess estrus cyclicity. Similarly, PND 23 male rats
are dosed daily until PND 53 and examined for the day that preputial separation occurs.
Both assays offer the possibility of other end points being determined at necropsy (e.g.,
serum hormones, histopathology, etc.). Another possible assay that is being promoted is the
15-Day Intact Adult Male Rats Assay, where PND 70 male rats are dosed for 15 consecutive days and where reproductive organ weights, serum hormones, and histopathology of
reproductive tissues are the end points.

If the combined data from the Tier 1 tests indicate that endocrine disruption is probable,
the chemical will need to be investigated further in Tier 2 tests, discussed next.

17.5.3 Tier 2 In Vivo Tests

In the Tier 2 battery of tests, there are nonmammalian two-generation assays that have
been proposed. The amphibian two-generation (frog), avian two-generation (Japanese
quail), the fish life-cycle two-generation (fathead minnows, Japanese medaka, zebrafish, or
sheepshead minnows) and the invertebrate life-cycle two-generation test (aquatic arthro-
pods) will provide data relevant to endocrine disruption relatively rapidly, but ultimately,

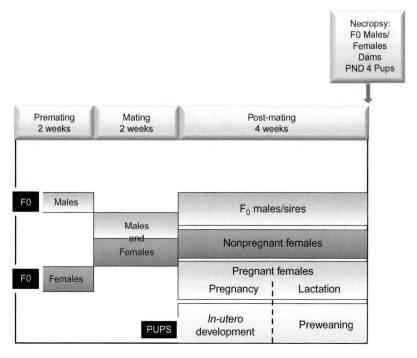

FIGURE 17.3   Scheme of the Reproductive Screening Test (OECD TG 421). Sexually mature male and female animals are exposed to the test substance continuously for a minimum of a 2-week premating period and a 2-week mating period. The parental (F0) males are further treated for at least another 2 weeks post-mating. Treatment of the F0 females is continued during pregnancy and lactation until termination after the weaning of their litters. For the pups, exposure to the test substance will occur only indirectly through the placenta and milk. *Source: Adapted from OECD TG 421 [61].*

mammalian tests that target particular stages in reproductive development will be necessary. The OECD has validated several guidelines for mammalian testing. Historically the gold standard for reproductive toxicity testing was the Two-Generation Reproduction Study (OECD Guideline 416), but this is being phased out due to the large number of animals needed to conduct the study and because the number of studies where the second generation showed an effect when the first generation did not are very few. The extended One-Generation Reproduction Study (OECD 443), which will eventually replace OECD 416, contains more reproductive end points and will provide an opportunity for the second generation to be conducted if the data from the first generation indicates that it is necessary.

Other OECD guidelines are shorter-term designs that examine toxic effects of chemicals at specific stages of reproductive development. For example, three OECD guidelines emphasize the effects of chemicals during fetal development. OECD 414 involves the dosing of pregnant dams from Gestational Day (GD) 5 immediately after implantation has occurred, to GD 20, shortly before parturition. Observations such as dam weight gain; survival; pregnancy loss; organ weights; numbers of live pups, dead pups. and resorptions for each litter; fetus weights; sex ratios; external malformations; and skeletal malformations are included. OECD Guidelines 421 (Figure 17.3) and 422 are more detailed and involve parental males and females being dosed before mating and females being dosed throughout pregnancy and up to PND 4. Parents and pups are examined for weight gain, number of pregnancies, organ weights, and other statistics, but the assessment of skeletal abnormalities is not required. The major difference between OECD 421 and 422 is that the latter includes more extensive clinical biochemistry and hematology end points. So, these relatively short assays can give much information about the toxicity of chemicals to fertility and fetal development.

A more detailed study of the effect of chemical toxicity is the One-Generation Reproduction Study (OECD 415). Here, parental males are dosed for a complete sperm cycle (70 days in the rat) and females are dosed for 14 days (three to four estrus cycles) before mating, and dams continue to be dosed throughout pregnancy and lactation until weaning. After delivery, pups are not dosed but are monitored until sacrifice. The end points to be reported include body weights, organ weights, number of pregnancies, and histopathology of the reproductive tissues. The requirements could be considered basic in comparison to the new Extended One-Generation Reproductive Toxicity Study (OECD 443; Figure 17.4), which has a similar experimental design except that the parental males are dosed for only 2–4 weeks prior to mating and then dosing continues for a complete sperm cycle, at which time histopathology and biochemical parameters are assessed. However, in OECD 443, the pups are dosed, and during their development, androgen- and estrogen-dependent end points such as ano-genital distance, the timing of vaginal opening, and time to first estrus and estrus cycle length for the females and the timing of preputial separation for the males are assessed. In addition, the guideline includes the possibility of assessing immunotoxicology end points and neurotoxicology end points. Since this design generates a considerable amount of data concerning the effect of the chemicals on the reproductive success of the parental generation and postnatal development of the pups, the decision can be made to produce a second generation by mating the pups when adult. These second-generation pregnancies would be sacrificed before parturition. Consequently, there is a better use of the animals used in this design than in both the One-Generation Reproductive Study (OECD 415) and the Two-Generation Reproduction Study (OECD 416); for this reason, this method is highly recommended for reproductive toxicity studies.

17.6 CONCLUSION AND FUTURE DIRECTIONS

In this chapter, we have provided some examples of EDCs that may get into foods by several different routes, such as from food-packaging materials; as a result of pesticide use, food processing, or veterinary practices; or from naturally occurring sources in the form of contaminants or components of food crops or natural health products. It should be noted that the existing testing protocols for endocrine disrupters that have been described are guidelines and will evolve over time with the addition of new end points. Recommendations for these revisions come from the scientific community as the state of the science and the knowledge base expands. Some emerging end points that have been suggested for inclusion in the reproductive tests are the retinoid signaling pathway, the peroxisome proliferator activated receptor (PPAR) pathway, vitamin D signaling, and enhanced functional assessment of the adrenal gland. The current assessment of the adrenal involves just the basic determination of the organ weight and its gross pathology [50,64]. Some

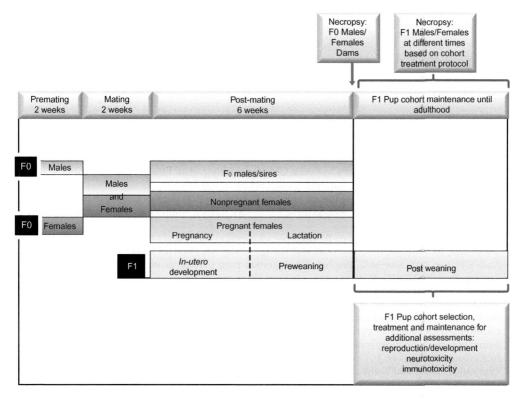

FIGURE 17.4 Scheme of the Extended One-Generation Reproductive Toxicity Study (OECD TG 443). Sexually mature male and female animals are exposed to the test substance administered continuously. The parental (F0) generation is dosed for a minimum of 2 weeks of pre-mating period and a 2-week mating period. F0 males are further treated at least until weaning of the F1. Treatment of the F0 females is continued during pregnancy and lactation until termination after the weaning of their litters. For the F1 offspring, exposure to the test substance will occur only indirectly through the placenta and milk until they receive direct treatment with the test substance from weaning to adulthood. For reproductive toxicity assessment, animals can be maintained on treatment beyond PND 90 and bred to obtain a F2 generation if necessary. *Source: Adapted from OECD TG 443 [61].*

research groups already incorporate genomics and proteomics approaches for the enhanced assessment of endocrine-disruptive effects in relevant organs exposed in vivo to chemicals in the OECD test guideline–based treatment protocols [65,66]. Furthermore, as we advance into the epigenomics era, one area on which future efforts will need to focus is the testing of epigenetic effects of endocrine disrupters, especially where trans-generational effects are suspected. Research on such epigenetic changes in humans is currently underway [67]. The gametes that made us were exposed to environmental chemicals when our grandmothers were pregnant with our parents. Consequently, there is a need to identify which epigenetic changes are likely to be of concern for endocrine disruption and then to validate markers for detecting changes in the epigenome and methyl transferase and histone acetylase activities so that these may be incorporated into existing assay protocols or possibly utilized in the design of novel protocols.

Acknowledgment

The authors would like to thank Joel Rotstein, Paul Rowsell, Michael Steller, Anastase Rulibikiye, and Mark Feeley for a critical review of this manuscript and helpful suggestions.

References

[1] Jurewicz J, Hanke W. Prenatal and childhood exposure to pesticides and neurobehavioral development: review of epidemiological studies. Int J Occ Med Envion Health 2008;21(2):212–32.

[2] Mnif W, Hassine AIH, Bouaziz A, Bertegi A, Thomas O, Roig B. Effect of endocrine disruptor pesticides: a review. Int J Environ Res Public Health 2011;8:2265–303.

[3] Adeeko A, Li D, Forsyth DS, Casey V, Cooke GM, Barthelemy J, et al. Effects of *in utero* tributyltin chloride exposure in the rat on pregnancy outcome. Toxicol Sci 2003;74(2):407–15.

[4] Cooke GM. Effect of organotins on human aromatase activity *in vitro*. Toxicol Lett 2002;126(2):121–30.

[5] PMRA. The Health Canada Pest Management Regulatory Agency, <http://www.hc-sc.gc.ca/cps-spc/pest/index-eng.php>.

[6] Bhunia K, Sablani SS, Tang J, Rasco B. Migration of chemical compounds from packaging polymers during microwave, conventional heat treatment, and storage. Comp Rev Food Sci Food Safety 2013;12:523–45.

[7] Nam S-H, Seo Y-M, Kim M-G. Bisphenol A migration from polycarbonate baby bottle with repeated use. Chemosphere 2010;79:949–52.

[8] Muncke J. Endocrine disrupting chemicals and other substances of concern in food contact materials: an updated review of exposure, effect and risk assessment. J Steroid Biochem Mol Biol 2011;127:118–27.

[9] Bradley EL, Honkalampi-Hämäläinen U, Weber A, Andersson MA, Bertaud F, Castle L, et al. The BIOSAFEPAPER project for *in vitro* toxicity assessments: preparation, detailed chemical characterisation and testing of extracts from paper and board samples. Food Chem Toxicol 2008;46:2498–509.

[10] Honkalampi-Hämäläinen U, Bradley EL, Castle L, Severin I, Dahbi L, Dahlman O, et al. Safety evaluation of food contact paper and board using chemical tests and *in vitro* bioassays: role of known and unknown substances. Food Addit Contam 2010;27(3):406–15.

[11] Ozaki A, Yamaguchi Y, Fujita T, Kuroda K, Endo G. Chemical analysis and genotoxicological safety assessment of paper and paperboard used for food packaging. Food Chem Toxicol 2004;42:1323–37.

[12] Ozaki A, Yamaguchi Y, Fujita T, Kuroda K, Endo G. Safety assessment of paper and board food packaging : chemical analysis and genotoxicity of possible contaminants in packaging. Food Addit Contam 2005;22(10):1053–60.

[13] Poças M-F, Hogg T. Exposure assessment of chemicals from packaging materials in foods: a review. Trends Food Sci Technol 2007;18:219–30.

[14] Muncke J, Myers JP, Scheringer M, Porta M. Food packaging and migration of food contact materials: will epidemiologists rise to the neotoxic challenge? J Epidemiol Community Health 2014;68(7):592–94.

[15] NTP. Toxicology and carcinogenesis studies of furan (CAS No. 110-00-9) in F344/N rats and B6C3F1 mice (gavage studies). Technical Report Series No. 402, NIH Publication No 93-2857. Research Triangle Park, NC and Bethesda, MD: US Department of health and Human Services, National Toxicology Program; 1993.

[16] Gill S, Bondy G, Lefebvre DE, Becalski A, Kavanagh M, Hou Y. Subchronic oral toxicity study of furan in Fischer-344 rats. Toxicol Pathol 2010;38:619–30.

[17] de Conti A, Kobets T, Escudero-Lourdes C, Montgomery B, Tryndyak V, Beland FA, et al. Dose- and time-dependent epigenetic changes in the livers of Fisher 344 rats exposed to Furan. Toxicol Sci 2014;139(2):371–80.

[18] Cooke GM, Taylor M, Bourque C, Curran I, Gurofsky S, Gill S. Effects of furan on male rat reproduction parameters in a 90-day gavage study. Reprod Toxicol 2014;46:85–90.

[19] Khan MA, Davis CA, Foley GL, Friedman MA, Hansen LG. Changes in thyroid gland morphology after acrylamide exposure. Toxicol Sci 1999;47:151–7.

[20] Bowyer JF, Latendresse JR, Delongchamp RR, Muskhelishvili L, Warbritton AR, Thomas M, et al. The effects of subchronic acrylamide exposure on gene expression, neurochemistry, hormones, and histopathology in the hypothalamus-pituitary-thyroid axis of male Fischer 344 rats. Toxicol Appl Pharmacol 2008;230:208–15.

[21] Scanlan RA. Formation and occurrence of nitrosamines in food. Cancer Res 1983;43(Suppl. 5):2435s–40s.

[22] Dietrich M, Block G, Pogoda JM, Buffler P, Hecht S, Preston-Martin S. A review: dietary and endogenously formed N-nitroso compounds and risk of childhood brain tumors. Cancer Causes Control 2005;16:619–35.

[23] Saegermann C, Pussemier L, Huyghebaert A, Scippo M-L, Berkvens D. On-farm contamination of animals with chemical contaminants. Rev Sci Tech 2006;25(2):655–73.

[24] Galbraith H. Hormones in international meat production: biological, sociological and consumer issues. Nutr Res Rev 2002;15:293–314.

[25] Health Canada, Setting standards for maximum residue limits (MRLs) of veterinary drugs used in food-producing animals, <http://www.hc-sc.gc.ca/dhp-mps/vet/mrl-lmr/mrl-lmr_levels-niveaux-eng.php>.

[26] CFIA, Government agencies and departments responsible for imported food, <http://www.inspection.gc.ca/food/imports/commercial-importers/importing-food-products/eng/1376515896184/1376515983781?chap=3>.

[27] Vromann V, Maghuin-Rogister G, Vleminckx C, Saegerman C, Pussemier L, Huyghebaert A. Risk ranking priority of carcinogenic and/or genotoxic environmental contaminants in food in Belgium. Food Add Contam Part A 2014;31(5):872–88.

[28] Needham LL, Grandjean P, Heinzow B, Jorgensen PJ, Nielson F, Patterson Jr DG, et al. Partition of environmental chemicals between maternal and fetal blood and tissues. Environ Sci Technol 2011;45:1121–6.

[29] Vahter M, Marafante E, Dencker L. Metabolism of arsenobetaine in mice, rats and rabbits. Sci Total Environ 1983;30:197–211.

[30] Taylor M, Lau BP, Feng SY, Bourque C, Buick J, Bondy GS, et al. Effects of oral exposure to arsenobetaine during pregnancy and lactation in Sprague-Dawley rats. J Toxicol Environ Health Part A 2013;76(24):1333–45.

[31] Jiménez-Ortega V, Barquilla PC, Fernández-Mateos P, Cardinali DP, Esquifino AI. Cadmium as an endocrine disruptor: correlation with anterior pituitary redox and circadian clock mechanisms and prevention by melatonin. Free Rad Biol Med 2012;53:2287–97.

[32] Lafeunte A. The hypothalamic-pituitary-gonadal axis is target of cadmium toxicity. An update of recent studies and potential therapeutic approaches. Food Chem Toxicol 2013;59:395–404.

[33] Canadian Grain Commission. The history of durum wheat breeding in Canada and summaries of recent research at the Canadian Grain Commission on factors associated with durum wheat processing, <http://www.grainscanada.gc.ca/research-recherche/dexter/hdwb-habd/hdwb-habd-2-eng.htm>.

[34] Adams NR. Detection of the effects of phytoestrogens on sheep and cattle. J Anim Sci 1995;73:1509–15.

[35] Riet-Correa F, Medeiros RMT, Schild AL. A review of poisonous plants that cause reproductive failure and malformations in the ruminants of Brazil. J Appl Toxicol 2012;32:245–54.

[36] Cederroth CR, Zimmermann C, Nef S. Soy, phytoestrogens and their impact on reproductive health. Mol Cell Endocrinol 2012;355:192–200.

[37] Cederroth CR, Auger J, Zimmermann C, Eustache F, Nef S. Soy, phytoestrogens and male reproductive function: a review. Int J Androl 2010;33:304–16.

[38] Neill AS, Ibiebele TI, Lahmann PH, Hughes MC, Nagle CM, Webb PM. Dietary phyto-estrogens and the risk of ovarian and endometrial cancers: findings from two Australian case-control studies. Br J Nutr 2014;111:1430–40.

[39] Boberg J, Mandrup KR, Jacobsen PR, Isling LK, Hadrup N, Berthelsen L, et al. Endocrine disruptive effects in rats perinatally exposed to a dietary relevant mixture of phytoestrogens. Reprod Toxicol 2013;40:41–51.

[40] Hilakivi-Clarke L, Andrade JE, Helferich W. Is soy consumption good or bad for the breast? J Nutr 2010;140:2326S–2334S.

[41] Morton MS, Arisaka O, Miyake N, Morgan LD, Evans BAJ. Phytoestrogen concentrations in serum from Japanese men and women over 40 years of age. J Nutr 2002;132:3168–71.

[42] Setchell KDR, Zimmer-Nechimias L, Cai J, Heubi JE. Exposure of infants to phytoestrogens from soybased infant formula. Lancet 1997;350:23–7.

[43] Cooke GM. A review of animal models used to investigate the health benefits of soy isoflavones. J AOAC Int 2006;89(4):1215–27.

[44] Messina M, Hilakivi-Clarke L. Early intake appears to be the key to the proposed protective effects of soy intake against breast cancer. Nutr Cancer 2009;61:792–8. http://dx.doi.org/10.1080/01635580903285015.

[45] Yang JH, Nakagawa H, Tsuta K, Tsubura A. Influence of perinatal genistein exposure on the development of MNU-induced mammary carcinoma in female Sprague-Dawley rats. Cancer Lett 2000;149:171–9.

[46] Hilakivi Clarke L, Cho E, Onojafe I, Raygada M, Clarke R. Maternal exposure to genistein during pregnancy increases carcinogen-induced mammary tumorigenesis in female rat offspring. Oncol Rep 1999;6:1089–95.

[47] Lamartiniere CA, Cotroneo MS, Fritz WA, Wang J, Mentor-Marcel R, Elgavish A. Genistein chemoprevention: timing and mechanisms of action in murine mammary and prostate. J Nutr 2002;132:552S–8S.

[48] Mehta R, Lok E, Caldwell D, Mueller R, Kapal K, Taylor M, et al. Mammary gland tumor promotion in F1 generation offspring from male and female rats exposed to soy isoflavones for a lifetime. J AOAC Int 2006;89(4):1197–206.

[49] Raju J, Bielecki A, Caldwell D, Lok E, Taylor M, Kapal K, et al. Soy isoflavones modulate azoxymethane-induced rat colon carcinogenesis exposed pre- and postnatally and inhibit growth of DLD-1 human colon adenocarcinoma cells by increasing the expression of estrogen receptor-β. J Nutr 2009;139:474–81.

[50] Alexander J, Benford D, Chaudhry Q, Hardy A, John Jeger M, Luttik R, et al. EFSA ScientificCommittee: scientific opinion on the hazard assessment of endocrine disrupters: scientific criteria for identification of endocrine disrupters and appropriateness of existing test methods for assessing effects mediated by these substances on human health and the environment. EFSA J 2013;11(3):3132;1–84.

[51] Vandenberg LN, Colborn T, Hayes TB, Heindel JJ, Jacobs Jr. DR, Lee DH, et al. Hormones and endocrine-disrupting chemicals: low-dose effects and nonmonotonic dose responses. Endocr Rev 2012;33:378–455.

[52] Health Canada, Foods marketed as natural health products, <http://www.hc-sc.gc.ca/fn-an/prodnatur/index-eng.php>.

[53] Health Canada, Natural Health Products, <http://www.hc-sc.gc.ca/dhp-mps/prodnatur/index-eng.php>.

[54] Bailey RL, Dodd KW, Gahche JL, Dwyer JT, McDowell MA, Yetley EA, et al. Total folate and folic acid intake from foods and dietary supplements in the United States:2003–2006. Am J Clin Nutr 2010;91:231–7.

[55] Tsang V, Fry RC, Niculescu MD, Rager JE, Saunders J, Paul DS, et al. The epigenetic effects of a high prenatal folate intake in mouse fetuses exposed in utero to arsenic. Toxicol Appl Pharmacol 2012;264(3):439–50.

[56] Shin S, Jang JY, Park D, Mon J-M, Baek I-J, Hwang BY, et al. Korean Red Ginseng extract does not cause embryo-fetal death or abnormalities in mice. Birth Defects Res (Part B) 2010;89:78–85.

[57] El-Tantawy WH, Temraz A, El-Ghindi OD. Free serum testosterone level in male rats treated with Tribulus alatus extracts. Int Braz J Urol 2007;33(4):544–59.

[58] Ralebona N, Sewani-Rusike CR, Nkeh-Chungag BN. Effects of ethanolic extract of Garcinia kola on sexual behaviour and sperm parameters in male Wistar rats. Afr J Pharm Pharmacol 2012;6(14):1077–82.

[59] Ratnasooriya WD, Fernando TSP. Effect of black tea brew of Camellia sinensis on sexual competence of male rats. J Ethnopharmacol 2008;118:373–7.

[60] Marx-Stoelting P, Nuemann L, Ritz V, Ulbrich B, Gall A, Hirsch-Ernst KI, et al. Assessment of three approaches for regulatory decision making on pesticides with endocrine disrupting properties. Reg Toxicol Pharmacol 2014 http://dx.doi.org/10.1016/j.yrtph.2014.09.001.

[61] OECD guidelines for the testing of chemicals, Section 4. Health effects, <http://www.oecd-ilibrary.org/environment/oecd-guidelines-for-the-testing-of-chemicals-section-4-health-effects_20745788>.

[62] OECD guidance document on the standardised test guidelines for evaluating chemicals for endocrine disruption: series on testing and assessment No 150. Paris, France. <http://www.oecd.org/chemicalsafety/testing/seriesontestingandassessmentpublicationsbynumber.htm>; 2012.

[63] US-EPA, Endocrine Disruption Screening Program. <http://www.epa.gov/endo/pubs/assayvalidation/status.htm>.

[64] Harvey PW, Everett DJ. Regulation of endocrine disrupting chemicals: critical overview and deficiencies in toxicology and risk assessment for human health. Best Pract Res Clin Endocrinol Metab 2006;20(1):145–65.

[65] McVey MJ, Cooke GM, Curran IHA. Altered testicular microsomal steroidogenic enzyme activities in rats with lifetime exposure to soy isoflavones. J Steroid Biochem Mol Biol 2004;92:435–46.

[66] Ferguson LR, Philpott M. Genetics, epigenetics and genomic technologies: importance and application to the study of endocrine-disrupting chemicals. In Endocrine Disrupting Chemicals in Food Shaw I, (ed.) Woodhead Publishing Series in Food Science, Technology and Nutrition. CRC Press: Boca Raton, NY; 2009. pp. 291–305. http://dx.doi.org/10.1533/9781845695743.3.291.

[67] Domingues-Salas P, Moore SE, Baker MS, Bergen AW, Cox SE, Dyer RA, et al. Maternal nutrition at conception modulates DNA methylation of human metastable epialleles. Nat Commun 2014;5:3746. http://dx.doi.org/10.1038/ncomms4746, <http://www.nature.com/ncomms/2014/140429/ncomms4746/full/ncomms4746.html>.

CHAPTER

18

Considerations of Endocrine Disrupters in Drinking Water

Rowena H. Gee, Leon S. Rockett and Paul C. Rumsby

OUTLINE

Abstract

The provision of "pure and wholesome" drinking water remains a priority for the protection of human health. This chapter investigates the potential concern to human health that could occur if endocrine-disrupting chemicals (EDCs) coming from a range of different industrial, agricultural, and household sources, reached our drinking water, and the processes and regulations in place to prevent such an occurrence. The passage of water from wastewater to drinking water includes treatment before release into environmental waters and further procedures after abstraction from rivers and other sources before drinking water is finally produced. These two stages of treatment are described and their effectiveness in the removal of EDCs assessed, including a summary of studies measuring the concentration of many EDCs in drinking water throughout the world. The use of standards and guidelines to control the concentrations of chemicals, including EDCs, in environmental and drinking waters are outlined, and finally some suggestions are made as to how the presence of EDCs in the environment could be limited.

Endocrine Disruption and Human Health.
DOI: http://dx.doi.org/10.1016/B978-0-12-801139-3.00018-1

319

18.1 INTRODUCTION

The provision of safe, wholesome water is vital to the health of the population. This chapter will consider how endocrine-disrupting chemicals (EDCs) that may be present in the environment could potentially reach drinking water, and how treatment processes, together with standards and monitoring, can protect water supplies against the presence of such contaminant chemicals. The examples in this chapter are taken mainly from the experience of water treatment in the United Kingdom and developed industrial and agricultural countries, where the treatment processes may be more sophisticated.

Figure 18.1 shows the basic treatment of water from the entry of sewage into wastewater treatment works (WwTWs) and the treatment of this wastewater before its entry into environmental water, followed by abstraction and treatment processes (including disinfection) to finished drinking water. These processes will be explained in detail later in this chapter.

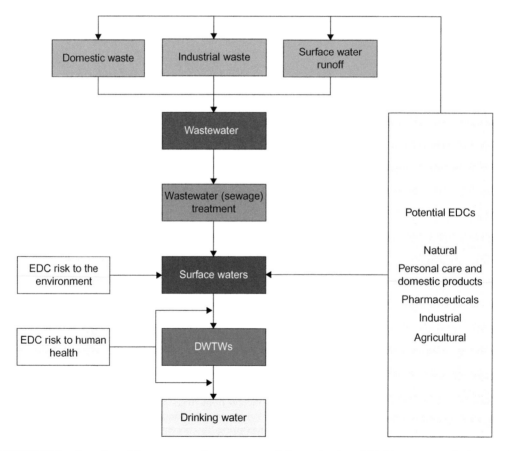

FIGURE 18.1 Overview of the treatment of wastewater and the production of drinking water, and where EDCs could potentially pose a risk to human health and the environment.

Chemicals with potential endocrine-disrupting properties (i.e., EDCs) may come from a variety of sources and enter the water cycle. These can include the following:

- Natural substances, such as steroid hormones
- Pharmaceuticals
- Industrial chemicals
- Agricultural chemicals
- Personal care and cleaning products

These chemicals can enter water systems in a number of ways, such as via sewage into the wastewater treatment and then into environmental waters. This would be the main route of entry for natural substances, pharmaceuticals, and personal care and cleaning products, while industrial and agricultural products could enter environmental waters by diffuse pollution (i.e., pollution from a wide area rather than a specific point of release into the environment) from the land. The presence of EDCs in environmental waters could be potentially damaging to aquatic organisms and perhaps to human health via recreational use of waters, while the presence of EDCs in final drinking water could also be a risk to human health.

18.2 STANDARDS AND GUIDELINES

There are a number of European regulations that control the presence of certain prioritized chemicals in environmental waters. These chemicals have been prioritized owing to their potential toxic effects on organisms in the environment. These regulations involve the requirement for monitoring and the setting of Environmental Quality Standards (EQSs), above which concentrations of these chemical should not rise, for a list of Priority Substances (33 in total, of which 20 are Priority Hazardous Substances), plus a further list of 8 chemicals. This list of chemicals contains several that are potential endocrine disrupters, such as di(2-ethylhexyl)phthalate (DEHP), nonylphenol and octaphenols, and a number of pesticides such as simazine, atrazine, and dichlorodiphenyltrichloroethane (DDT), although none of these pesticides are currently registered for use in the European Union (EU). Recently, there has been the need for a Watch List of three chemicals for which further monitoring data are required; these include the steroid estrogens (SEs), 17α-ethinylestradiol (EE2) and 17β-estradiol (E2), and diclofenac, an anti-inflammatory pharmaceutical. Owing to the effects of estrogenic compounds on aquatic organisms at low concentrations, it has proved difficult to set achievable EQSs for the natural estrogen, E2, and the oral contraceptive component, EE2, which are widely present in the environment.

Encouraged by the World Health Organization (WHO), regulators and water companies around the world are increasingly using drinking water safety plans to identify risks to drinking water from chemicals and microorganisms which may be present in the area around abstraction and drinking water treatment works (DWTWs), due to activities such as industries, agriculture, or hospitals. Suitable treatment processes can then be used to minimize the risk of chemicals reaching final drinking water.

The Drinking Water Inspectorate (DWI), which regulates the provision of drinking water in the United Kingdom, declares that the drinking water provided must be "wholesome." This is a carryover from the first provision in the Waterworks Clauses Act of 1947 that drinking water must be "pure and wholesome," and this is defined in law by standards for a wide range of substances, organisms, and properties of water in regulations. The standards are set to protect public health, and the definition of *wholesome* reflects the importance of ensuring that water quality is acceptable to consumers. There is good agreement worldwide on the science behind the setting of health-based standards for drinking water, and this expert evidence is documented by WHO in their Guidelines for Drinking-water Quality (GDWQ). The legal standards in the United Kingdom are those which are set in Europe in the Drinking Water Directive 1998, together with national standards set to maintain the high quality of water already achieved. The standards are strict and include wide safety margins. They cover

- Microorganisms
- Chemicals such as nitrate and pesticides
- Metals such as lead and copper
- The way water looks and how it tastes

This being the case, there is also the proviso that the water must not contain any substance or microorganism at a concentration or value that would constitute a potential danger to human health. The potential presence of EDCs in drinking water would be covered by this statement and may also include chemicals such as pesticides that may have endocrine-disrupting properties. The standard set for individual pesticides is $0.1\,\mu g/L$ and the sum of all pesticides is $0.5\,\mu g/L$. This is not a health-based standard, however; rather, it constitutes a desire to have pesticide-free drinking water.

18.3 OVERVIEW OF SEWAGE TREATMENT

Sewage can refer to domestic and industrial waste. Domestic sewage includes toilet water, bath and shower water, and water from clothes and dish washing. As a result, domestic sewage can be a complex mixture of human waste, cleaning chemicals, skin, hair, and improperly discarded medications. Industrial waste is a nebulous term that includes waste from offices and commercial businesses, as well as large chemical and industrial plants. Some industries may be subject to discharge consents agreed with regulatory bodies; i.e., releases of waste are monitored, typically at a designated point within a sewage treatment works, and concentrations of specific chemicals must remain within an acceptable level. In addition, some sewerage systems combine surface water runoff, such as rain from roads, with sewage. Therefore, since sewage is such a complex mixture of chemicals and microorganisms from a diverse range of sources, there is significant potential for chemicals with effects on the human endocrine system to enter sewage treatment works.

Sewage treatment works can vary considerably in design and in the complexity of removal processes, depending on the typical waste load entering the works. As a result, different sewage treatment works will have varying capabilities with regard to the removal of EDCs. Figure 18.2 provides an overview of sewage treatment processes at an activated sludge plant (ASP). In general, sewage treatment works can be divided into the following stages of treatment. However, it should be noted that not all sewage treatment works will have all of these stages:

- Preliminary screening to remove grit
- Primary treatment (solid removal)

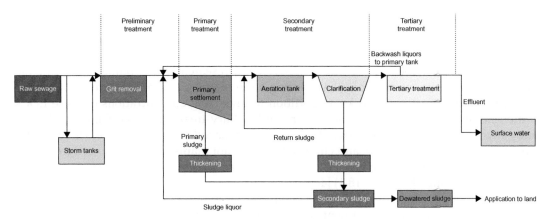

FIGURE 18.2   Overview of sewage treatment processes. Between inflow into a sewage treatment works and discharge to surface water, sewage undergoes a number of treatment processes designed to remove visible debris and chemicals.

- Secondary treatment (biological oxidation processes), e.g.,
  - Non-nitrifying or partially nitrifying ASPs
  - ASPs
  - Biofilters
- Tertiary treatment (further oxidative treatment processes), e.g.,
  - Sand filters
  - ASPs
  - Biological aerated flooded filters (BAFFs)

18.4 FATE OF SEs DURING SEWAGE TREATMENT

Sewage is a complex mixture of chemicals that have the potential for endocrine disruption, including pharmaceuticals, industrial chemicals, and personal care and cleaning products. However, the majority of studies on the fate of EDCs during sewage treatment have focused on the natural SEs, estrone (E1) and E2, and the synthetic estrogen EE2, the active ingredient of the contraceptive pill, as these are likely to be the common and the most potent EDCs in wastewater. Therefore, the following sections of this chapter focus on these three SEs. However, it should be noted that there are also numerous examples of other potential EDCs detected in wastewater, including in many of the papers referenced throughout this chapter, and this topic is not discussed here.

It is worth noting that SEs are eliminated in the urine and feces of humans primarily as inactive gluocuronide or sulfated conjugates. Sewage treatment processes are biological processes, therefore, the presence of bacterial populations in sewage that are capable of producing β-glucuronidase and arylsulfatase enzymes may result in the deconjugation of SEs to their free and active forms [1,2]. Conjugated material may represent a significant proportion of the total SEs within a sewage treatment works; in one study, conjugated estrogens accounted for approximately 50% of total SE [3].

18.5 REMOVAL OF EDCs DURING SEWAGE TREATMENT

In a large review of the effectiveness of sewage treatment processes in the United Kingdom, UK Water Industry Research (UKWIR), a research body comprising all of the UK water companies, conducted a monitoring study of the concentrations of E1, E2, and EE2 at 14 sewage treatment works. In addition to reviewing concentrations of these EDCs in the raw sewage and following secondary and tertiary treatments (see Figure 18.2), this study investigated the effectiveness of additional advanced treatment processes [granular activated carbon (GAC), ozone, and chlorine] at two pilot plants. These advanced treatment processes are typically used in DWTWs, where they are used to remove and treat a range of chemicals, including SEs (Table 18.1) [4–6].

This study demonstrated a wide range of efficiencies in removal with regard to these SEs, particularly with secondary treatment, where in general, non-nitrifying or partially nitrifying ASPs demonstrated lower removal efficiencies than other treatment processes, and nitrifying ASP provided treatment comparable to some tertiary treatment processes.

The advanced treatment processes demonstrated very high removal of naturally occurring SEs, with average removal rates of 96.2% and 97.9% for E1 and E2, respectively. Removal of EE2 varied but also generally demonstrated good removal (average removal of 68.9%). A similar level of removal was obtained from nitrifying ASPs, with average removal rates of 93.8% and 96.5% for E1 and E2, respectively, and variable removal of EE2 (average removal of 53.9%). Average removals of E1 and E2 across nitrifying biofilters were 40.2% and 75.5%, respectively. Non-nitrifying ASPs tended to show the poorest removal of SEs (average of 17.9% and 62.5% removal for E1 and E2, respectively) [4–6].

Other studies have been published on the removal of SEs during wastewater treatment, and these results are summarized in Table 18.2. It is notable that in these studies,

TABLE 18.1 Overview of the Occurrence of E1, E2, and EE2 in Crude Sewage and Following Different Treatment Processes During the UKWIR EDC Demonstration Programme [4–6]

Treatment Stage	Treatment process[a]	Concentration (mean and upper 95 percentile) (ng/L)		
		E1	E2	EE2
Crude influent	None	37.90 (69.07)	13.52 (28.90)	0.78 (2.10)
Secondary treatments	Non-nitrifying or partially nitrifying ASP	46.55 (107.99)	6.50 (15.42)	1.30 (2.43)
	Nitrifying biofilter	20.16 (31.79)	2.95 (5.46)	0.73 (2.07)
	Nitrifying ASP	2.33 (4.60)	0.49 (1.23)	0.34 (0.84)
Tertiary treatments	[Nitrifying biofilter] Sand filter	6.13 (13.31)	0.83 (1.94)	0.53 (0.82)
	[Non-nitrifying or partially nitrifying ASP] ASP and BAFF	2.60 (5.85)	0.60 (1.19)	0.80 (1.19)
	[Nitrifying ASP] Disc filters	0.76 (2.35)	0.20 (0.61)	0.23 (0.71)
Advanced treatments	[Nitrifying ASP], [Tertiary treatment] GAC, ozone, or chlorine dioxide	0.19 (0.64)	0.12 (0.30)	0.13 (0.44)

[a]Process described in brackets is the preceding treatment.

TABLE 18.2 Reported Concentrations of E1, E2, and EE2 in Sewage Influent and Effluent and, Where Available, the Reported Removal Efficiency of the Sewage Treatment Works

Location	E1			E2			EE2			Reference
	Influent (ng/L)	Effluent (ng/L)	Removal (%)	Influent (ng/L)	Effluent (ng/L)	Removal (%)	Influent (ng/L)	Effluent (ng/L)	Removal (%)	
Rio Penha WwTW (Brazil)	40	7	83	21	<1.0	95.0	5	1	78	[7]
Frankfurt WwTW (Germany)	27	9	66.7	15	<2.0	>86.7	1.5	1	33.3	[7]
Corbia (Italy)	71.0 + 35.5	9.6 + 5.1	86.0 + 6.1	16.1 + 7.5	1.5 + 1.0	88.9 + 9.7	3.9 + 5.1	0.5 + 0.3	70.1 + 23.4	[8]
Fregene (Italy)	67.0 + 17.8	4.1 + 1.5	93.9 + 1.6	9.2 + 5.1	0.9 + 0.7	87.6 + 11.3	3.4 + 2.3	0.6 + 0.6	70.6 + 27.4	[8]
Ostia (Italy)	50.6 + 12.8	44.6 + 25.0	17.6 + 29.5	14.7 + 7.0	2.4 + 1.2	83.6 + 3.0	2.5 + 1.8	0.6 + 0.3	67.9 + 19.2	[8]
Roma Est (Italy)	50.4 + 14.3	7.7 + 2.6	83.8 + 8.1	9.3 + 2.0	0.8 + 0.04	91.2 + 1.7	2.3 + 1.6	0.4 + 0.2	70.8 + 26.4	[8]
Roma Nord (Italy)	36.8 + 8.4	13.9 + 14.7	64.3 + 33.3	11.5 + 3.2	1.0 + 0.5	91.7 + 3.1	3.0 + 2.3	0.4 + 0.1	74.0 + 22.9	[8]
Roma Sud (Italy)	35.2 + 9.6	30.3 + 16.3	8.8 + 43.1	8.6 + 2.3	1.9 + 0.9	76.2 + 13.1	2.9 + 2.1	0.6 + 0.4	69.0 + 24.9	[8]
Languedoc-Rusillon (France) (October)	6–119 (ND–18)[a]	2–8 (<1)[a]	NR	23–28 (3–4)[a]	ND–2 (<1)[a]	NR	5–20 (ND –11)[a]	2 (1)[a]	NR	[3]
Languedoc-Rusillon (France) (April)	52–97 (8–20)[a]	1–3 (<1)[a]	NR	13–25 (4–5)[a]	2–3 (<1)[a]	NR	ND-2 (ND)[a]	ND (ND)[a]	NR	[3]
Calaf (Spain)	<2.5–115	<2.5–8.1	NR	11.0–30.4	<5.0	NR	<5.0	<5.0	NR	[9]
Igualada (Spain)	<2.5–8.1	<2.5–2.7	NR	<5.0	<5.0–7.6	NR	<5.0	<5.0	NR	[9]
Piera (Spain)	<2.5–13.1	<2.5	NR	<5.0	<5.0	NR	<5.0	<5.0	NR	[9]
Manresa (Spain)	29.0–56.5	<2.5–7.2	NR	<5.0–14.5	<5.0	NR	<5.0	<5.0	NR	[9]

ND, not detected; NR, not reported.

[a]As conjugated material.

the concentration of EE2 in the influent is higher than that observed in the UK study. The authors of the UK study suggested that this was due to the use of a preservative during the UK sampling, which was not used in the earlier studies. This preservative prevented the deconjugation of EE2 metabolites to free EE2 during the sampling, transport, and storage of these samples, preventing erroneously high levels of free EE2 being reported.

18.6 OVERVIEW OF DRINKING WATER TREATMENT

The discharge of effluents from wastewater treatment into rivers and other bodies of water that may potentially be used as sources of drinking water, as well as the occurrence of EDCs in these waters, has given rise to the question of whether these EDCs can get into drinking water [10], therefore affecting human health.

Drinking water for human consumption is generally of good quality since before reaching the tap, it undergoes thorough treatment via a number of sequential processes (Figure 18.3). These processes are designed to remove visible debris, as well as microorganisms and chemicals that may be present in environmental waters, where the different treatment processes are efficient at removing different substances.

The initial process of withdrawing water from a source in order to produce drinking water is known as *abstraction*, where this abstracted water is frequently referred to as *raw water* prior to treatment. Sources used for abstraction can be separated into groundwater (e.g., springs and wells) and surface water (e.g., streams, lakes, rivers, reservoirs, and stored rainwater), where groundwater is likely to be less polluted than surface water [11], although leaching of pesticides into groundwater can occur depending on the environmental fate and behavior of the chemical [12]. A process of assessment, monitoring, or both is used to inform decision making on what processes are necessary for the production of clean water. Basic treatment processes include screening, coagulation, clarification, filtration, and disinfection. In addition, where specific pollution is known to be or may potentially be present, a number of other processes may be used on certain DWTWs, including air stripping, for the removal of volatile compounds; filtration using GAC or powdered activated carbon (PAC) [13] and advanced oxidation processes (AOPs) using treatment with various combinations of ozone, ultraviolet (UV) light, titanium dioxide (TiO_2), and hydrogen peroxide (H_2O_2) [14].

18.7 REMOVAL OF EDCs DURING DRINKING WATER TREATMENT

Due to the large number and diverse nature of chemicals that are considered to have endocrine-disrupting potential, it is not possible here to provide a comprehensive description of the removal of every EDC during drinking water treatment processes. However, this section will aim to provide an overview of EDC removal, as well as mentioning a number of the key studies and reviews that have been conducted in this area to date. It should be noted that the fact that a chemical can be removed by drinking water treatment does not necessarily indicate that the chemical will be present in raw water.

In 1996, a preliminary laboratory investigation was undertaken by WRc, on behalf of UKWIR, into the removal of a range of steroids (E1, mestranol, E2, EE2, norethistrone, ethistrone, and

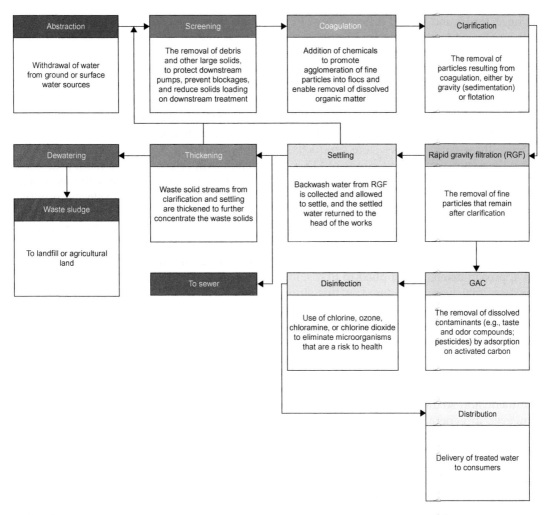

FIGURE 18.3 Overview of drinking water treatment processes. Between abstraction and human consumption, water undergoes a number of treatment processes designed to remove visible debris, microorganisms, and chemicals.

estriol) and a commercial mixture of nonylphenols by chlorination, ozonation, coagulation, and PAC from spiked borehole water (i.e., groundwater) [15]. Coagulation using aluminum sulfate was shown to have only a limited effect under the conditions of the study, whereas chlorine and ozone effectively removed all of the steroids and nonylphenols, respectively. PAC also effectively removed the steroids and removed approximately 65% of the nonylphenols.

A further study in 1997, conducted by WRc on behalf of UKWIR and DWI [10], confirmed these results. In this study, six DWTWs, using a number of different treatment processes (ranging from basic coagulation and chlorination to ozone and GAC treatment), were sampled, each on three separate occasions, and the concentrations of E1, E2, and EE2 were measured. A sensitive analytical method was used that allowed detection down to concentrations of

0.2 ng/L for E1 and E2 and 0.4 ng/L for EE2, but in all cases, the concentrations of these steroids was found to be below these limits of detection. Laboratory-scale studies using borehole water, designed to repeat the previous 1996 study but using the improved analytical method, indicated that chlorination, ozonation, and PAC treatment effectively reduced the concentrations of the three steroids (>95% removal), but that coagulation and filtration were ineffective. The authors noted that the results from the coagulation tests are limited, and that there may be greater removal from surface water, which contains higher organic matter content, due to the adsorption of the lipophilic steroids to the particulate matter.

Since these early studies were conducted, a large number of other studies have investigated the removal of a wider range of EDCs by different drinking water treatment processes. Table 18.3 summarizes a small number of these investigations and indicates the treatment processes that have been shown to be effective or ineffective at removing a selected number of EDCs. In addition, where experimental or field data are not available, it is possible to estimate the likely removal of chemicals by drinking water treatment processes based on their physicochemical properties, and the best current scientific and technical understanding of the chemical mechanisms and effectiveness of these various treatment processes. This was the approach taken, and applied to EDCs, in a study funded by DWI in 2012 [12]. Treatment processes that were considered in this study were coagulation/filtration, ozone, activated carbon, and chlorine, and some of these data are included in the table.

The selected chemicals listed in Table 18.3 have a range of different uses, including as industrial chemicals, pharmaceuticals, pesticides, and plasticizers, and have an array of different chemical structures, indicating the diverse nature of chemicals that are considered to have endocrine-disrupting potential. This diversity means that there are vast differences in the efficiencies of different processes in removing these chemicals during drinking water treatment; and so there is no one process that will remove all chemicals of potential concern. However, in general, the use of processes such as activated carbon filtration (PAC, GAC), UV irradiation, nanofiltration, and AOPs has been shown to result in effective removal, whereas processes such as simple coagulation and filtration are ineffective at removing many EDCs. The risk assessment and risk management approach to creating drinking water safety plans, as recommended by WHO and DWI [65,66], should identify any contaminants of particular concern for a specific water supply chain and take this into account when planning the treatment for that area.

18.8 OCCURRENCE OF EDCs IN DRINKING WATER

Studies at DWTWs have demonstrated that in many cases, chemicals that are detected in the source water to the works are no longer detected in the final water after treatment. A study at two DWTWs in Germany (published in 2002), reported trace (ng/L) concentrations of the pharmaceuticals clofibric acid and diclofenac in source waters to the works, but these same pharmaceuticals were not detected following the final stage of treatment. The first DWTW in this study used pre-ozonation, flocculation, ozonation, and GAC as treatment processes, and the second DWTW used flocculation, GAC, bank filtration, and slow sand filtration [67].

Similar data are available from research on a number of other EDCs. In a study reported in 2000, high concentrations of bisphenol A (BPA) were reported in the rivers Rhine and

TABLE 18.3   Overview of Removal of Selected EDCs by Drinking Water Treatment Processes

Chemical	Nature of chemical	Treatment process		
		Effective removal*[a]	Moderately effective*	Ineffective*[b]
Bisphenol A	Industrial chemical	Ozone, chlorine, chlorine dioxide [16] Nanofiltration [17]	–	UV light [18]
Clofibrate (clofibric acid)[c]	Pharmaceutical (lipid regulator)	Nanofiltration [19] UV light + TiO_2 [20]	Chlorine dioxide [21] UV + H_2O_2 [22]	Coagulation (iron), ozone, GAC [23]
Diclofenac	Pharmaceutical (NSAID)	GAC [24] Chlorine ozone [25] UV light + H_2O_2 [26] Chlorine dioxide [21] Nanofiltration [19]	Coagulation (ferric sulfate) [24]	Coagulation (aluminum sulfate) [24]
DDT[d]	Organochlorine insecticide	Coagulation, sedimentation, filtration [27] Combination of ozone and UV light [28] UV irradiation [29] PAC [30], GAC [31] Reverse osmosis [32]	Ozonation [27]	Chlorination [27]
Estrogenic steroids	Natural or synthetic hormones	Chlorine, ozone, PAC [10,15]	–	Coagulation, filtration [10,15]
Ibuprofen	Pharmaceutical (NSAID)	Ozone + H_2O_2 [33]	Chlorine [26] PAC [26] Ozone [34] Nanofiltration [19]	Coagulation [34] Ultrafiltration [35]
Iodinated contrast media	Pharmaceutical	UV light + TiO_2 [36,37] UV light + H_2O_2 [38] Nanofiltration[l]	Ozone, PAC [39]	Coagulation, sedimentation, filtration, chlorination, GAC [40]
MTBE	Petrol additive	Aeration [41] Ozone + H_2O_2 [42] Photocatalytic degradation using TiO_2 [43]	Ozone alone [42]	GAC [42]
Nonylphenols[e]	Industrial chemicals	Chlorine, ozone [15] Chlorine dioxide [16]	PAC [15]	Coagulation, filtration [15]
Nonylphenol ethoxylates[f]	Industrial chemicals	PAC [44] Ozonation [45]	–	–
Organotins[g]	PVC stabilizers, pesticides, anti-fouling	No data; generally considered to be removed with particulate matter [46]	–	–

(Continued)

4. PUBLIC POLICY AND REGULATORY CONSIDERATIONS

TABLE 18.3   (Continued)

Chemical	Nature of chemical	Treatment Process		
		Effective removal*[a]	Moderately effective*	Ineffective*[b]
Parabens[h,i]	Preservatives	Ozone [12]	Activated carbon, chlorine [12]	Coagulation [12]
Pesticides (atrazine and simazine)[j]	Triazine herbicides	UV light [47,48] Nanofiltration [49]	Ozone [30,50] Chlorine [30] PAC [30,51] GAC [52,53]	Coagulation and filtration [53,54]
Phthalates	Plasticizers	Activated carbon, PAC [55] UV light, ozone, and combinations [56]	–	–
Styrene[k]	Industrial chemical	Ozone, aeration, chlorine dioxide [57]	GAC [57]	Potassium permanganate, H_2O_2 [58]
Triclosan	Anti-bacterials	Coagulation, filtration and chlorination [59] Ozone [60] GAC [61] UV light + TiO_2 [62]	Nanofiltration [63]	UV light or TiO_2 alone [62]

Note: Chemicals included cover a range of different chemical classes and representative uses.

DDT, dichlorodiphenyltrichloroethane; GAC, granular activated carbon; H_2O_2, hydrogen peroxide; MTBE, methyl *tert*-butyl ether; NSAID, nonsteroidal anti-inflammatory drug; PAC, powdered activated carbon; TiO_2, titanium dioxide; UV, ultraviolet.

*Under the test conditions.
[a]*Generally less than 10% removal (where quantitative information available).*
[b]*Generally greater than or equal to 70% removal (where quantitative information available).*
[c]*Now less commonly prescribed due to long-term side effects.*
[d]*Now banned for all uses other than malaria control [64].*
[e]*Use is currently severely restricted in the EU.*
[f]*Now banned for use in domestic detergents in Europe.*
[g]*Use is now severely restricted, particularly as anti-fouling agents.*
[h]*Benzyl-, butyl-, ethyl-, methyl-, and propylparaben.*
[i]*Estimated based on the physico-chemical properties.*
[j]*Atrazine and simazine are no longer approved for use in the EU, although both are still approved for use in the United States and Australia.*
[k]*Considered to be a potential endocrine disrupter [an].*
[l]*pers comm.*

Meuse, but concentrations were below the limit of detection (8.8 or 11 ng/L) in drinking waters derived from these rivers at three DWTWs [40].

In 2003, as part of a European study, four DWTWs (in England, the Netherlands, France, and Germany) were monitored for a number of EDCs, including synthetic and natural estrogens, alkylphenols and alkylphenol ethoxylates, BPA, and organotin compounds. The four works included used a variety of different treatment processes and raw water sources. Concentrations of synthetic and natural estrogens were found to be below the limits of detection (0.050 ng/L for both E2 and EE2, and 0.25 ng/L for E1) at all four works, leading to a conclusion in the report that within the works in this case study, the occurrence of these estrogens in drinking water is not problematic. In general, in this study, low concentrations of EDCs, close to the limits of quantification, were detected in final drinking water in only a few cases, and it was concluded that although raw waters frequently contain EDCs, common drinking water treatment processes should be effective in removing EDCs [40].

The report from this European study discussed the possibility that even if EDCs are efficiently removed during the drinking water treatment processes, certain EDCs may still be present in final drinking water as a result of contamination due to leaching from plastic pipes or tubing in parts of the works [40]. In support of this theory, styrene was detected at a higher concentration in drinking water at the works than in raw waters. Styrene is an intermediate used in the manufacture of plastics and resins [68] and is suspected of being an endocrine disrupter [40,68,69]. In addition to leaching from plastics in the works themselves, certain chemicals may leach slightly over time from plastic pipes used in drinking water distribution. Phthalates are used as plasticizers, particularly in polyvinyl chloride (PVC) plastics where they impart flexibility, and it may be possible that they could leach from plastics over time into the drinking water supply; however, it has also been reported that few plastics used in contact with drinking water are likely to be plasticized with phthalates [70]. Equally, dialkyltins are used as stabilizers in PVC plastic pipes [46], and there is some evidence that although they migrate only slightly from rigid PVC [71], they can leach into drinking water from plastic pipes and can be present at low concentrations [46]. For this reason, PVC pipes are now less commonly used for drinking water distribution in the United Kingdom, and polyethylene pipes are the most widely used. In 2001, a study was conducted for DWI that investigated the exposure to EDCs via materials in contact with drinking water, and the conclusion was that the risk to consumers was negligible following correctly installed or refurbished water storage tanks [69]. However, PVC pipes are still commonly used in other countries, such as the United States and Canada [72], and in 2004, it was reported that 78% of drinking water pipes in the United States were made of PVC [73].

Another area of current interest is whether the process of natural gas extraction via hydraulic fracking could affect the levels of EDCs in the environment, and the subsequent potential for EDCs to contaminate water sources, including those that may be used for drinking water abstraction. The process of fracking involves the underground injection of a mixture of water, chemicals, and suspended solids under pressure, where more than 100 out of the 750 chemicals reportedly used in the process of fracking are known or suspected EDCs [74]. One study has shown higher levels of estrogenic, anti-estrogenic, androgenic, and anti-androgenic activity (as measured using reporter gene assays in human cell lines) in groundwater and surface water samples collected from a drilling-dense region of Colorado compared to control samples from the Colorado River [74]. The importance of these findings in terms of drinking water quality is unclear at present, but may have implications when planning potential sites for either hydraulic fracking or for drinking water abstraction. In the United Kingdom, the current position of Public Health England, an executive agency of the Department of Health, is that contamination of groundwater from the fracking process itself is unlikely, and that reported problems typically occur as a result of operational failure or poor regulation; and as a result, good on-site management and appropriate regulation are necessary for minimizing the risk to the environment and public health [75].

In general, reported levels of EDCs in finished drinking water are low (in the ng/L range) as shown in Table 18.4, which summarizes data from a number of monitoring studies, and

TABLE 18.4 Reported Concentrations of Selected EDCs in Finished Drinking Water

Chemical	Concentration (ng/L)	Sample Details	Countries/Regions	References
BPA	128 (maximum), 10.8 (median)	Detected in 60 out of 62 DWTWs from 31 major cities	China (reported in 2013)	[76]
	ND-44.3 (median: 2.7)	Detected 50% of samples from a DWTW	The United States (reported in 2013)	[77]
	3.7–50.3 (median: 14.8)	Detected in six tap water samples from private residences	Spain (2012)	[78]
	ND (raw water: 6.1–6.3)	Detected in tap water from four DWTWs	Europe[a] (reported in 2003)	[40]
	120	Detected at one of five DWTWs that monitored for bisphenol A	Europe[b] (2001)	[40]
	0.5–2	Detected in drinking water derived from groundwater and surface waters	Country not specified (reported in 2001)	[40]
	<LOD (raw water: 39–21 220[c])	Detected in drinking water derived from the river Rhine and Meuse	Belgium, Germany, and the The Netherlands (reported in 2000)	[40]
Clofibrate (clofibric acid)	19	Average concentration, detected in five out of eight tap waters	Spain (2012)	[79]
	5.3	Maximum concentration detected	Italy (reported in 2005)	[67]
	N/A	Detected but concentration not reported	The United Kingdom (reported in 2005)	[67]
	170	Maximum concentration in samples from 1 of 14 DWTWs	Germany (reported in 1996)	[67,80]
	<75	Concentrations in samples from the remaining 13 DWTWs (samples for two were below the limit of detection)		
Diclofenac	ND-9.4	Detected in 25% of samples from a DWTW	The United States (reported in 2013)	[77]
	18	Average concentration, detected in three out of eight tap waters	Spain (2012)	[79]
	ND (raw water: 76.3)	Maximum concentrations detected in a 12-month monitoring study at four DWTWs	The United Kingdom (2010)	[81]
	6	Maximum concentration detected	Germany (reported in 2005)	[67]
DDT	848.2, 275.3, and 115.9	Mean concentrations detected in drinking water samples from three rural areas	India (reported in 2012)	[82]
	6.5	Mean concentration detected in drinking water	South Africa (reported in 2009)	[83]
	3	Mean concentration detected in drinking water samples	Ottawa, Canada (1976)	[84]

Compound	Concentration	Description	Location	Reference
Estrogenic steroids	1.7 (maximum), 0.3 (median)	Detected in 53 out of 62 DWTWs from 31 major cities (estrone)	China (reported in 2013)	[76]
	0.1 (maximum), 0.04 (median)	Detected in 31 out of 62 DWTWs from 31 major cities (17β-estradiol)		
Ibuprofen	<LOD	Tap water from four DWTWs	Europe[a] (reported in 2003)	[40]
	ND-10.2	Detected in 13% of samples from a DWTW	The United States (reported in 2013)	[77]
	39	Average concentration, detected in seven out of eight tap waters	Spain (2012)	[79]
	3.07 (raw water: 38.4)	Maximum concentrations detected in a 12-month monitoring study at 4 DWTWs	The United Kingdom (2010)	[81]
	3	Maximum concentration detected	Germany (reported in 2005)	[67]
Iodinated contrast media		Tap water from four DWTWs:	Europe[a] (reported in 2003)	[40]
	180	Iopamidol		
	29	Iopromide		
	18-100	Diatrizoate		
	12	Iomeprol		
	ND	Iothalamic acid, ioxithalamic acid and iohexol		
MTBE	20	Median concentration detected in 45 drinking water samples	The Netherlands (2001)	[85]
	43-100	Concentration detected in drinking water samples	Germany (1999-2001)	[86]
Nonylphenols	558 (maximum), 27 (median)	Detected in 55 out of 62 DWTWs from 31 major cities	China (reported in 2013)	[76]
	12.4-60.6 (median: 19.5)	Detected in all samples from a DWTW	The United States (reported in 2013)	[77]
	2.5-20.5 (median: 7.3)	Detected in six tap water samples from private residences	Spain (2012)	[78]
	ND (raw water: 21-59 ng/L)	Tap water from four DWTWs	Europe[a] (reported in 2003)	[40]
	2.1 (raw water: 15-8000)	Detected at four out of five DWTWs that monitored for nonylphenol (maximum)	Europe[b] (2001)	[40]
	8	Mean reported concentration	Germany (2000)	[87]
	2.5-16	Concentration range		

(Continued)

TABLE 18.4 (Continued)

Chemical	Concentration (ng/L)	Sample Details	Countries/Regions	References
Nonylphenol ethoxylates	2.1–15 (median: 2.6)	Detected in six tap water samples from private residences (nonylphenol diethoxylate)	Spain (2012)	[78]
	2.6 (raw water: 0.9–12 ng/L)	Detected in the tap water from one out of four DWTWs (4-nonylphenol monoethoxylate)	Europe[a] (reported in 2003)	[40]
	8–110 (raw water: 180–1100)	Detected at one DWTW that monitored for nonylphenol ethoxylates	Europe[b] (2001)	[40]
Organotins	1.1 (raw water: ND–4.1)	Detected in the tap water from one out of four DWTWs (monobutyltin)	Europe[a] (reported in 2003)	[40]
	0.5–257	Detected in 10 out of 22 houses located on distribution lines where PVC pipes had recently been installed in five municipalities: methyltin	Canada (1996)	[88]
	0.5–6.5	Dimethyltin		
	0.49–8.1	Detected in a small number of drinking water supplies: methyltin	Florida, United States (1979)	[89]
	0.4–2.2	Dimethyltin		
Parabens	8.9–17.5 (median: 13.2)	Detected in six tap water samples from private residences: methylparaben	Spain (2012)	[78]
	0.97	Ethylparaben		
	7.12–17.2 (median: 11.9)	Propylparaben		
Pesticides (atrazine and simazine)	0.6–14.8 (median: 3.7)	Detected in all samples from a DWTW (atrazine)	The United States (reported in 2013)	[77]
	11.4	Detected in one sample from a UK-based water company (atrazine)	The United Kingdom (2009)	[90]
	<LOQ–43 (raw water: 10–390)	Detected in 10 out of 51 DWTWs that monitored for simazine	Europe[b] (2001)	[40]
	<LOQ–20 (raw water: 10–500)	Detected in 10 out of 51 DWTWs that monitored for atrazine		
	>100	Detected in a small percentage of samples from nine UK-based water companies (0.1–50.3% of samples, depending on the company) (atrazine)	The United Kingdom (1990)	[91]

	Concentration	Detection note	Location (year)	Reference
Phthalates	60 (raw water: 160)	Detected at the one DWTW that monitored for diisobutyl phthalate	Europe[b] (2001)	[40]
	100 (raw water: 290)	Detected at the one DWTW that monitored for dibutyl phthalate		
	7–289 (raw water: 13–840)	Detected at the two DWTWs that monitored for benzylbutyl phthalate		
	920–1200 (raw water: 1100–2900)	Detected at the one DWTW that monitored for bis(2-ethylhexyl)phthalate		
	50–9000	Detected in a drinking water supply (specific phthalates not reported)	Canada (1977)	[92]
	130–270	Detected at three DWTWs in New Orleans (dimethyl phthalate)	The United States (year not reported)	[93]
	Not reported	Detected by WRc at low μg/L levels in drinking water[d]	The United Kingdom (year not reported)	[94]
Styrene	193 (raw water: 70)	Maximum concentration detected in tap water from four DWTWs	Europe[a] (reported in 2003)	[40]
Triclosan	ND-59.6 (median: 1.4)	Detected in 63% of samples from a DWTW	The United States (reported in 2013)	[77]
	0.6–14.5	Detected in drinking water	China (reported in 2010)	[95]
	6.4	Maximum concentration detected in drinking water	The United States (reported in 2009)	
	<0.2–4	Detected in drinking water	Europe (reported in 2007)	

DDT, dichlorodiphenyltrichloroethane; LOD, limit of detection; LOQ, limit of quantification; MTBE, methyl tert-butyl ether; ND, not detected; PVC, polyvinyl chloride.

Note: Data from a range of studies have been included, including monitoring studies of tap water from private homes and at DWTWs, where these studies span a number of countries in order to be representative.

[a]One DWTWs from each of the following European countries: England, the Netherlands, France, and Germany, in an EU monitoring study.

[b]Completed study questionnaires were received from 51 DWTWs from five European countries (Spain, Germany, the United Kingdom, Belgium, and the Netherlands).

[c]The authors considered the maximum concentration to be unrealistically high and expressed some doubts about the validity of that result.

[d]A range of phthalates (dibenzyl phthalate, DEHP, butylbenzyl phthalate, diethyl phthalate, dimethyl phthalate, and dioctyl phthalates).

exposure to EDCs via drinking water is considered to be of minor importance in comparison to total exposure to these chemicals from all sources [40].

In 2012, a DWI-funded report was published that aimed to assess the likelihood of consumer exposure to chemicals with endocrine-disrupting potential of relevance to human health via drinking water. An initial literature search identified a candidate list of 325 possible EDCs that could be present in water bodies of relevance. Following prioritization and a multistage modeling process, 35 chemicals were predicted to have highest (worst-case) concentrations of greater than or equal to 100 ng/L in drinking water following conventional treatment processes. The extent of the risk posed was determined for these chemicals by establishing the margin of safety (MOS) between the estimated worst-case intake via drinking water and an established authoritative health-base value, or by deriving a limit using available hazard data, where an MOS greater than 100 was considered to indicate no appreciable risk. Only six chemicals with an MOS of less than or equal to 10 were identified; three industrial chemicals (p-benzylphenol, dibutyl phthalate, and 4-nitrophenol) and three pharmaceuticals (digoxin, fluticasone, and salbutamol). However, the report concluded that even at the predicted worst-case EDC concentrations, there would be no significant risk to human health from drinking water consumption (when expressed in terms of an equivalent E2 intake) [12].

18.9 CONCLUSIONS

Two treatment stages are generally in place to treat wastewater (sewage) through to drinking water. These stages are generally referred to as *wastewater treatment* and *drinking water treatment*. In addition, there is generally significant distance (and therefore dilution) between points of discharge from a sewage treatment works and abstraction of water at a DWTW.

Sewage is a complex mixture of materials that can refer to domestic and industrial waste, with sources including toilet water, bath and shower water, water from clothes and dish washing, and waste from offices and commercial businesses, as well as large chemical and industrial plants. Consequently, there is significant potential for chemicals with effects on the human endocrine system, including pharmaceuticals, industrial chemicals, and personal care and cleaning products, to enter sewage treatment works.

Sewage treatment works can also vary considerably in their design and complexity of removal processes, depending on the typical waste load entering the works. As a result, different sewage treatment works will have varying capabilities with regard to the removal of EDCs, which may vary widely in their chemical structures. However, taking the SEs as example of EDCs, sewage treatment works are generally more effective at removing the natural steroid estrogens E1 and E2 than the synthetic estrogen (and active ingredient of the contraceptive pill) EE2.

Drinking water treatment is, in general, more stringent than wastewater in removing chemicals, due to the potential risk to human health through ingestion of drinking water and its use in showering and bathing, and so on. The processes are based on the likely chemicals identified in the area due to, for example, industrial use of chemicals or pesticides used in agriculture. These processes may include the use of oxidative processes, UV light (which may break double bonds in organic chemicals, as well as kill microorganisms) and absorption by activated carbon. Generally, studies throughout the world indicate that EDCs, if present at all in drinking water, are detected at trace (ng/L) concentrations. While this concentration of the natural steroid hormone E2 may have estrogenic effects, most EDCs are of a much lower potency.

Countries may use a number of standards and guidelines derived using methods and studies accepted worldwide, in order to control the concentration of certain hazardous chemicals in both environmental and drinking water. At present, these controls are limited for EDCs as regulators continue to deal with problems related to hazard versus risk, mechanisms of action and potency as regards a recognized toxicological end point. However, a number of chemicals that may have endocrine-disrupting properties may be subject to a chemical-specific standard. In addition, in the EU, as well as standards for specific chemicals, there is a "catch-all" requirement for "wholesomeness" of drinking water that requires that the water to be free of a concentration of any chemical that may be of harm to human health.

Any potential risk to human health and the environment from exposure to EDCs in environmental and drinking water could be further reduced by societal and personal control of release of these chemicals. This includes the control of large-scale processes; for example, increasing knowledge of the toxicology, chemical properties and fate and behavior of industrial chemicals, such as that required by the EU Registration, Evaluation, Authorisation, and restriction of CHemicals (REACH) regulations, and increasing information about and control of pesticides used on agricultural land around water courses. However, it also involves personal everyday behavior such as the appropriate disposal of domestic cleaning agents, pesticides and pharmaceuticals and not simply flushing them down the sink, drain, or toilet.

Acknowledgments

The authors would like to thank Dave Shepherd, Glenn Dillon, and Rod Palfrey for their helpful discussions.

References

[1] Belfroid AC, Van des Horst A, Vethaak AD, Schäfer AJ, Rijs GBJ, Wegener J, et al. Analysis and occurrence of estrogenic hormones and their glucuronides in surface water and wastewater in the Netherlands. Sci Total Environ 1999;225:101–8.

[2] D'Ascenzo G, Di Corcia A, Gentili A, Mancini R, Mastropasqua R, Nazzari M, et al. Fate of natural estrogen conjugates in municipal sewage transport and treatment facilities. Sci Total Environ 2003;302:199–209.

[3] Muller M, Rabenoelina F, Balaguer P, Patureau D, Lemenach K, Budzinski H, et al. Chemical and biological analysis of endocrine-disrupting hormones and estrogenic activity in an advanced sewage treatment plant. Environ Toxicol Chem 2008;27:1649–58.

[4] Butwell AJ, Gardner M, Johnson I, Rockett L. Endocrine disrupting chemicals national demonstration programme logistical support project—assessment of the performance of the removal of oestrogenic substances at WwTWs—Final report. UKWIR TX04B; 2008.

[5] UKWIR Endocrine Disrupting Chemicals National Demonstration Programme: Assessment of the performance of WwTW in removing oestrogenic substances (09/TX/04/16). ISBN: 1 84057 525 5; 2009. Available from: <http://www.ukwir.org/ukwirlibrary/92721>.

[6] UKWIR Assessment of the performance of wastewater treatment works in removing oestrogenic substances (10/TX/04/17). ISBN: 1 84057 562 X; 2010. Available from: <https://www.ukwir.org/web/ukwirlibrary/93361>.

[7] Ternes TA, Stumpf M, Mueller J, Haberer K, Wilken R-D, Servos M. Behaviour and occurrence of estrogens in municipal sewage treatment plants—I. Investigations in Germany, Canada and Brazil. Sci Total Environ 1999;225:81–90.

[8] Baronti C, Curini R, D'Ascenzo G, Di Corcia A, Gentili A, Samperi R. Monitoring natural and synthetic estrogens at activated sludge treatment plants and in a receiving river water. Environ Sci Technol 2000;34:5059–66.

[9] Petrovic M, Solé M, López De Alda M, Barcelo D. Endocrine disruptors in sewage treatment plants, receiving river waters, and sediments: integration of chemical analysis and biological effects in feral carp. Environ Toxicol Chem 2002;21:2146–56.

[10] James H.A., Fielding M., Franklin O., Williams D., Lunt D. Steroid concentrations in treated sewage effluents and water courses—implications for water supplies. Final report to the Department of Environment and UK Water Industry Research Ltd. Report No. DWI 4323; 1997.

[11] Vigneswaren S, Visvanathan C. Water treatment processes. Simple options: CRC Press LLC.; 1995. ISBN-0-8493-8283-1.

[12] Bevan R, Harrison P, Youngs L, Whelan M, Golsan E, Macadam J, et al. A review of latest endocrine disrupting chemicals research implications for drinking water. Final report DWI 70/2/266. Available from: <www.dwi.gov.uk>; 2012.

[13] WRc. Water treatment processes and practices. ISBN-0-902156-87X; 1992.

[14] Linden KG, Rosenfeldt EJ, Kullman SW. UV/H2O2 degradation of endocrine-disrupting chemicals in water evaluated via toxicity assays. Water Sci Technol 2007;55:313–9.

[15] UKWIR. Effect of water treatment processes on oestrogenic chemicals. UKWIR; Report DW-05/10 Final. ISBN: 1-84057-006-7; 1996. Available from: <https://www.ukwir.org/web/ukwirlibrary/435>.

[16] Lenz K, Beck V, Fuerhacker M. Behaviour of bisphenol A (BPA), 4-nonylphenol (4-NP) and 4-nonylphenol ethoxylates (4-NP1EO, 4-NP2EO) in oxidative water treatment processes. Water Sci Technol 2004;50:141–7.

[17] Bing-zhi D, Lin W, Nai-yun G. The removal of bisphenol A by ultrafiltration. Desalination 2008;221:312–7.

[18] Zhou D, Wu F, Deng N, Xiang W. Photooxidation of bisphenol A (BPA) in water in the presence of ferric and carboxylic salts. Water Res 2004;38:4107–16.

[19] Verliefde A, Heijman D, Cornellisen E, Amy G, Van der Bruggen B, Van Dijk J. Influence of electrostatic interaction on the rejection with NF and assessment of the removal efficiency during NF/GAC treatment of pharmaceutically active compounds in surface water. Water Res 2007;41:3227–40.

[20] Doll TE, Frimmel FH. Kinetic study of photocatalytic degradation of carbamazepine, clofibric acid, iomeprol and iopromide assisted by different TiO2 materials-determination of intermediates and reaction pathways. Water Res 2004;38:955–64.

[21] Huber MM, Korhonene S, Ternes TA, Von Gunten U. Oxidation of pharmaceuticals during water treatment with chlorine dioxide. Water Res 2005;39:3607–17.

[22] Pereira V, Linden K, Weinberg H. Evaluation of UV irradiation for photolytic and oxidative degradation of pharmaceutical compounds in water. Water Res 2007;41:4413–23.

[23] Ternes TA, Meisenheimer M, McDowell D, Sacher F, Brauch H-J, Haiste-Gulde B, et al. Removal of pharmaceuticals during water treatment. Environ Sci Technol 2002;36:3855–63.

[24] Vieno N, Tuhkanen T, Kronberg L. Removal of pharmaceuticals in drinking water treatment: effect of chemical coagulation. Environ Technol 2006;27:183–92.

[25] Westerhoff P, Yoon Y, Snyder S, Wert E. Fate of endocrine-disruptor, pharmaceutical and personal care products during simulated drinking water treatment processes. Environ Sci Technol 2005;39:6649–63.

[26] Vogna D, Marotta R, Napolitano A, Andreozzi R, d'Ischia M. Advanced oxidation of the pharmaceutical drug diclofenac with UV/H2O2 and ozone. Water Res 2004;38:414–22.

[27] Robeck GG, Dostal KA, Cohen JM, Kreissed JF. Effectiveness of water treatment processes in pesticide removal. J Am Water Works Assoc 1965;57:181–200.

[28] Mauk CE. Oxidation of pesticides by ozone and ultra-violet light: US Department of Commerce, National Technical Information Service; 1976. A)-A028 306, July.

[29] Burrows H, Canle M, Santaballa J, Steenken S. Reaction pathways and mechanisms of photodegradation of pesticides. J Photochem Photobiol B 2002;67:71–108.

[30] Ormad MP, Miguel N, Claver A, Matesanz JM, Ovelleiro JL. Pesticide removal in the process of drinking water production. Chemosphere 2008;71:97–106.

[31] Thakkar N, Muthal P. Granular activated carbon in pesticide removal. Indian J Environ Health 1980;22:124–9.

[32] Bennet PJ. Removal of organic pesticides by reverse osmosis. 23rd industrial waste water conference, part 2; 1968. p. 1000–1017.

[33] Zweiner C, Frimmel FH. Oxidative treatment of pharmaceuticals in water. Water Res 2000;34:1881–5.

[34] Ternes TA, Stuber J, Hermann N, McDowell D, Reid A, Kampmann M, et al. Ozonation: a tool for removal of pharmaceuticals, contrast media and musk fragrances from wastewater? Water Res 2003;37:1976–82.

[35] Snyder SA, Adham S, Redding AM, Cannon FS, DeCarolis J, Oppenheimer J, et al. Role of membranes and activated carbon in the removal of endocrine disruptors and pharmaceuticals. Desalination 2007;202:156–81.

[36] Doll T, Frimmel F. Removal of selected persistent organic pollutants by heterogeneous photocatalysis in water. Catal Today 2005;101:195–202.

[37] Doll TE, Frimmel FH. Photocatalytic degradation of carbamazepine, clofibric acid and iomeprol with P25 and Hombikat UV100 in the presence of natural organic matter (NOM) and other organic water constituents. Water Res 2005;39:403–11.

[38] Sprehe M, Geissen S-U, Vogelpohl A. Photochemical oxidation of iodized X-ray contrast media (XRC) in hospital wastewater. Water Sci Technol 2001;44:317–23.

[39] Magdeburg A, Stalter D, Schlusener M, Ternes T, Oehlmann J. Evaluating the efficiency of advanced wastewater treatment: target analysis of organic contaminants and (geno-) toxicity assessment tell a different story. Water Res 2014;50:35–47.

[40] Wenzel A, Muller J, Ternes T. Env.D.1/ETU/200/0083 Study of endocrine disruptors in drinking water. Schmallenberg and Wiesbaden: Fraunhofer IME; 2003.

[41] McKinnon R, Dyksen J. Removing organics from groundwater through aeration plus GAC. J Am Water Works Assoc 1984;76:42–7.

[42] Dyksen JE, Ford R, Raman K, Schaefer JK, Fung L, Schwartz B, et al. In-line ozone and hydrogen peroxide treatment for removal of organic chemicals. AWWA Res Found Am Water Works Assoc 1992.

[43] Barreto RD, Gray KA, Anders K. Photocatalytic degradation of methyl-*tert*-butyl ether in TiO$_2$ slurries: a proposed reaction scheme. Water Res 1995;29:1243–8.

[44] Narkis N, Ben-David B. Adsorption of non-ionic surfactants on activated carbon and mineral clay. Water Res 1985;19:815–24.

[45] Delanghe B, Mekras C, Graham N. Aqueous ozonation of surfactants: a review. Ozone Sci Eng 1991;13:639–73.

[46] WHO. Dialkyltins in drinking-water. Background document for development of WHO Guidelines for Drinking-Water Quality. World Health Organization. WHO/SDE/WSH/03.04/109; 2004. Available from: <http://www.who.int/water_sanitation_health/dwq/chemicals/dialkyltins.pdf?ua=1>.

[47] Le Brun O, Merlet M, Croue JP, Dore M. Photolytic decomposition of pesticides in an aqueous medium. Sci Tech Eau 1993;26:97–101.

[48] Bourgine FP, Chapman JI, Keral H, Duval JL, Green JG, Hamilton D. The degradation of atrazine and other pesticides by photolysis. Water Environ Manage 1995;9:417–23.

[49] Hofman JAMH, Noij THM, Kruithof JC, Schippers JC. Removal of pesticides and other micropollutants with membrane filtration. Water Supply 1993;11:259–69.

[50] Duguet JP, Bernazeau F, Bruchet A. Occurrence of pesticides in natural waters and removal during drinking water treatment processes. Water Supply 1994;12:111–5.

[51] Haist-Gulde B, Baldauf G, Brauch HJ. Removal of pesticides from raw waters. Water Supply 1993;11:187–96.

[52] Croll B, Chadwick B, Knight B. The removal of atrazine and other herbicides from water using granular activated carbon. Water Supply 1992;10:111–20.

[53] Normann S, Haberer K, Oehmichen U. Behaviour of nitrogen containing plant protection agents (herbicides) during drinking water purification. Vom Wasser 1987;69:233–49.

[54] Van Hoof F, Ackermans P, Celens JN. Herbicides in the River Meuse Basin in Belgium and their behaviour during water treatment. Water Supply 1992;10:81–8.

[55] Shahmansouri A, Bellona C. Application of quantitative structure-property relationships (QSPRs) to predict the rejection of organic solutes by nanofiltration. Sep Purif Technol 2013;118:627–38.

[56] Oh BS, Jung YJ, Oh YJ, Yoo YS, Kang JW. Application of ozone, UV and ozone/UV processes to reduce diethyl phthalate and its estrogenic activity. Sci Total Environ 2006;367:681–93.

[57] US EPA. Reviews of environmental contamination and toxicology, vol. 107. 1989.

[58] Kun Z, Hui C, Guanghe L, Zhaochang L. *In situ* remediation of petroleum compounds in groundwater aquifer with chlorine dioxide. Water Res 1998;32:1471–80.

[59] Azzouz A, Ballesteros E. Influence of seasonal climate differences on the pharmaceutical, hormone and personal care product removal efficiency of a drinking water plant. Chemosphere 2013;93:2046–54.

[60] Suarez S, Dodd MC, Omil F, von Gunten U. Kinetics of triclosan oxidation by aqueous ozone and consequent loss of antimicrobial activity: relevance to municipal wastewater ozonation. Water Res 2007;41:2481–90.

[61] Behera SK, Oh SY, Park HS. Sorption of triclosan onto activated carbon, kaolinite and montmorillonite: effects of pH, ionic strength and humic acid. J Hazard Mater 2010;179:684–91.

[62] Yu JC, Kwong TY, Luo Q, Cai Z. Photocatalytic oxidation of triclosan. Chemosphere 2006;65:390–9.

[63] Whitaker AF, Moore AT. Pilot scale investigations on the removal of volatile organics and phthalates from electronics manufacturing wastewater. Proceedings of the 38th industrial waste conference. Purdue University; 1983. p. 579–589.

[64] US EPA Pesticides. Topical & chemical fact sheets. DDT—a brief history and status. Available from: <http://www.epa.gov/pesticides/factsheets/chemicals/ddt-brief-history-status.htm>.

[65] WHO Water safety plans. Managing drinking-water quality from catchment to consumer. World Health Organization. WHO/SDE/WSH/05.06; 2005. Available from: <http://www.who.int/water_sanitation_health/dwq/wsp170805.pdf>.

[66] DWI. A brief guide to drinking water safety plans. UK Drinking Water Inspectorate. Available from: <http://dwi.defra.gov.uk/stakeholders/guidance-and-codes-of-practice/Water%20Safety%20Plans.pdf>; 2005.

[67] Watts C, Maycock D, Crane M, Fawell J, Goslan E. Desk based review of current knowledge on pharmaceuticals in drinking water and estimation of potential levels: Watts and Crane Associates and Cranfield University; 2007. Defra Project Code: CSA 7184/WT02046/DWI70/2/213. Available from: <http://dwi.defra.gov.uk/research/completed-research/reports/dwi70-2-213.pdf>.

[68] Centre for Food Safety. Endocrine disrupting chemicals in food. Risk assessment studies report no. 48. Food and Environmental Hygiene Department, The Government of the Hong King Special Administrative Region. Available from: <http://www.cfs.gov.hk/english/programme/programme_rafs/files/programme_rafs_fc_01_32_EDC_in_food_Report.pdf>; 2012.

[69] Duckham C, Abery B. Exposure to endocrine disruptors via materials in contact with drinking water—phase 2. Final report to DEFRA/DWI. DWI 70/2/88(II); 2001. Available from: <http://dwi.defra.gov.uk/research/completed-research/reports/DWI70_2_88_ed.pdf>.

[70] Fatoki OS, Vernon F. Phthalate esters in rivers of the Greater Manchester area U.K. Sci Total Environ 1990;95:227–32.

[71] Gachter R, Muller H, editors. Plastics additives handbook. Stabilizers, processing aids, plasticizers, fillers, reinforcements, colourants for thermoplastics. Munich, Vienna, New York: Hanser Publishers; 1985.

[72] Rahman S. Thermoplastics at work: a comprehensive review of municipal PVC piping products. Underground construction; 2004. p. 56–61.

[73] Rahman S. PVC Pipe & fittings: underground solutions for water and sewer systems in North America. 2nd Brazilian PVC Congress. Sao Paulo, Brazil; June 19–20, 2007.

[74] Kassotis CD, Tillitt DE, Davis JW, Hormann AM, Nagel SC. Estrogen and androgen receptor activities of hydraulic fracturing chemicals and surface and ground water in a drilling-dense region. Endocrinology 2014;155:897–907.

[75] Kibble A, Cabianca T, Daraktchieva Z, Gooding T, Smithard J, Kowalczk G, et al. Review of the potential public health impacts of exposures to chemical and radioactive pollutants as a result of the shale gas extraction process. Radiation: PHE-CRCE report series. Centre for Radiation, Chemical and Environmental Hazards, Public Health England. 2014. ISBN 978-0-85951-752-2. Available from: <https://www.gov.uk/government/uploads/system/uploads/attachment_data/file/332837/PHE-CRCE-009_3-7-14.pdf>.

[76] Fan Z, Hu J, An W, Yang M. Detection and occurrence of chlorinated by-products of bisphenol A, nonylphenol and estrogens in drinking water of China: comparison to the parent compounds. Environ Sci Technol 2013;47:10841–10850.

[77] Padhye LP, Yao H, Kung'u FT, Huang CH. Year-long evaluation on the occurrence and fate of pharmaceuticals, personal care products, and endocrine disrupting chemicals in an urban drinking water treatment plant. Water Res 2014;51:266–76.

[78] Esteban S, Gorga M, González-Alonso S, Petrovic M, Barceló D, Valcárcel Y. Monitoring endocrine disrupting compounds and estrogenic activity in tap water from Central Spain. Environ Sci Pollut Res Int 2014;21(15):9297–310.

[79] Carmona E, Andreu V, Picó Y. Occurrence of acidic pharmaceuticals and personal care products in Turia River Basin: from waste to drinking water. Sci Total Environ 2014;484:53–63.

[80] Heberer T, Stan HJ. Occurrence of polar organic contaminants in Berlin drinking water. Vom Wasser 1996;86:19–31.

[81] Boxall ABA, Monteiro SC, Fussell R, Williams RJ, Brumer J, Greenwood R, et al. Targeted monitoring for human pharmaceuticals in vulnerable source and final waters. Drinking Water Inspectorate; 2011. Project No. WD0805 (Ref DWI 70/2/231). Available from: <http://dwi.defra.gov.uk/research/completed-research/reports/DWI70_2_231.pdf>.

[82] Kaushik CP, Sharma HR, Kaushik A. Organochlorine pesticide residues in drinking water in the rural areas of Haryana, India. Environ Monit Assess 2012;184:103–12.

[83] Sereda B, Bouwman H, Kylin H. Comparing water, bovine milk, and indoor residual spraying as possible sources of DDT and pyrethroid residues in breast milk. J Toxicol Environ Health, Part A 2009;72:842–51.

[84] Williams DT, Benoit FM, McNeil EE, Otson R. Organochlorine pesticide levels in Ottawa drinking water, 1976. Pestic Monit J 1978;12:163.

[85] Morgenstern P, Versteegh AF, de Korte GA, Hoogerbrugge R, Mooibroek D, Bannink A, et al. Survey of the occurrence of residues of methyl tertiary butyl ether (MTBE) in Dutch drinking water sources and drinking water. J Environ Monit 2003;5:885–90.

[86] Achten C, Kolb A, Püttmann W. Occurrence of methyl *tert*-butyl ether (MTBE) in riverbank filtered water and drinking water produced by riverbank filtration. 2. Environ Sci Technol 2002;36:3662–70.

[87] Kuch HM, Ballschmiter K. Determination of endocrine-disrupting phenolic compounds and estrogens in surface and drinking water by HRGC-(NCI)-MS in the picogram per liter range. Environ Sci Technol 2001;35:3201–6.

[88] Sadiki A-I, Williams DT, Carrier R, Thomas B. Pilot study on the contamination of drinking water by organotin compounds from PVC materials. Chemosphere 1996;32:2389–98.

[89] Braman RS, Tompkins MA. Separation and determination of nanogram amounts of inorganic tin and methyltin compounds in the environment. Anal Chem 1979;51:12–19.

[90] DWI. Report by the Chief inspector of drinking water. UK Drinking Water Inspectorate. DWI report 2009. Available from: <http://webarchive.nationalarchives.gov.uk/20120906081707/http:/dwi.defra.gov.uk/about/annual-report/2009/index.htm>.

[91] PSD. Pesticides 2003. Electronic guide to approved pesticides. Pesticides Safety Directorate (an executive agency of the Ministry of Agriculture, Fisheries and Food) and the Health and Safety Directorate. HMSO. Available from: <http://www.pesticides.gov.uk/>; 1992.

[92] Leah TD. The production use and distribution of phthalic acid esters in Canada. Inland Waters Directorate, Ontario Region, Water Planning and Management Branch; 1977.

[93] EC IUCLID datasheet on dimethyl phthalate. International uniform chemical information dataset: European Commission, European Chemicals Bureau; 2000.

[94] Lewis S, Howe AJ, Comber S, Reynolds P, Mascarenhas R, Sutton A, et al. Proposed environmental quality standards for phthalates in water. Final report to the Department of the Environment, Transport and the Regions. DoE 3929/3 (P); 1998.

[95] Bedoux G, Roig B, Thomas O, Dupont V, Le Bot B. Occurrence and toxicity of antimicrobial triclosan and by-products in the environment. Environ Sci Pollut Res Int 2012;19:1044–65.

Regulatory Considerations for Dermal Application of Endocrine Disrupters in Personal Care Products

Philippa D. Darbre and Philip W. Harvey

OUTLINE

Endocrine Disruption and Human Health.
DOI: http://dx.doi.org/10.1016/B978-0-12-801139-3.00019-3

Abstract

This chapter provides an overview of the chemical components of personal care products (PCPs) that possess endocrine-disrupting activity, and cites evidence that such endocrine-disrupting chemicals (EDCs) can be absorbed from application to human skin. Reported cases are described where absorption of EDCs from PCPs has affected human endocrine health. The use of PCPs presents high dermal exposure to multiple EDCs on a daily basis, and many of these EDCs have been measured in human tissue. Although it is not possible to identify the source of each EDC measured in human tissue, many of these chemicals are used only in PCPs, and several studies have found an association between concentrations measured in the tissue and self-reported use of PCPs. Dermal application of PCPs as a source of EDCs is an emerging issue, and national and international regulatory bodies are moving toward greater regulation of the component chemicals.

19.1 INTRODUCTION

Personal care products (PCPs) applied to the human body as lotions, creams, or sprays are a source of high exposure to endocrine-disrupting chemicals (EDCs). A majority of exposures are dermal, although there is the potential for inhalation from sprays [1], as well as for oral exposure from compounds such as triclosan, which is used in toothpaste and mouthwash [2]. Table 19.1 illustrates the range of products that are used, not only by women, but also by men, young children, and babies. In addition, use of such products by pregnant women presents the potential for placental transfer to the baby in utero. Intensive advertising and social pressures ensure conformity to using a range of these products, and not only are multiple products used every day, but many of these products are reapplied multiple times each day [3]. Presumably, increasing sales of PCPs would indicate increased exposure, and total personal care expenditure by the UK population continues to increase, from 12.9 billion pounds in 1997 to 26.7 billion pounds in 2013 [4].

Some products are washed off, but many are left on the skin for extended periods, which allows component chemicals to be absorbed at low doses over the long term and deposited into underlying tissues. Many of the formulations contain ingredients designed specifically to aid the even spread of the chemicals over the skin surface and to increase penetration. Some products, such as underarm cosmetics and aftershave lotions, are applied after shaving, and since shaving can damage the skin [5], this practice can allow for a greater uptake of chemicals than through intact skin (see Section 19.3).

The link between EDCs and reproductive abnormalities in aquatic wildlife has been attributed to the near-continuous exposure of these organisms to the chemicals in the water in which they live (see Chapter 1). The use of leave-on PCPs provides an analogous situation for the human body, exposing various proportions of the skin for prolonged time periods to chemicals, some of which possess endocrine-disrupting properties. This final section describes the accumulating evidence that PCPs provide a significant exposure to EDCs for the human body, and that greater regulation of their use is an appropriate precaution to protect human health.

TABLE 19.1   Exposure Routes for PCPs

Products	Rinse-off products	Leave-on products
DERMAL EXPOSURE		
Skin-care products	Soaps	Creams, lotions, powder
Underarm products		Deodorants, antiperspirants
Makeup		Eyes, facial, nails
Hair products	Shampoos	Colors, conditioners, creams, gels, lotions, perms, sprays, waxes
Fragrances		Lotions, sprays
Shaving products	Shaving creams and foams	Aftershave lotions
Sun-care products		Creams, lotions, oils
Bath products	Bubble baths, gels, oils, salts	
Feminine hygiene		Personal lubricants, creams
DERMAL EXPOSURE WITH INHALATION		
Underarm products		Deodorants, antiperspirants in spray formats
Hair products		Colors, conditioners, lotions, perms in spray formats
Fragrances		Perfume and cologne sprays
Shaving and sun-care products		Sprays
DERMAL WITH ORAL EXPOSURE		
Makeup		Lipstick
Oral hygiene	Mouthwash, toothpaste	
DERMAL EXPOSURE IN EARLY LIFE		
Baby care	Soaps, shampoos, bath products	Baby wipes, creams, lotions, powders (especially in the diaper area)

19.2 WHERE ARE EDCs FOUND IN PCPs?

Chemical constituents of PCPs are added for a variety of functional reasons, and many components have now been found to possess endocrine-disrupting properties, as illustrated in Figure 19.1. This breadth of products gives the potential for dermal exposure to a mixture of EDCs on a daily basis.

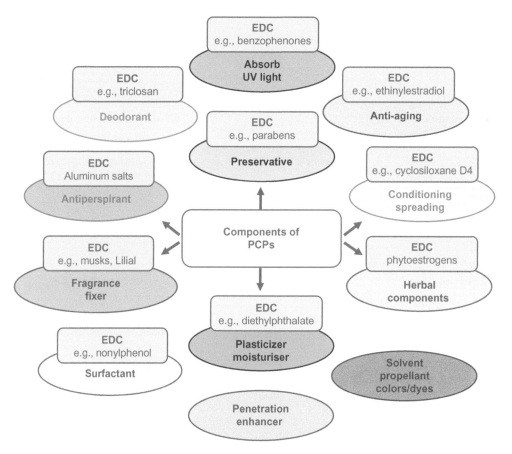

FIGURE 19.1   Components of PCPs that possess endocrine-disrupting ability. References documenting the endocrine-disrupting activity of the example compounds are given in the text.

Preservatives are added in order to prevent microbial or fungal growth during storage of the product, and the alkyl esters of *p*-hydroxybenzoic acid (parabens), which are frequently used for this purpose, have been shown to possess estrogenic and antiandrogenic activity [6,7], thyroid hormone–disrupting activity [8,9], and obesogenic properties [10].

Deodorants are used to mask, modify, or prevent body odor. Since undesirable smells are generated through the action of bacteria on sweat on the skin surface, a variety of phenolic compounds, often chlorinated, are added as antimicrobials to kill the bacteria. Triclosan (5-chloro-2-(2,4-dichlorophenoxy)phenol) is one such compound that is used frequently as both a deodorant and a preservative. Triclosan has known endocrine-disrupting activities [2], including estrogenic and androgenic activity [11], and thyroid hormone-disrupting activity [9]. Fragrances are used to mask any smell generated.

Antiperspirant agents are added to prevent perspiration, particularly in underarm cosmetics [12]. These are principally aluminum-based salts, aluminum chloride, aluminum chlorohydrate, or aluminum zirconium chlorohydrate glycine complexes [12]. Their mechanism of action is thought to involve the formation of a physical plug at the top of the sweat duct, which then prevents the escape of sweat onto the body surface [12]. Aluminum is a metalloestrogen [13].

Chemical components are added to PCPs to absorb ultraviolet-A (UVA; 315–400nm) or ultraviolet-B (UVB; 280–315nm) radiation. These are used in sunscreen products to protect the user from sunburn, but also in other products to protect the product itself from ultraviolet (UV) damage during storage. Many different chemical compounds are used as UV filters, but frequently used chemicals with known endocrine-disrupting properties include benzophenone-2 (BP-2), benzophenone-3 (BP-3), octylmethoxycinnamate (OMC), 4-methylbenzilidene-camphor (4-MBC), and homosalate (HS) [14].

Fragrances are added to most PCPs, and fragrance fixers are added to extend the life of the fragrance. Nitromusks and polycyclic musk fragrances are used in many cosmetics, perfumes, and laundry detergents, and several possess estrogenic activity [15,16]. Benzyl salicylate and butylphenylmethylpropional (Lilial) also possess estrogenic activity [17].

Cyclosiloxanes [18] have been incorporated widely as spreading and conditioning agents. Octamethylcyclotetrasiloxane (D4) is a low-molecular-weight cyclic siloxane with high lipid solubility and is permitted in PCPs up to 40–60% by weight [19]. D4 has long been known to interfere with the female reproductive system in animal models [20], and it possesses estrogenic activity in both in vitro models and in vivo uterotropic assays [21,22].

Diethyl phthalate (DEP) is used in cosmetics as a plasticizer, a solvent, and a carrier for fragrance [23]. A 2011 survey in Canada confirmed that it is the most frequently used phthalate in PCPs, contained in 103 out of 252 products surveyed, and with the highest levels found in fragrances [24]. In the United States, dibutyl phthalate (DBP) was found, as well as DEP, most frequently in perfumes (detection frequency of 100% for DEP, 67% for DBP), skin toners (90% for DEP), and nail polishes (90% for DBP) [25]. DEP and DBP are known to possess estrogenic activity [26], and increased concentrations of the metabolite monoethylphthalate in human urine has been associated with obesity [27,28].

Nonylphenol ethoxylates and nonylphenol are nonionic surfactants used in laundry detergents and cosmetics for cleansing purposes. Both nonylphenol ethoxylates and nonylphenol possess endocrine-disrupting properties [29].

In contrast to the compounds added to PCPs and subsequently found to possess endocrine-disrupting activity, some components are added to cosmetic products and cosmeceuticals specifically for their endocrine properties. The synthetic estrogen ethinylestradiol is added to anti-aging creams to extend a youthful phenotype to skin. Extracts containing phytoestrogens from hop or from *Pueraria mirifica* are added to increase bust size and contain the phytoestrogens 8-prenylnaringenin and mirestrol/deoxymirestrol [30], respectively. Extracts of *Aloe vera* are added widely for their skin-healing properties, but anthraquinones do possess estrogenic activity [31]. Lavender oil and tea-tree oils are also added to cosmetics, and they contain estrogenic components [32].

19.3 EVIDENCE THAT EDCs CAN BE ABSORBED FROM DERMAL APPLICATION OF COSMETICS

The principle that EDCs contained in cosmetic creams can be absorbed from dermal application in human subjects has been established by Janjua et al. in Denmark using human volunteers. The rates of absorption of three dermally applied sunscreens (BP-3, 4MBC, and OMC) were measured in 32 healthy volunteers (15 men and 17 women). None of the sunscreens were detectable before the first application, but after dermal application, all three were detectable in plasma after 2 h and in urine after 24 h [33]. In a separate study, systemic absorption of dermally applied DEP, DBP, and butylparaben was demonstrated in 26 healthy male volunteers with levels measurable in blood after 1 h [34] and in urine after 8–12 h [35]. Studies of triclosan applied at 2% as a cream to six volunteers showed that an average of $5.9 \pm 2.1\%$ of the dose had penetrated the skin within 48 h [36].

Studies of the ability of cosmetic chemicals to be absorbed through human skin can be performed in vitro using a Franz diffusion cell. The Franz cell consists of two chambers separated by a membrane, which can be human skin. The test product is applied to the skin through the top chamber and samples can be taken for analysis from the bottom chamber which is fluid-filled. Such studies have confirmed that parabens can be absorbed through human skin as intact esters [37]. Although it had been assumed that unbroken skin would provide a barrier to the transdermal uptake of aluminum from its application as antiperspirant salts to the underarm, using Al^{26} as a tracer of the aluminum, Flarend et al. [38] demonstrated in 2001 that aluminum can penetrate the skin from application as aluminum chlorohydrate to the underarm. In vitro studies using a Franz diffusion cell have confirmed that aluminum can be absorbed through human skin from application of antiperspirant salts and can be absorbed to a greater extent through stripped (a procedure equivalent to shaving) than through intact skin [39]. Comparison of aluminum chlorohydrate from a stick formulation showed aluminum absorption of $1.81 \mu g/cm^2$ for intact skin, but this value increased to $11.5 \mu g/cm^2$ for stripped skin [39]. Percutaneous absorption studies of octamethylcyclotetrasiloxane (D4) using the human skin/nude mouse model have shown that dermal absorption is low, but nevertheless, of the 0.02% of the applied dose that remained in the skin after 24 h, 29% could be retained in the dermis and 10% in the subcutaneous adipose tissue [40].

19.4 REPORTED CASES WHERE ABSORPTION OF EDCs FROM PCPs HAS AFFECTED HUMAN ENDOCRINE HEALTH

Several reports now testify to endocrine abnormalities following topical exposure to products containing hormonally active substances. One of the most cited cases is "The Mortician's Mystery," published in the *New England Journal of Medicine* in 1988 [41]. This paper describes the case of an embalmer who presented with gynecomastia and hypogonadotropic hypogonadism, but with undetectable levels of endogenous estrogens. His pubertal development had been uneventful, and he had fathered seven children, but over the previous 10 years, he had suffered progressive loss of libido, decrease in testicular size, and marked breast development. Over these 10 years, he had been working as an embalmer applying creams to corpses without wearing gloves. The paper gives evidence that the cream contained estrogenic components, and that after a year of the cessation of exposure to the embalming cream through wearing gloves, the symptoms had reversed, including increase in the size of his testes. This demonstrates a case where long-term topical exposure of the hands to embalming creams can result in endocrine disruption in the human body, and following other similar findings in other morticians, this syndrome has been termed "the embalmer's curse" [42].

Endocrine disruption has now been reported in women as well as men following inappropriate exposure to topical estrogenic chemicals in PCPs. A case in Italy reports premature breast development (thelarche), menstruation, and uterus enlargement in a 36-month-old girl following exposure to hair lotion containing estrogenic components used by her mother [43]. Youth enhancement in a 46-year-old woman was noted after 4 weeks of use of an estrogen-containing skin moisturizer, which was noted to be of concern because she had presented with estrogen receptor (ER)–positive breast cancer [44]. Long-term use of an ethinylestradiol-containing body-care cream in a 93-year-old woman was reported as associated with abnormal genital bleeding, endometrial hyperplasia, and development of breast cancer [45]. On the other hand, prepubertal gynecomastia has been reported in three boys (28 months, 33 months, and 8 years of age) following indirect exposure to topical estrogen-containing creams used by their mothers [46] and in a prepubertal boy following exposure to an estrogen-containing hair cream [47]. In this context, natural products are also not without effect, and cosmetics containing lavender oil and tea-tree oil have been reported to expand breast tissue, giving rise to gynecomastia in men [32].

By contrast, some topical creams can contain androgenic or anabolic substances, and these have also been reported to cause endocrine disruption in women and men. Two women have been reported to develop symptoms of virility following exposure to androgen-containing cream, one (aged 44 years) associated with dysphonia and one (aged 52 years) with facial acneiform eruption and hypertrichosis [48]. In the same report, three men were reported with endocrine problems following exposure to topical anabolic cream, one man (31 years) had gynecomastia, one man (35 years) had symptoms of erectile dysfunction, loss of libido and infertility, and a third man (26 years) had striae distensae and acne [48].

Another equally poignant case was described in the *American Journal of Medicine* in 2004, where a female patient presented with bone pain and extreme fatigue recognized as being associated with the previous four years of aluminum-based antiperspirant use [49]. Aluminum levels in her plasma were measured as 4 mM, but after discontinuing antiperspirant use, the levels returned to the normal range (0.1–0.3 mM) within 8 months, and the associated symptoms disappeared. Again, this demonstrates a case where a topically applied cosmetic can penetrate the skin and give rise to adverse physiological consequences.

Nowadays, the administration of hormone replacement therapy (HRT) by skin patches relies on the ability of the hormones to be absorbed from a patch through the skin and to then have a physiological impact on menopausal symptoms. Similarly, contraceptives can also be administered by skin patch. This, therefore, poses serious questions as to whether daily application of multiple cosmetic products containing a variety of chemicals with endocrine-disrupting properties could result in low-level absorption of many different chemicals, which together might be generating adverse endocrine responses over the long term.

19.5 DERMAL EXPOSURE AND MEASUREMENT IN HUMAN TISSUE

EDCs applied in PCPs present a high level of exposure to human skin, and despite low-level absorption from each application, there can still be the potential that low doses will be retained in underlying tissues from long-term usage, especially from leave-on products. Although it is not possible to identify the specific source of chemicals measured in human tissue, many of the EDCs used in PCPs have been measured widely in urine, blood, or both from across the general population. Some studies have specifically correlated higher concentrations of some EDCs with greater usage of PCPs. Table 19.2 summarizes some of the EDCs in PCPs and their detection in human tissues.

19.5.1 Parabens

Although some exposure to parabens may come through their use as preservatives in medical products, in paper products, or through their presence in indoor air, the main routes of exposure are oral (from food) or dermal (from topical application of PCPs) [6,7]. On the basis of paraben concentrations measured in foods and per-capita daily ingestion rates of foods in the United States, a recent estimated daily intake of total parabens has been calculated as 940, 879, 470, and 307 ng/kg/day for infants, toddlers, children, and adults, respectively [75]. However, on the basis of the amount and frequency of use of PCPs and measured median paraben concentrations in products, the total dermal intake doses of parabens have been calculated to be 31.0 μg/kg/day for adult females and between 58.6 and 766 μg/kg/day for infants and toddlers [25], suggesting that exposure through PCPs can be substantial. A similar conclusion was also reached through calculations showing that a significant estrogenic challenge to breast tissue could be achieved from dermal absorption of total parabens [76] or even single-paraben esters [7] in one application of a body-care lotion to the breast/chest area. Using no more than maximal current European Union (EU)–recommended levels, the estrogenic stimulus generated from a single application of lotion is biologically meaningful; values in Table 19.3 shown in bold are those greater than 20% of the endogenous estrogen levels of 55.3 pg/mL/g in tissue [81]. From comparison to the concentrations of each of the paraben esters measured in human breast tissue [51] as converted to estrogen equivalents, it can be seen that even the highest concentrations measured in the human breast tissue could be achieved by very few such applications of lotion (Table 19.3). This needs to be considered in the context of exposure of a large global population where, on average, each consumer would use not one but multiple PCPs on a daily basis [3].

Since the first detection of parabens in human breast tumor tissue in 2004 [52], further measurements have confirmed their presence in all regions of the human breast [51] and in human milk [53,54], opening a debate on their potential involvement in breast cancer development [6,7]. They have also been measured ubiquitously in urine samples of the general US [59,60] and European populations [57,61]. A Norwegian study reported that paraben esters can be measured in over 60% of blood samples taken from the general population, and that there was a significant association between blood paraben concentration and self-reported use of PCPs [50]. In the US urine survey, differences in paraben concentrations across demographic groups, especially sex and race/ethnicity, were also suggested to reflect different patterns of cosmetic use [60]. Other studies have found parabens in human semen in Denmark [57] and in the United States [58], which has opened a debate on possible involvement in sperm DNA damage and male reproductive health [58], especially in view of previously reported reproductive toxicity in male animal models [82–85].

TABLE 19.2   Components of PCPs with Endocrine-Disrupting Activity: Evidence That They Can Be Absorbed from Topical Application and Measurement in Human Tissue

Component chemicals	Function in the product	Endocrine-disrupting activity	Systemic absorption into humans from topical application	Measurement in human tissue
Parabens (methyl-, ethyl-, n-propyl-, isopropyl, n-butyl-, isobutyl, benzyl)	Preservative	Estrogenic and antiandrogenic [6], thyroid disruption [8,9], obesogenic [10]	Dorsal skin into blood [34] and urine [35]	Blood [50], breast tissue [51,52], milk [53,54], placenta [55,56], semen [57,58], urine [57,59–61]
Triclosan	Deodorant/preservative	endocrine disrupting [2] including estrogenic and androgenic [11] and thyroid-disrupting activities [9]	Dermal cream into blood [36]	Blood [62], milk [53,63,64], urine [65]
BP-3, BP-2, octyl-methoxycinnamate, 4-MBC, HS	Absorb UV light	In vitro and in vivo rodent uterotrophic [14]	Dorsal skin into blood and urine [33]	Milk [54], urine [66,67]
Aluminum salts (aluminum chlorohydrate)	Antiperspirant	Metalloestrogen [13]	Underarm skin into blood [38,49]	Breast tissue [68], breast cyst fluid [69], nipple aspirate fluid [70]
Polycyclic musks (HHCB, AHTN)	Fragrance	In vitro [15,16]		Adipose tissue [71], milk [54,72]
Nitromusks (musk xylene, musk ketone)	Fragrance	In vitro [15]		Milk [54]
Benzyl salicylate, butylphenyl methylpropional (Lilial)	Fragrance	In vitro [17]		
Benzyl benzoate	Fragrance fixer, acaricide	In vitro [17]		
Octamethylcyclotetrasiloxane	Conditioning, spreading	In vitro and in animal models [20–22]		Blood [73]
Nonylphenol	Surfactant	In vitro and in rodent uterotrophic assay [29]		Urine [74]
Diethylphthalate, dibutylphthalate	Plasticizer, solvent, fragrance carrier	Estrogenic [26]	Dorsal skin into blood [34] and urine [35]	Urine [27]
Ethinylestradiol	Anti-aging	Synthetic estrogen	Physiological effects from cosmetic cream [45]	
Anthraquinones (A. vera)	Herbal additive—wound healing	In vitro [31]		
8-Prenylnaringenin (Hop)	Herbal additive—enhance breast size	In vitro [30]		
Deoxymiroestrol/miroestrol (Pueraria)	Herbal additive—enhance breast size	In vitro [30]		
Lavender oil, tea-tree oil	Herbal additive	Gynecomastia [32]	Gynecomastia from cosmetic use [32]	

TABLE 19.3　Calculated Potential for Human Dermal Absorption of Parabens in a PCP Lotion and Potency of Estrogenic Action Determined from the Published Relative Binding Affinity to ER [77]

Application		Absorption	Relative estrogenic potency	Estrogen equivalents absorbed		Range of concentrations measured in human breast tissue [51]	
Paraben content of lotion (maximum permitted by EU) [78–80]	Paraben in one daily application of 4.2 mL (mg)	Dermal absorption (10% of application) (mg) [76]	Relative binding affinity to ER (fold lower than estradiol) [77]	Estrogen equivalents of absorbed paraben (ng)	Estrogen equivalents absorbed per day, assuming an area 500 cm^2 (pg/g)	ng/g measured [51]	Estrogen equivalents of measured paraben (pg/g)
0.87% Mixed parabens	36.3	3.6	100,000	36	72		
0.4% Methylparaben	16.8	1.7	1,000,000	1.7	3.4	0–5102.9	0–5.1
0.4% Ethylparaben	16.8	1.7	167,000	10.1	20.1	0–499.7	0–3.0
0.19% Propylparaben	8	0.8	100,000	8	16.0	0–2052.7	0–20.5
0.19% Butylparaben	8	0.8	33,000	24.2	48.5	0–95.4	0–2.9
0.19% Isobutylparaben	8	0.8	13,000	61.5	123.1	0–802.9	0–61.8

Calculations are as published by Harvey and Everett [76] and Darbre and Harvey [7]; calculated values are given in estrogen equivalents and compared to measured concentrations in human breast tissue [51]. Application assumes a 125-mL bottle of lotion is used in 1 month by one application of 4.2 mL per day. Values in bold are greater than 20% of the estrogen in normal tissue [81].

19.5.2　Triclosan

The main route of human exposure to triclosan is thought to be through PCPs, and the concentration of triclosan in these products is typically in the range of 0.1–0.3% [2]. Absorption studies with human skin in vitro have shown a penetration of 6.3% of the dose by 24 h [86], which is in good agreement with the 5.9% of the dose observed to be absorbed after topical application to human volunteers [36]. However, triclosan is also used in oral hygiene products and has been shown to be absorbed from oral ingestion [87]. Triclosan has been measured in 74.6% of urine samples of the general US population in the National Health and Nutrition Examination Survey (NHANES) at concentrations ranging from 2.4–3790 µg/L [65]. Triclosan has been measured in human milk [53,63], and concentrations in the milk have been related to use of triclosan-containing PCPs [64]. Triclosan has been measured in blood with serum concentrations up to twofold higher in Australia than in Sweden, which is a country that discourages consumer use of triclosan [62].

19.5.3 Aluminum Salts

Aluminum-based antiperspirant salts, aluminum chloride, aluminum chlorohydrate, or aluminum zirconium chlorohydrate glycine complexes are recommended in the EU for over-the-counter use at concentrations of up to 15%, 20%, or 25% by weight, respectively [78], which provides high exposure to the skin surface. Both the Food and Drug Administration (FDA) of the United States [88] and the EU [78] include statements that these products should not be applied to broken, damaged, or irritated skin, but current cultural practices can include shaving before antiperspirant application, a procedure which can create abrasions in the skin, loss of stratum corneum, and irritation from hair removal [5], thereby negating the specific warning by the FDA and EU [78,88]. Studies using human breast tissue have shown that aluminum can be measured in a range of breast structures at levels that are higher than in blood, including breast tissue [68], breast cyst fluid [69], and nipple aspirate fluid [70]. Although the human population is exposed to aluminum in many ways in everyday living, including diet, use of antacids, and adjuvants in vaccinations, measurements of aluminum at high levels in breast structures has sparked debate concerning the connection of antiperspirant application with breast cancer, not least because the majority of breast cancers originate in the upper outer quadrant of the breast [89], which is close to the site of underarm application of antiperspirant [90].

19.5.4 UV Filters

Many different compounds are used as UV filters, and several have been detected in human milk samples [54]. Mean values for 54 milk samples were 27.5 ng/g lipid for 2-ethylhexyl-4-methoxy cinnamate, 30.2 ng/g lipid for octocrylene, 22.1 ng/g lipid for 4-MBC, 29.4 ng/g lipid for HS, 52.2 ng/g lipid for BP-3, and 49.0 ng/g lipid for octyl-dimethyl-p-aminobenzoic acid [54]. A significant correlation was found between the amount of UV filters measured and self-reported use of cosmetic products [54].

BP-3, one of the most widely used UV filters, is found in products at levels up to 5–6% in the United States and Japan, and 10% in Europe [91]. On the basis of concentrations measured in products and daily usage rates of PCPs, the daily geometric mean intake of BP-3 was estimated to be 0.98 µg in China and 24.4 µg in the United States [92]. BP-3 has been found in 96.8% of urine samples from the US population (NHANES 2003–2004) with a geometric mean concentration of 22.9 µg/L and a 95th-percentile value of 1040 µg/L [66]. Differences between values by gender and race/ethnicity were suggested to reflect variations in the use of PCPs containing BP-3 [66]. BP-3 has been detected in urine samples from pregnant women in Puerto Rico at levels even higher than in the United States, with a median concentration of 31.3 ng/mL and values correlated with self-reported cosmetic use [67].

19.5.5 Musk Fragrances

Synthetic polycyclic musks are added to most soaps, perfumes, and cosmetics [93], and 7-acetyl-1,1,3,4,4,6-hexamethyl-1,2,3,4-tetrahydronapthalene (AHTN) and 1,3,4,6,7,8-hexahydro-4,6,6,7,8,8-hexamethylcyclopenta[g]-2-benzopyran (HHCB) have become high-production-volume chemicals produced at quantities greater than 100 metric tons annually.

Cosmetics contain varied levels of AHTN (<5ng/g to 451µg/g) or HHCB (<5ng/g to >4000µg/g), with the highest levels found in perfume, body cream, body lotion, and deodorant [93]. AHTN and HHCB have been measured in human adipose tissue at concentrations of less than 5–134 and 12–798ng/g lipid, respectively [71]. In Danish human milk samples, HHCB has been measured with a median concentration of 147µg/kg fat [72]. In human milk samples from Switzerland, HHCB has been found to have a mean concentration of 55.0ng/g lipid, and AHTN a mean concentration of 14.0ng/g lipid [54].

Synthetic nitromusks include musk ketone (4-*tert*-butyl-2,6-dimethyl-3,5-dinitroacetophenone) and musk xylene (1-*tert*-butyl-,5-dimethyl-2,4,6-trinitrobenzene). Musk xylene is the most widely used, but it is being phased out in Europe as a substance of very great concern due to its persistence in the environment and ability to bioaccumulate [94]. Musk xylene and musk ketone have both been detected in human milk samples at mean concentrations of 2.9 and 1.6ng/g lipid, respectively [54].

19.5.6 Cyclosiloxanes

Cyclosiloxanes are incorporated widely into PCPs, often as a blended mixture of octamethylcyclotetrasiloxane (D4) and decamethylcyclopentasiloxane (D5), which is termed *cyclomethicone* at concentrations ranging from 0.06% to 89% [18]. Hexamethylcyclotrisiloxane (D3) is a contaminant of D4 and is also found in cosmetic products [18]. Dermal application of D4 and D5 to axilla skin of three women and three men has shown that D4 and D5 can be detected in the blood within 1h, and maximal absorption of D4 was 0.12% of the dose for men/0.3% for women, and for D5 was 0.05% for both men and women [95]. Due to their ubiquitous use in consumer products, they can now be measured in indoor air [96]. A study in Norway has reported the detection of D4 in 85% of adult female human plasma samples, with a median value of 4.8ng/mL (range 2.9–12.7ng/mL) [73].

19.5.7 Phthalates

DEP and DBP are the most frequently used phthalates in PCPs in Canada [24] and the United States [25]. Survey in Canada in 2011 reported that the highest levels (up to 2.6%) were found in fragrances [24]. DEP and DBP were found most frequently in perfumes, skin toners, and nail polishes, with the highest levels reaching 1000µg/g of product [25]. Daily exposure to DEP from PCP use in the Netherlands was estimated using a product data survey of 512 Dutch adults (210 male and 302 female) for 32 PCPs; the results found a median value of 4.1µg/kg, but with a wide range from 0 to 467.0µg/kg. The median value for the women (5.4µg/kg) was higher than for the men (2.3µg/kg) [97]. In Canada, based on general patterns of use of 252 PCPs, maximum daily exposure for female adults was estimated to be 78µg/kg/day [24]. Measurements in urine samples of the general US population (NHANES) showed mean levels of the metabolites monoethyl phthalate (MEP) to be 771 ± 67µg/g creatinine and monobutyl phthalate (MBP) to be 33.8 ± 1.6µg/g creatinine [27], but exposure to phthalates may be from other sources than PCPs.

19.5.8 Nonylphenol

Dermal exposure to nonylphenol from cosmetics is estimated as 0.1 μg/kg/day [29]. However, although nonylphenol has been detected in human urine samples [74], it is not known how much specifically originates from PCPs.

19.6 THE POTENTIAL FOR PLACENTAL TRANSFER AND EXPOSURE IN UTERO FROM DERMALLY APPLIED COSMETICS

Parabens [61] and benzophenone [67] have been measured in the urine of pregnant women, indicating the potential for placental transfer to babies. Direct measurements of parabens in placental tissue [55] and in paired placental tissue and cord blood samples [56] demonstrates that these compounds can be transferred from the mother to the fetus in utero. The reported correlation between urinary levels of parabens in mother and child pairs in rural and urban regions of Denmark [98] and between mothers and their newborn infants in South Korea [99] is also indicative of an environmental link within families. This should be an emerging area of concern for risk assessment.

19.7 REGULATORY CONSIDERATIONS FOR COSMETIC PRODUCTS

Until relatively recently, chemicals used in cosmetic products have received considerably less regulatory attention than other chemicals to which the human population is exposed, probably because of the long-held view that absorption from external surfaces into the human body was negligible. Cosmetics are broadly defined as those products applied only to external parts of the human body (skin, hair, and nails, and also including the teeth and inside of the mouth) used for purposes of protection, altering odor, changing appearance, cleansing, moisturizing, exfoliating, or drying. However, formulations are becoming increasingly sophisticated and exposure of the skin is at very high levels. Increasing numbers of EDCs used in PCPs have been measured in human body tissues, and although specific products cannot be identified as the source, many of these chemicals are mainly used in PCPs and so are most likely to have originated from them. The traditional framework of recommendation has therefore moved over recent years toward regulation. Within the EU, the Cosmetics Directive was set up in 1976 [78], which allowed the recommendation and ongoing review of excipient chemicals, with opinions published regularly from the Scientific Committee on Consumer Safety (SCCS) [formerly Scientific Committee on Consumer Products (SCCP)] by the European Commission. However, in 2013, this was replaced by the EU Cosmetics Products Regulation (Regulation EC No1223/2009) and applies to all countries of the EU, as well as Iceland, Norway, and Switzerland. Under this new legislation, manufacturers, retailers, and importers of cosmetics in the EU are all given "Responsible Person" status, being legally required to comply with regulations and to hold dossiers of product safety. In the United States, regulation of cosmetic products falls under the FDA following section 201 of the federal Food, Drug, and Cosmetic Act (FD&C Act), and in

Australia, cosmetics are regulated under the National Industrial Chemicals Notification and Assessment Scheme (NICNAS) of the federal government.

At the current time, most assessment concerns the use of single chemicals or groups of related chemicals in cosmetic products. EU opinions have been published by the SCCP/SCCS for many cosmetic ingredients over recent years, some recommending maintenance of the status quo and others recommending adjustments. Recent reviews of the use of parabens have recommended reduction in levels from a total of 0.8% with a maximum of 0.4% of any one ester [78] down to a combined maximum concentration of 0.19% for n-propylparaben and n-butylparaben and no recommendation for isopropylparaben or isobutylparaben [79,80]. The use of aluminum salts as an antiperspirant agent has been subject to more recent reviews in which safety concerns were expressed, but lack of data impeded risk assessment [100]. Review of triclosan approved the recommendation of a maximal level of 0.3%, but only for some cosmetic products, not all products [101]. Reviews are ongoing for the individual UV filters HS [102], BP-3 [103], and 4-MBC [104].

However, since PCPs contain complex mixtures of chemicals and multiple products are used on a daily basis [3], there is a need for assessment of mixtures of cosmetic chemicals rather than considering single chemicals in isolation from one another. The ban on testing cosmetics on animals in the EU has provided a significant barrier to hazard and risk assessment. Testing on animals for eye and skin irritancy has caused outcry from animal rights campaigners over many years, but the imposition of a complete ban on testing cosmetics on animals now prevents any testing for other concerns for human health. Nevertheless, there are significant concerns that exposure to mixtures of EDCs from PCPs may have long-term effects on human endocrine health, and assessment of their potential involvement in male and female reproductive health problems and endocrine cancers needs to continue.

As final considerations, many of the chemicals used in PCPs are old, with an incomplete and aged toxicology data package (e.g., parabens), and the studies that do exist fall far short of modern regulatory standards. For example, studies of parabens have administered them by the oral route which, because of rapid metabolism by esterases [6], does not produce the same exposure profile to intact molecules as the dermal route (or, indeed, local biological responses) and cannot provide all data that is actually necessary for dermal hazard and risk assessment. Understanding the limitations of the data set is vital to appreciate risk assessment conclusions and often unstated deficiencies in scope. Specifically, the current data set on parabens cannot provide any information on whether there is any effect on mammary tumorigenesis from local dermal application of these compounds. Thus, in order to model exposure and effect properly, there is a need to conduct safety studies on materials used in PCPs by the actual route of human exposure, which is the usual procedure for all other regulated materials (e.g., pharmaceuticals and agrochemicals) to which individuals and populations are exposed.

References

[1] Steiling W, Bascompta M, Carthew P, Catalano G, Corea N, D'Haese A, et al. Principle considerations for the risk assessment of sprayed consumer products. Toxicol Lett 2014;227:41–9.
[2] Dann AB, Hontela A. Triclosan: environmental exposure, toxicity and mechanisms of action. J Appl Toxicol 2011;31:285–311.

[3] Biesterbos JW, Dudzina T, Delmaar CJ, Bakker MI, Russel FG, von Goetz N, et al. Usage patterns of personal care products: important factors for exposure assessment. Food Chem Toxicol 2013;55:8–17.

[4] Office of National Statistics, UK: Household final consumption expenditure. 12.1 Personal care. Published 30th September 2014, <http://www.ons.gov.uk>.

[5] Turner GA, Moore AE, Marti VPJ, Paterson SE, James AG. Impact of shaving and anti-perspirant use on the axillary vault. Int J Cosmet Sci 2007;29:31–8.

[6] Darbre PD, Harvey PW. Paraben esters: review of recent studies of endocrine toxicity, absorption, esterase and human exposure, and discussion of potential human health risks. J Appl Toxicol 2008;28:561–78.

[7] Darbre PD, Harvey PW. Parabens can enable hallmarks and characteristics of cancer in human breast epithelial cells: a review of the literature with reference to new exposure data and regulatory status. J Appl Toxicol 2014;34:925–38.

[8] Taxvig C, Vinggaard AM, Hass U, Axelstad M, Boberg J, Hansen PR, et al. Do parabens have the ability to interfere with steroidogenesis? Toxicol Sci 2008;106:206–13.

[9] Koeppe ES, Ferguson KK, Colacino JA, Meeker JD. Relationship between urinary triclosan and paraben concentrations and serum thyroid measures in NHANES 2007–2008. Sci Total Environ 2013;445–446:299–305.

[10] Hu P, Chen X, Whitener RJ, Boder ET, Jones JO, Porollo A, et al. Effects of parabens on adipocyte differentiation. Toxicol Sci 2013;131:56–70.

[11] Gee RH, Charles A, Taylor N, Darbre PD. Oestrogenic and androgenic activity of triclosan in breast cancer cells. J Appl Toxicol 2008;28:78–91.

[12] Laden K, Felger CB. Antiperspirants and deodorants. Cosmetic science and technology series, vol 7. New York, NY: Marcel Dekker; 1988.

[13] Darbre PD. Metalloestrogens: an emerging class of inorganic xenoestrogens with potential to add to the oestrogenic burden of the human breast. J Appl Toxicol 2006;26:191–7.

[14] Schlumpf M, Cotton B, Conscience M, Haller V, Steinmann B, Lichtensteiger W. In vitro and in vivo estrogenicity of UV screens. Environ Health Perspect 2001;109:239–44.

[15] Gomez E, Pillon A, Fenet H, Rosain D, Duchesne MJ, Nicolas JC, et al. Estrogenic activity of cosmetic components in reporter cell lines: parabens, UV screens and musks. J Toxicol Environ Health Part A 2005;68:239–51.

[16] Burg B, Schreurs R, Linden S, Seinen W, Brouwer A, Sonneveld E. Endocrine effects of polycyclic musks: do we smell a rat? Int J Androl 2008;31:188–93.

[17] Charles AK, Darbre PD. Oestrogenic activity of benzyl salicylate, benzyl benzoate and butylphenylmethylpropional (Lilial) in MCF7 human breast cancer cells in vitro. J Appl Toxicol 2009;29:422–34.

[18] Johnson Jr W, Bergfeld WF, Belsito DV, Hill RA, Klaassen CD, Liebler DC, et al. Safety assessment of cyclomethicone, cyclotetrasiloxane, cyclopentasiloxane, cyclohexasiloxane, and cycloheptasiloxane. Int J Toxicol 2011;30(Suppl. 3):149S–227S.

[19] Luu HMD, Hutter JC. Bioavailability of octamethylcyclotetracyclosiloxane (D4) after exposure to silicones by inhalation and implantation. Environ Health Perspect 2001;109:1095–101.

[20] Hayden JF, Barlow SA. Structure–activity relationships of organosiloxanes and the female reproductive system. Toxicol Appl Pharmacol 1972;21:68–79.

[21] McKim JM, Wilga PC, Breslin WJ, et al. Potential estrogenic and antiestrogenic activity of the cyclic siloxane ocatamethylcyclotetrasiloxane (D4) and the linear siloxane hexamethyldisiloxane (HMDS) in immature rats using the uterotrophic assay. Toxicol Sci 2001;63:37–46.

[22] He B, Rhodes-Brower S, Miller MR, et al. Octamethylcyclotetrasiloxane exhibits estrogenic activity in mice via ERa. Toxicol Appl Pharmacol 2003;192:254–61.

[23] Api AM. Toxicological profile of diethyl phthalate: a vehicle for fragrance and cosmetic ingredients. Food Chem Toxicol 2001;39:97–108.

[24] Koniecki D, Wang R, Moody RP, Zhu J. Phthalates in cosmetic and personal care products: concentrations and possible dermal exposure. Environ Res 2011;111:329–36.

[25] Guo Y, Kannan K. A survey of phthalates and parabens in personal care products from the United States and its implications for human exposure. Environ Sci Technol 2013;47:14442–9.

[26] Harris CA, Henttu P, Parker MG, Sumpter JP. The estrogenic activity of phthalate esters in vitro. Environ Health Perspect 1997;105:802–11.

[27] Stahlhut RW, van Wijngaarden E, Dye TD, Cook S, Swan SH. Concentrations of urinary phthalate metabolites are associated with increased waist circumference and insulin resistance in adult U.S. males. Environ Health Perspect 2007;115:876–82.

[28] Hatch EE, Nelson JW, Qureshi MM, Weinberg J, Moore LL, Singer M, et al. Association of urinary phthalate metabolite concentrations with body mass index and waist circumference: a cross-sectional study of NHANES data, 1999–2002. Environ Health 2008;7:27.

[29] World Health Organisation International programme on chemical safety: integrated risk assessment: nonylphenol case study. Geneva, Switzerland: WHO; 2004.

[30] Matsumura A, Ghosh A, Pope GS, Darbre PD. Comparative study of oestrogenic properties of eight phytoestrogens in MCF7 human breast cancer cells. J Steroid Biochem Mol Biol 2005;94:431–43.

[31] Matsuda H, Shimoda H, Morikawa T, Yoshikawa M. Phytoestrogens from the roots of *Polygonum cuspidatum* (polygonaceae): structure-requirement of hydroxyanthraquinones for estrogenic activity. Bioorg Med Chem Lett 2001;11:1839–42.

[32] Henley DV, Lipson N, Korach KS, Bloch CA. Prepubertal gynecomastia linked to lavender and tea tree oils. New Engl J Med 2007;356:479–85.

[33] Janjua NR, Kongshoj B, Andersson AM, Wulf HC. Sunscreens in human plasma and urine after repeated whole-body topical application. JEADV 2008;22:456–61.

[34] Janjua NR, Mortensen GK, Andersson AM, Kongshoj B, Skakkebaek NE, Wulf HC. Systemic uptake of diethyl phthalate, dibutyl phthalate, and butyl paraben following whole-body topical application and reproductive and thyroid hormone levels in humans. Environ Sci Technol 2007;41:5564–70.

[35] Janjua NR, Frederiksen H, Skakkebaek NE, Wulff HC, Andersson AM. Urinary excretion of phthalates and paraben after repeated whole-body topical application in humans. Int J Androl 2008;31:118–30.

[36] Queckenberg C, Meins J, Wachall B, Doroshyenko O, Tomalik-Scharte D, Bastian B, et al. Absorption, pharmacokinetics, and safety of triclosan after dermal administration. Antimicrob Agents Chemother 2010;54: 570–2.

[37] El Hussein S, Muret P, Berard M, Makki S, Humbert P. Assessment of principal parabens used in cosmetics after their passage through human epidermis-dermis layers (*ex-vivo* study). Exp Dermatol 2007;16:830–6.

[38] Flarend R, Bin T, Elmore D, Hem SL. A preliminary study of the dermal absorption of aluminium from antiperspirants using aluminium-26. Food Chem Toxicol 2001;39:163–8.

[39] Pineau A, Guillard O, Fauconneau B, Favreau F, Marty MH, Gaudin A, et al. *In vitro* study of percutaneous absorption of aluminium from antiperspriants through human skin in the FranzTM diffusion cell. J Inorg Biochem 2012;110:21–6.

[40] Zareba G, Gelein R, Morrow PE, Utell MJ. Percutaneous absorption studies of octamethylcyclotetrasiloxane using the human skin/nude mouse model. Skin Pharmacol Appl Skin Physiol 2002;15:184–94.

[41] Finkelstein JS, McCully WF, MacLaughlin DT, Godine JE, Crowley WF. The mortician's Mystery. New Engl J Med 1988;318:961–5.

[42] Bhat N, Rosato EF, Gupta PK. Gynecomastia in a mortician. A case report. Acta Cytol 1990;34:31–4.

[43] Guaneri MP, Brambilla G, Loizzo A, Colombo I, Chiumello G. Estrogen exposure in a child from hair lotion used by her mother: clinical and hair analysis data. Clin Toxicol 2008;46:762–4.

[44] Olsen AC, Link JS, Waisman JR, Kupiec TC. Breast cancer patients unknowingly dosing themselves with estrogen by using topical moisturizers. J Clin Oncol 2009;27:103–4.

[45] Komori S, Ito Y, Nakamura Y, Aoki M, Takashi T, Kinuta T, et al. A long-term user of cosmetic cream containing estrogen developed breast cancer and endometrial hyperplasia. Menopause 2008;15:1191–2.

[46] Felner EI, White PC. Prepubertal gynecomastia: indirect exposure to estrogen cream. Pediatrics 2000;105(e55):1–3.

[47] Edidin DV, Levitsky LL. Prepubertal gynecomastia associated with estrogen-containing hair cream. Am J Dis Child 1982;136:587–8.

[48] Wollina U, Pabst F, Schonlebe J, Abdel-Naser MB, Konrad H, Gruner M, et al. Side-effects of topical androgenic and anabolic substances and steroids. A short review. Acta Dermatoven 2007;16:117–22.

[49] Guillard O, Fauconneau B, Olichon D, et al. Hyperaluminemia in a woman using an aluminium-containing antiperspirant for 4 years. Am J Med 2004;117:956–9.

[50] Sandanger TM, Huber S, Moe MK, Braathen T, Leknes H, Lund E. Plasma concentrations of parabens in postmenopausal women and self-reported use of personal care products: the NOWAC postgenome study. J Exp Sci Environ Epidemiol 2011;21:595–600.

[51] Barr L, Metaxas G, Harbach CAJ, Savoy LA, Darbre PD. Measurement of paraben concentrations in human breast tissue at serial locations across the breast from axilla to sternum. J Appl Toxicol 2012;32:219–32.

[52] Darbre PD, Aljarrah A, Miller WR, Coldham NG, Sauer MJ, Pope GS. Concentrations of parabens in human breast tumours. J Appl Toxicol 2004;24:5–13.

[53] Ye X, Bishop AM, Needham LL, Calafat AM. Automated on-line column-switching HPLC-MS/MS method with peak focusing for measuring parabens, triclosan, and other environmental phenols in human milk. Anal Chim Acta 2008;622:150–6.

[54] Schlumpf M, Kypke K, Wittassek M, Angerer J, Mascher H, Mascher D, et al. Exposure patterns of UV filters, fragrances, parabens, phthalates, organochlorpesticides, PBDEs and PCBs in human milk: correlation of UV filters with use of cosmetics. Chemosphere 2010;81:1171–83.

[55] Jimenez-Diaz I, Vela-Soria F, Zafra-Gomez A, Navalon A, Ballesteros O, Navea N, et al. A new liquid chromatography-tandem mass spectrometry method for determination of parabens in human placental tissue samples. Talanta 2011;84:702–9.

[56] Towers CV, Chambers W, Lewis D, Howard B, Chen J, Terry P. Transplacental passage of antimicrobial paraben preservatives. Obstet Gynecol 2014;123(Suppl. 1):175S–6S.

[57] Frederiksen H, Jorgensen N, Andersson AM. Parabens in urine, serum and seminal plasma from healthy Danish men determined by liquid chromatography–tandem mass spectrometry (LC-MS/MS). J Exp Sci Environ Epidemiol 2011;21:262–71.

[58] Meeker JD, Yang T, Ye X, Calafat AM, Hauser R. Urinary concentrations of parabens and serum hormone levels, semen quality parameters, and sperm DNA damage. Environ Health Perspect 2011;119:252–7.

[59] Ye X, Bishop AM, Reidy JA, Needham LL, Calafat AM. Parabens as urinary biomarkers of exposure in humans. Environ Health Perspect 2006;114:1843–6.

[60] Calafat AM, Ye X, Wong LY, Bishop AM, Needham LL. Urinary concentrations of four parabens in the U.S. population: NHANES 2005–2006. Environ Health Perspect 2010;118:679–85.

[61] Casas L, Fernandez MF, Llop S, Guxens M, Ballester F, Olea N, et al. Urinary concentrations of phthalates and phenols in a population of Spanish pregnant women and children. Environ Int 2011;37:858–66.

[62] Allmyr M, Harden F, Toms LM, Mueller JF, McLachlan MS, Adolfsson-Erici M, et al. The influence of age and gender on triclosan concentrations in Australian human blood serum. Sci Tot Environ 2008;393:162–7.

[63] Adolfsson-Erici M, Petersson M, Parkkonen J, Sturve J. Triclosan, a commonly used bacteriocide found in human milk and in the aquatic environment in Sweden. Chemosphere 2002;46:1485–9.

[64] Allmyr M, Adolfsson-Erici M, McLachlan MS, Sandborgh-Englund G. Triclosan in plasma and milk from Swedish nursing mothers and their exposure via personal care products. Sci Tot Environ 2006;372:87–93.

[65] Calafat AM, Ye X, Wong LY, Reidy JA, Needham LL. Urinary concentrations of triclosan in the US population: 2003–2004. Environ Health Perspect 2008;116:303–7.

[66] Calafat AM, Wong LY, Ye X, Reidy JA, Needham LL. Concentrations of the sunscreen agent benzophenone-3 in residents of the United States: national health and nutrition examination survey 2003–2004. Environ Health Perspect 2008;116:893–7.

[67] Meeker JD, Cantonwine DE, Rivera-González LO, Ferguson KK, Mukherjee B, Calafat AM, et al. Distribution, variability, and predictors of urinary concentrations of phenols and parabens among pregnant women in Puerto Rico. Environ Sci Technol 2013;47:3439–47.

[68] Exley C, Charles LM, Barr L, Martin C, Polwart A, Darbre PD. Aluminium in human breast tissue. J Inorg Biochem 2007;101:1344–6.

[69] Mannello F, Tonti GA, Darbre PD, John Wiley & Sons, Ltd Concentration of aluminium in breast cyst fluids collected from women affected by gross cystic breast disease. J Appl Toxicol 2009;29:1–6.

[70] Mannello F, Tonti GA, Medda V, Simone P, Darbre PD. Analysis of aluminium content and iron homeostasis in nipple aspirate fluids from healthy women and breast cancer-affected patients. J Appl Toxicol 2011;31:262–9.

[71] Kannan K, Reiner JL, Yun SH, Perrotta EE, Tao L, Johnson-Restrepo B, et al. Polycyclic musk compounds in higher trophic level aquatic organisms and humans from the United States. Chemosphere 2005;61:693–700.

[72] Duedahl-Olesen L, Cederberg T, Pedersen KH, Hojgard A. Synthetic musk fragrances in trout from Danish fish farms and human milk. Chemosphere 2005;61:422–31.

[73] Hanssen L, Warner NA, Braathen T, Odland JO, Lund E, Nieboer E, et al. Plasma concentrations of cyclic volatile methylsiloxanes (cVMS) in pregnant and postmenopausal Norwegian women and self-reported use of personal care products (PCPs). Environ Int 2013;51:82–7.

[74] Calafat AM, Kuklenyik Z, Reidy JA, Caudill SP, Ekong J, Needham LL. Urinary concentrations of bisphenol A and 4-nonylphenol in a human reference population. Environ Health Perspect 2005;113:391–5.

[75] Liao C, Liu F, Kannan K. Occurrence of and dietary exposure to parabens in foodstuffs from the United States. Environ Sci Technol 2013;47:3918–25.

[76] Harvey PW, Everett DJ. Regulation of endocrine-disrupting chemicals: critical overview and deficiencies in toxicology and risk assessment for human health. Best Pract Res Clin Endocrinol Metab 2006;20:145–65.

[77] Darbre PD. Environmental oestrogens, cosmetics and breast cancer. Best Pract Res Clin Endocrinol Metab 2006;20:121–43.

[78] EU Cosmetics Directive 76/768/EEC, <http://eur-lex.europa.eu/LexUriServ/LexUriServ.do?uri=CONSLEG:1976L0768:20100301:en:PDF>.

[79] SCCS. Scientific Committee on Consumer Safety. Opinion on parabens. COLIPA No. P82. SCCS/1348/10. European Commission, Directorate-General for Health and Consumers; 2010.

[80] SCCS. Scientific Committee on Consumer Safety. Opinion on parabens. COLIPA No. P82. SCCS/1514/13. European Commission, Directorate-General for Health and Consumers; 2013.

[81] Clarke R, Leonessa F, Welch JN, Skaar TC. Cellular and molecular pharmacology of antiestrogen action and resistance. Pharmacol Rev 2001;53:25–72.

[82] Oishi S. Effects of butylparaben on the male reproductive system in rats. Toxicol Ind Health 2001;17:31–9.

[83] Oishi S. Effects of propylparaben on the male reproductive system. Food Chem Toxicol 2002;40:1807–13.

[84] Oishi S. Effects of butylparaben on the male reproductive system in mice. Arch Toxicol 2002;76:423–9.

[85] Oishi S. Lack of spermatotoxic effects of methyl and ethyl esters of p-hydroxybenzoic acid in rats. Food Chem Toxicol 2004;42:1845–9.

[86] Moss T, Howes D, Williams FM. Percutaneous penetration and dermal metabolism of triclosan (2,4,4-tri-chloro-2-hydroxydiphenyl ether). Food Chem Toxicol 2000;38:361–70.

[87] Sandborgh-Englund G, Adolfsson-Erici M, Odham G, Ekstrand J. Pharmacokinetics of triclosan following oral ingestion in humans. J Toxicol Environ Health Part A 2006;69:1861–73.

[88] Food and Drug Administration. Fed Regist 1982;47(162):36492–505, <http://www.fda.gov/downloads/Drugs/DevelopmentApprovalProcess/DevelopmentResources/Over-the-CounterOTCDrugs/StatusofOTCRulemakings/ucm110643.pdf>.

[89] Darbre PD. Recorded quadrant incidence of female breast cancer in Great Britain suggests a disproportionate increase in the upper outer quadrant of the breast. Anticancer Res 2005;25:2543–50.

[90] Darbre PD, Mannello F, Exley C. Aluminium and breast cancer: sources of exposure, tissue measurements and mechanisms of toxicological actions on breast biology. J Inorg Biochem 2013;128:257–61.

[91] Kim S, Choi K. Occurrences, toxicities, and ecological risks of benzophenone-3, a common component of organic sunscreen products: a mini-review. Environ Int 2014;70:143–57.

[92] Liao C, Kannan K. Widespread occurrence of benzophenone-type UV light filters in personal care products from China and the United States: an assessment of human exposure. Environ Sci Technol 2014;48:4103–9.

[93] Reiner JL, Kannan K. A survey of polycyclic musks in selected household commodities from the United States. Chemosphere 2006;62:867–73.

[94] Taylor KM, Weisskopf M, Shine J. Human exposure to nitro musks and the evaluation of their potential toxicity: an overview. Environ Health 2014;13(e14):1–7.

[95] Reddy MB, Looney RJ, Utell MJ, Plotzke KP, Andersen ME. Modeling of human dermal absorption of octa-methylcyclotetrasiloxane (D4) and decamethylcyclopentasiloxane (D5). Toxicol Sci 2007;99:422–31.

[96] Pieri F, Katsoyiannis A, Martellini T, Hughes D, Jones KC, Cincinelli A. Occurrence of linear and cyclic vola-tile methyl siloxanes in indoor air samples (UK and Italy) and their isotopic characterization. Environ Int 2013;59:363–71.

[97] Delmaar C, Bokkers B, Burg W, Schuur G. Validation of an aggregate exposure model for substances in consumer products: a case study of diethyl phthalate in personal care products. J Exp Sci Environ Epidemiol 2014:1–7. [EPub ahead of print].

[98] Frederiksen H, Nielsen JKS, Morck TA, Hansen PW, Jensen JF, Nielsen O, et al. Urinary excretion of phthalate metabolites, phenols and parabens in rural and urban Danish mother–child pairs. Int J Hyg Environ Health 2013;216:772–83.

[99] Kang S, Kim S, Park J, Kim HJ, Lee J, Choi G, et al. Urinary paraben concentrations among pregnant women and their matching newborn infants of Korea, and the association with oxidative stress biomarkers. Sci Total Environ 2013;461–462:214–21.

[100] SCCS. Scientific Committee on Consumer Safety. Opinion on the safety of aluminium in cosmetic products. SCCS/1525/14. European Commission, Directorate-General for Health and Consumers; 2014.

[101] SCCS. Scientific Committee on Consumer Safety. Opinion on triclosan. COLIPA No. P32. SCCS/1414/11. European Commission, Directorate-General for Health and Consumers; 2011.

[102] SCCP. Scientific Committee on Consumer Products. Opinion on homosalate. COLIPA No. S12. SCCP/1086/07. European Commission, Directorate-General for Health and Consumers; 2007.

[103] SCCP. Scientific Committee on Consumer Products. Opinion on benzophenone-3. COLIPA No. S38. SCCP/1201/08. European Commission, Directorate-General for Health and Consumers; 2008.

[104] SCCP. Scientific Committee on Consumer Products. Opinion on 4-methylbenzilidene camphor (4-MBC). COLIPA No. S60. SCCP/1184/08. European Commission, Directorate-General for Health and Consumers; 2008.

Appendix

LIST OF ABBREVIATIONS

ACTH	Adrenocorticotrophic hormone
ADHD	Attention-deficit hyperactivity disorder
ADME	Absorption, distribution, metabolism, and excretion
AGD	Anogenital distance
AhR	Aryl hydrocarbon receptor
AHRE	Aryl hydrocarbon receptor response element
AHTN	7-Acetyl-1,1,3,4,4,6-hexamethyl-1,2,3,4-tetrahydronapthalene
AKR1C3	Aldo-keto reductase 1C3
AKR1D1	Steroid 5β-reductase
AMA	Amphibian Metamorphosis Assay
AMH	Anti-Müllerian hormone
AOP	Adverse outcome pathway
AOP	Advanced oxidation process
API	Anal position index
AR	Androgen receptor (NR3C4)
ARE	Androgen-response element
ARNT	Aryl hydrocarbon receptor nuclear translocator
ART	Assisted reproductive technology
ASD	Autism spectrum disorder
ASP	Activated sludge plant
AVP	Arginine vasopressin
BAFF	Biological aerated flooded filter
BaP	Benzo[a]pyrene
BBP	Butylbenzylphthalate
BE	2-Butoxyethanol
β-GAL	β-Galactosidase
BFR	Brominated flame retardant
bHLH/PAS	Basic helix-loop-helix/period AhR nuclear translocator single-minded
BMI	Body mass index
BOO	Bladder outlet obstruction
BP-3	Benzophenone-3
BPA	Bisphenol A
BPH	Benign prostatic hyperplasia
BRCA1/2	Breast cancer (susceptibility/early onset) gene/protein type 1/2
CAR	Constitutive androstane receptor
CAT	Chloramphenicol acetyl transferase
CBG	Corticosteroid-binding globulin
CF	Conceptual Framework (OECD—for the screening and testing of endocrine disrupting chemicals)
CNS	Central nervous system
COX-1/-2	Cyclooxygenase 1/2
CPT	Conner's continuous performance test
CRH	Corticotrophin-releasing hormone
CVD	Cardiovascular disease
CYP	Cytochrome P450 (enzyme)
CYP11A	Cytochrome P45011A
D3	Hexamethylcyclotrisiloxane
D4	Octamethylcyclotetrasiloxane
D5	Decamethylcyclopentasiloxane
DBD	DNA-binding domain
DBP	Dibutyl phthalate
DDE	Dichlorodiphenyldichloroethylene
DDT	Dichlorodiphenyltrichloroethane
DEHP	Di(2-ethylhexyl) phthalate
DEP	Diethyl phthalate
DES	Diethylstilbestrol
DHEA	Dehydroepiandrosterone
DHT	Dihydrotestosterone
DIDP	Diisodecyl phthalate
DINP	Diisononyl phthalate
DIT	Diiodotyrosine
DNA	Deoxyribonucleic acid
DNCB	2,4-Dinitrochlorobenzene
DRE	Dioxin response element

DWI	Drinking Water Inspectorate (UK)	H_2O_2	Hydrogen peroxide
DWTW	Drinking water treatment works	HPA	Hypothalamo-pituitary-adrenocortical (axis)
E1	Estrone	HPG	Hypothalamus-pituitary-gonad (axis)
E2	17β-Estradiol		
E3	Estriol	HPT	Hypothalamic-pituitary-thyroid (axis)
ECHA	European Chemicals Agency		
ED	Endocrine disruptor	HPV	High-production-volume
EDC	Endocrine-disrupting chemical	HPV	Human papillomavirus
EDSP	Endocrine Disrupter Screening Program (U.S. EPA)	HRT	Hormone replacement therapy
		HS	Homosalate
EE2	17α-Ethinylestradiol	HSD	Hydroxysteroid dehydrogenase
EFA	Essential fatty acid	HSD3B2	3-β Dehydrosteroid dehydrogenase type 2
EPA	Environmental Protection Agency (USA)	HSD11B2	11-β Hydroxysteroid dehydrogenase type 2
EQS	Environmental Quality Standard	HSD17B3	17-β Hydroxysteroid dehydrogenase type 3
ER	Estrogen receptor		
ER+	Estrogen receptor positive (containing estrogen receptor)	HSP	Heat shock protein
		IARC	International Agency for Research on Cancer
ERα	Estrogen receptor alpha (NR3A1)		
ERβ	Estrogen receptor beta (NR3A2)	IC_{50}	Inhibitory concentration 50% (concentration causing 50% inhibition)
ERE	Estrogen response element		
EU	European Union		
EWG	Environmental Working Group	IDDM	Insulin-dependent diabetes mellitus
F0/F1/F2	Filial generation (of offspring) (F0 parental; F1/F2 first/second filial generation)	IFN-g	Interferon gamma
		Ig	Immunoglobulin
		IL	Interleukin
FDA	Food and Drug Administration (USA)	Insl3	Insulin-like factor-3
		IQ	Intelligence quotient
FSH	Follicle-stimulating hormone	KD	Kilodalton
GAC	Granular activated carbon	LBD	Ligand-binding domain
GD	Gestation Day	LBW	Low birth weight
GDWQ	Guidelines for Drinking-water Quality (WHO)	LD_{50}	Lethal dose at which 50% of the animals die
GFP	Green fluorescent protein		
GH	Growth hormone	LH	Luteinizing hormone
GnRH	Gonadotropin-releasing hormone	LLNA	Local lymph node assay
GPER	G-protein coupled estrogen receptor	LOAEL	Lowest observed adverse effect level
GR	Glucocorticoid receptor (NR3C1)	LOEC	Lowest observed effect concentration
GRE	Glucocorticoid response element		
HCB	Hexachlorobenzene	LUTS	Lower urinary tract symptoms
hCG	Human chorionic gonadotropin	MAPK	Mitogen-activated protein kinase
HEK	Human embryonic kidney	mAR	Membrane-bound form of androgen receptor
HEPA	High-efficiency particulate air (filter)		
HHCB	1,3,4,6,7,8-Hexahydro-4,6,6,7,8,8-hexamethylcyclopenta[g]-2-benzopyran	4-MBC	3-(4-Methylbenzilidene) camphor
		MBP	Monobutyl phthalate
		MBzP	Monobenzyl phthalate

MDR1	Multidrug resistance protein 1	PCR	Polymerase chain reaction
ME	2-Methoxyethanol	PE	Polyethylene
MEHP	Mono-(2-ethylhexyl)phthalate	PFC	Plaque-forming cell (assay)
MEP	Monoethyl phthalate	PFC	Perfluorinated compound
MIE	Molecular initiating event	PFOA	Perfluorooctanoic acid
MIT	Monoiodotyrosine	PFOS	Perfluorooctanesulphonic acid
MMI	Methimazole	PHE	Public Health England (UK)
MMTV-LTR	Mouse mammary tumor virus long terminal repeat	PI3K	Phosphatidyl-inositol-3-kinase
		PKC	Protein kinase C
MOF	Multioocyte follicle	PMRA	Pest Management Regulatory Agency (Canada)
MOS	Margin of safety		
MR	Mineralocorticoid receptor (NR3C2)	POF	Premature ovarian failure
		POP	Persistent organic pollutant
MRL	Maximum residue limit	PPAR	Peroxisome proliferator-activated receptor
MSC	Multipotent stromal cell		
MTD	Maximum tolerated dose	PPARα	Peroxisome proliferator-activated receptor alpha (NR1C1)
MXC	Methoxychlor		
NAS	National Academy of Sciences	PPARβ/δ	Peroxisome proliferator-activated receptor beta/delta (NR1C2)
NCoR	Nuclear receptor co-repressor 1		
NGO	Nongovernmental organization	PPARγ	Peroxisome proliferator-activated receptor gamma (NR1C3)
NHANES	National Health and Nutrition Examination Survey (USA)		
		PPRE	Peroxisome proliferator response element
NICU	Neonatal intensive care unit		
NIDDM	Non-insulin-dependent diabetes mellitus	PR	Progesterone receptor (NR3C3)
		PRE	Progesterone response element
NIS	Sodium–iodide symporter	PRL	Prolactin
NK	Natural killer (cell)	PTU	Propylthiouracil
NMDRCs	Nonmonotonic dose response curves	PVC	Polyvinyl chloride
		PVN	Paraventricular nucleus
NOAEL	No observed adverse effect level	PXR	Pregnane X receptor
NOEC	No-observed-effect concentration	RAR	Retinoid acid receptor
NSAID	Non-steroidal anti-inflammatory drug	RARα	Retinoid acid receptor alpha (NR1B1)
		RARβ	Retinoid acid receptor beta (NR1B2)
OC	Organochlorine		
OECD	Organisation for Economic Cooperation and Development	RARγ	Retinoid acid receptor gamma (NR1B3)
		RNA/mRNA	Ribonucleic acid/messenger ribonucleic acid
OMC	2-Ethylhexyl 4-methoxy cinnamate		
OP	Organophosphate	rT3	Reverse triiodothyronine
PAC	Powdered activated carbon	RXR	Retinoid X receptor
PAD	Peripheral arterial disease	RXRα	Retinoid X receptor alpha (NR2B1)
PAH	Polycyclic aromatic hydrocarbon		
PBB	Polybrominated biphenyl	RXRβ	Retinoid X receptor beta (NR2B2)
PBDE	Polybrominated diphenyl ether	RXRγ	Retinoid X receptor gamma (NR2B3)
PCDD	Polychlorinated dibenzodioxin		
PCDF	Polychlorinated dibenzofuran	REACH	Registration, Evaluation, Authorization, and restriction of CHemicals (EU)
PCB	Polychlorinated biphenyl		
PCOS	Polycystic ovary syndrome		
PCP	Personal care product		

RTPCR	Reverse transcriptase polymerase chain reaction	TEARS	Thyroid Epidemiology Audit and Research Study
SCCP	Scientific Committee on Consumer Products (European Commission)	TGCT	Testicular germ cell tumor
		TiO_2	Titanium dioxide
		TNF	Tumor necrosis factor
SCCS	Scientific Committee on Consumer Safety (European Commission)	TPO	Thyroperoxidase
		TR	Thyroid hormone receptor
		TRα	Thyroid hormone receptor alpha (NR1A1)
SE	Steroid estrogen		
SEER	Surveillance, Epidemiology and End Results (National Cancer Institute, USA)	TRβ	Thyroid hormone receptor beta (NR1A2)
		TRH	Thyrotropin-releasing hormone
SERM	Selective Estrogen Receptor Modulator	TSH	Thyroid-stimulating hormone (thyrotropin)
SHBG	Steroid hormone binding globulin	TTR	Transthyretin
		TZD	Thiazolidinedione
SMRT	Silencing mediator of retinoic acid and thyroid hormone receptor	UDP-GT	Uridine diphosphate glucuronyltransferase
		UK	United Kingdom
SRD5A	Steroid 5α-reductase	UKWIR	United Kingdom Water Industry Research
SRY	Sex-determining region of the Y chromosome		
		UNEP	United Nations Environment Programme
StAR	Steroid acute regulatory protein	UOQ	Upper outer quadrant
SULT	Sulphotransferase	US/USA	United States/United States of America
SVHC	Substances of Very High Concern		
		UV	Ultraviolet
T3	Triiodothyronine	VCD	4-Vinylcyclohexene diepoxide
T4	Thyroxine	VOC	Volatile organic compound
TBG	Thyroxine-binding globulin/protein	WHO	World Health Organization
		WISC	Wechsler Intelligence Scale for Children
TBT	Tributyltin		
TCDD	2,3,7,8-Tetrachlorodibenzo-p-dioxin	WWF	World Wildlife Fund
		WwTW	Wastewater treatment works
TDS	Testicular dysgenesis syndrome	XRE	Xenobiotic response element

Index

Note: Page numbers followed by "*f*" and "*t*" refer to figures and tables, respectively.

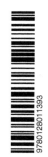